PREVENTION

PREVENTION

The Science and Art of Promoting Healthy Child and Adolescent Development

edited by

John G. Borkowski, Ph.D.

and

Chelsea M. Weaver, M.A., M.Ed.

University of Notre Dame
Notre Dame, Indiana

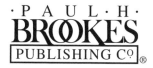

·P A U L·H·
BROOKES
PUBLISHING CO ®

Baltimore • London • Sydney

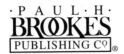

Paul H . Brookes Publishing Co.
Post Office Box 10624
Baltimore, Maryland 21285-0624

www.brookespublishing.com

Typeset by Auburn Associates, Inc., Baltimore, Maryland.
Manufactured in the United States of America by
Versa Press, Inc., East Peoria, Illinois.

The case studies in this book are fictional accounts and are not
related in any way to real families.

Library of Congress Cataloging-in-Publication Data

Prevention : the science and art of promoting healthy child and adolescent development /
[edited] by John G. Borkowski and Chelsea M. Weaver
   p.   cm.
Includes bibliographical references and index.
ISBN-13: 978-1-55766-868-4 (alk. paper)
ISBN-10: 1-55766-868-X (alk. paper)
   1. Children—Services for. 2. Youth—Services for. 3. Child development. 4. Youth
development. 5. Child welfare. 6. Developmental disabilities—Prevention. I. Borkowski,
John G., 1938- II. Weaver, Chelsea M. III. Title: The science and art of promoting healthy child
and adolescent development.

HV713.P734 2006
362.7—dc22   2006020959

British Library Cataloguing in Publication data are available from the British Library.

CONTENTS

About the Editors

John G. Borkowski, Ph.D., Andrew J. McKenna Family Chair of Psychology, University of Notre Dame, 114B Haggar Hall, Notre Dame, Indiana 46556

Professor Borkowski is recipient of the Career Research Scientist Award from the Academy on Mental Retardation, the Edgar Doll Award from the American Psychological Association, and Notre Dame's Faculty and Research Achievement Awards. He is currently engaged in two multisite longitudinal projects designed to understand and reduce the incidence of child abuse and neglect in at-risk mothers. A third major longitudinal project undertaken by Professor Borkowski has followed children born to adolescent mothers in the late 1980s as they enter their turbulent teenage years. His research programs on adolescent parenting and child neglect are supported by the National Institute of Child Health and Human Development. Professor Borkowski has published more than 150 research papers and chapters and is the co-author of six psychology texts, including *Interwoven Lives: Adolescent Mothers and Their Children* (Lawrence Erlbaum Associates, 2001) and *Parenting and the Child's World* (Lawrence Erlbaum Associates, 2002).

Chelsea M. Weaver, M.A., M.Ed., Research Associate, University of Notre Dame, Department of Psychology, 118 Haggar Hall, Notre Dame, Indiana 46556

Ms. Weaver is a doctoral candidate in developmental psychology at the University of Notre Dame. She received an M.A. in developmental psychology from Notre Dame and an M.Ed. in early intervention from the University of Pittsburgh. Her research has focused on the effects of exposure to violence on the development of delinquency and violent behaviors among children of adolescent mothers, as well as on the risk and protective factors that serve to mitigate or exacerbate these relationships. Ms. Weaver is interested in the effects of parenting and family dynamics on infant development and adjustment during early childhood with a specific focus on the suitability of using latent growth mixture modeling to approach research from a developmental psychopathology perspective. She also is currently a project director at the University of Pittsburgh for a multisite, family-based early intervention program designed to promote positive adjustment among high-risk children and their families.

CONTRIBUTORS

Carol E. Akai, M.A.
Research Associate
University of Notre Dame
118 Haggar Hall
Notre Dame, IN 46556

Elizabeth H. Blodgett, M.A.
Research Associate
University of Notre Dame
118 Haggar Hall
Notre Dame, IN 46556

Shannon S. Carothers, Ph.D.
Postdoctoral Fellow
Georgetown University
3700 Reservoir Road, NW
Washington, DC 20057

W. Brad Faircloth, Ph.D.
Research Associate
University of Notre Dame
118 Haggar Hall
Notre Dame, IN 46556

Amber M. Grundy, M.A.
Research Associate
University of Notre Dame
118 Haggar Hall
Notre Dame, IN 46556

Kimberly S. Howard, Ph.D
Research Associate
University of Notre Dame
118 Haggar Hall
Notre Dame, IN 46556

Peggy S. Keller, Ph.D.
Research Associate
University of Notre Dame
118 Haggar Hall
Notre Dame, IN 46556

Patricia M. Mitchell, M. Phil.
Research Associate
University of Notre Dame
118 Haggar Hall
Notre Dame, IN 46556

Jody S. Nicholson, M.A.
Research Associate
University of Notre Dame
118 Haggar Hall
Notre Dame, IN 46556

Julie N. Schatz, M.A.
Research Associate
University of Notre Dame
118 Haggar Hall
Notre Dame, IN 46556

Stacey B. Scott, M.A.
Research Associate
University of Notre Dame
118 Haggar Hall
Notre Dame, IN 46556

Leann E. Smith, M.A.
Research Associate
University of Notre Dame
118 Haggar Hall
Notre Dame, IN 46556

Lane E. Volpe, M.A.
Project Director, Mother-Baby
  Behavioral Sleep Lab
University of Notre Dame
118 Haggar Hall
Notre Dame, IN 46556

Willow A. Wetherall, M.A.
Parent Facilitator, My Baby and Me
University of Notre Dame
118 Haggar Hall
Notre Dame, IN 46556

FOREWORD

Every community shares a vision that its young people will have an opportunity to be healthy and successful and will contribute to the development of the next generation of its citizens. Unfortunately, a large proportion of children will not have that opportunity and will never become productive, successful adults. We know, for example, that 30% of young people in high school engage in high-risk behaviors linked to substance abuse, delinquency, and violence that can jeopardize their potential for life success (Dryfoos, 1997).

Taking to heart the adage "An ounce of prevention is worth a pound of cure," wise communities are investing in prevention programs that discourage their teenage population from participating in risky behaviors. By focusing on prevention, communities are avoiding the pay-later approach, ultimately saving the communities the much higher costs of juvenile correction and adult prisons, foster care, public assistance, and other expensive programs. Examples of the cost-effectiveness of prevention are numerous. In the health field, for instance, we know that for every dollar spent in early childhood immunizations against measles, mumps, and rubella, we save $16 on medical costs to treat those illnesses (Hatziandreu, Brown, & Halpern, 1994). Prevention programs result in similar cost savings when they address social risks; for example:

- Every $1 invested in intensive home visits saves $3 later in government assistance and criminal justice costs (Olds, Henderson, Chamberlin, & Tatelbaum, 1986).
- Every $1 invested in children's early care and education saves $7 by increasing the likelihood that children will become literate and employed rather than school dropouts, delinquents, welfare-dependent, or criminals (Karoly, Kilburn, & Cannon, 2005).
- Every $1 invested in substance abuse prevention saves $5.50 later in costs for needed health care, incarceration, and law enforcement (Caulkins, Everingham, Rydell, Chiesa, & Bushway, 1999).

Communities are looking for ways to optimize the well-being and development of their children and young people and prevent later adverse outcomes. They want to know what works. *Prevention: The Science and Art of Promoting Healthy Child and Adolescent Development* takes an innovative and much needed approach to examining prevention programs. Responding to the reality that an understanding of what is most effective in prevention relies on a description of program components and the science on which they are based, the authors create a marriage of these two critical aspects of prevention research. While prevention programs are often discipline-specific, the authors have crossed these disciplinary divides and described programs from many fields that address issues of infant growth and development, developmental delays, child maltreatment, risky sexual behavior, youth violence, adolescent substance abuse, dating violence, and marital conflict and divorce. In each of these areas, the authors showcase a few of the most effective prevention programs and discuss some of the factors that contribute to the programs' success. In each chapter, the authors critically analyze each program against characteristics consistently associated with effective prevention (Nation et al., 2003) and bring these essential features to life in their description of a model program. These models are enhanced through case examples illustrating how a child and family would move through the program.

What makes this volume unique is the blending of descriptions of good programs and good science in prevention. Individuals who are serious about expanding their knowledge and practice of prevention require both of these elements. An analysis of the scientific literature in each of the prevention areas outlined in this book clearly reveals a wide range of types of programs. What is noteworthy, however, is that the best programs share some common features: 1) they are based on theory; 2) they use a comprehensive set of intervention components instead of focusing narrowly on a risk or concern; 3) they employ varied teaching methods that maximize the engagement of a diverse range of participants and associated learning styles; 4) they rely on the establishment of high-quality, positive relationships between intervention staff and participants; 5) they are relevant to the cultural values of participants; and 6) they are implemented at sufficient levels of intensity, with high levels of fidelity, and at a time in a participant's life with the best hope of success.

All of these program features have been linked to promising outcomes and should maximize the likelihood of good outcomes. But besides understanding the content of programs, we also must understand the science behind them. Many prevention programs may be based on sound practices but they lack studies that demonstrate both the internal and external validity of their findings. If communities are to make wise choices among programs, they need to evaluate the strength of the evidence on which the programs are based. This book allows a community to examine how a program is put together and to understand whether the program has been rigorously tested. Understanding programmatic and methodological features is essential both to the researcher who is creating new prevention programs and to the community member who is searching for the most promising programs to replicate.

In *Prevention: The Science and Art of Promoting Healthy Child and Adolescent Development,* the reader will discover a wealth of information about how to prevent some of the most serious problems facing children and families today. The research is there demonstrating not only that these programs can make a difference in promoting better outcomes, but also that ultimately they are tremendous money savers for communities and the nation. It is worth noting that many of these programs and much of this knowledge has been around for more than a decade, yet communities investing in prevention programs such as these are the exception. Why is the implementation of prevention practices still so far behind our knowledge of what constitutes effective prevention? First, many communities are still unaware that there is a science of prevention and that research can give them a preemptive means of dealing with issues such as violence, substance abuse, and delinquency. Volumes such as this can shed light on the science of prevention using information that communities can access and providing examples that illustrate how programs can truly affect families' lives. Second, prevention researchers and program implementers often live in separate worlds. As a result, programs that are rigorously tested and proven to be effective often are missing some of the features necessary for their long-term sustenance in communities where caseloads are large, staff have limited skills, salaries are low, turnover is high, and time for training and supervision is a luxury. Being able to implement the programmatic features known to ensure successful outcomes such as high fidelity, adequate dosage, and quality relationships is challenging in the environment of community programs. Prevention researchers need to spend more time working with community partners in creating programs that can be maintained successfully in the realities of communities. Third, policy makers must become more attuned to the fact that prevention makes sense and is a wise investment. Stronger advocacy of this view will be promoted by science that informs programs and by programs that work together with researchers to build a knowledge and practice base promoting better outcomes for children and families. I applaud the authors of this book for creating a resource that contributes to continued research, practice, and policy making regarding prevention issues. This volume will be invaluable in assisting our communities in using an ounce of prevention early on instead of relying on a "pound of cure" later for enhancing the well-being of children and families.

Judith Carta, Ph.D.
Senior Scientist and Professor
Juniper Gardens Children's Project
Schiefelbusch Institute for Life Span Studies
University of Kansas

REFERENCES

Caulkins, J.P., Everingham, S.S., Rydell, C.P., Chiesa, J., & Bushway, S. (1999). *An ounce of prevention, a pound of uncertainty: The cost-effectiveness of school-based drug prevention programs.* Santa Monica, CA: RAND Corporation.

Dryfoos, J.G. (1997). The prevalence of problem behaviors: Implications for programs. In R.P. Weissberg, T.P. Gullotta, R.L. Hampton, B.S. Ryan, & G.R. Adams (Eds.), *Healthy children 2010: Enhancing children's wellness* (pp.17–26). Thousand Oaks, CA: Sage.

Hatziandreu E.J., Brown R.E., & Halpern, M.T. (1994). *A cost benefit analysis of the measles mumps rubella (MMR) vaccine.* Final report prepared for National Immunization

Program, Centers for Disease Control and Prevention. Arlington, VA: Center for Public Health Research and Evaluation, Battelle Memorial Institute.

Karoly, L.A., Kilburn, R., & Cannon, J.S. (2005). *Early childhood interventions: Proven results, future promise.* Santa Monica, CA: RAND Corporation.

Nation, M., Crusto, C., Wandersman, A., Kumpfer, K.L., Seybolt, D., Morrisey-Kane, E., et al. (2003). What works in prevention: Principles of effective prevention programs. *American Psychologist,* 58, 449–456.

Olds, D., Henderson, C., Chamberlin, R., & Tatelbaum, R. (1986). Preventing child abuse and neglect: A randomized trial of nurse home visitation. *Pediatrics,* 78(1), 65–78.

PREFACE

During the last quarter of the 20th century, the social landscape of the United States was altered in dramatic and often unforeseen ways. Instability in family life, inequalities in public education, a rapid rise in risky behaviors and violence in the lives of our youth, a decline in middle-class numbers, and entrenched poverty have isolated many Americans from the economic mainstream. As these events cascaded onto the American scene, overburdened and often perplexed state and federal agencies as well as local communities began to launch formal campaigns to forestall the insidious advance of these new social problems. Within this context, research on prevention emerged.

The growing importance of prevention research for modern society was articulated in an important address by George Albee in 1991. A past president of the American Psychological Association and the father of the prevention research movement, Albee argued that scientists and society at large usually fail to consider the importance of prevention, instead focusing on individualized interventions and remediation only after a problem has already emerged in its full-blown state. Individual treatment programs, although well meaning and necessary, are sometimes too late and almost always insufficient in bringing about far-reaching social change. This is because remediation only treats the symptoms associated with a problem. In contrast, prevention holds the power to revolutionize the culture of intervention by forestalling problems not just for a few individuals but also for entire at-risk populations. A shift in emphasis from remediation to prevention has the potential to affect not only future research directions and their funding sources but also the successful functioning of society as a whole as it raises its children and adolescents in increasingly complex environments.

Prevention: The Science and Art of Promoting Healthy Child and Adolescent Development represents the first synthesis of research accomplishments and methodological approaches across multiple problem areas affecting America's youth. Its main goals are to understand the state of prevention research at the outset of the 21st century and to chart a course for an overall improvement in the quality, and potential impact, of preventions targeted toward children and adolescents. Successful preventions represent a form of art, bridging the gap between the needs of society and the wealth of knowledge science offers. This form of inquiry requires investigators to skillfully balance rigorous methodologies with the practical demands of working in often politically turbulent, complex, and underfunded community contexts. In this book, we focus on the reciprocal relationship between science and practice in prevention research. In our scenario, science informs and is the foundation for community programs, and, at the same time, individuals targeted for prevention programs influence the format, operation, and focus of research-based interventions. The concept of art within science adds elements of respect and common sense to scientific research on prevention.

It is from this unique perspective—prevention research as both science and art—that this book is based. In Chapter 1, we identify a set of principles that are at the heart of effective prevention programs: comprehensiveness, varied teaching methods, sufficient treatment dosage, appropriately timed interventions, sociocultural relevance, thorough evaluations, and highly trained staff. This analytic framework is then used to review and critique the prevention literature in eight important areas: infancy and early development, childhood developmental delays, child maltreatment, youth violence, substance abuse, risky sexual behavior, dating violence, and the negative consequences of marital conflict and divorce.

Each of the content chapters is structured similarly, beginning with a review of the major prevention projects in nine carefully selected domains of research and ending with an illustration of a model program appropriate for community-based implementation. Within each chapter's review of the core literature, coverage is selective rather than exhaustive, focusing on well-designed, skillfully conducted, and rigorously evaluated projects that produce important statistical and/or clinical effects. Next, each set of studies is analyzed in terms of the characteristics of successful prevention research, as developed in Chapter 1. These characteristics—in addition to those mentioned previously—include the role of theory in designing prevention programs, the nature and scope of an intervention's multiple components as prerequisite for the successful generalization of results across time and settings, issues of sampling and attrition, treatment fidelity, and assessment of effect sizes and the extent of clinical impact. A distinctive feature of each chapter is an elaborate illustration of how *best practices* can be translated into community contexts in terms of a model prevention program.

The final chapter of the book provides a summary of the principles of successful prevention programs relative to the eight important domains of infant, child, and adolescent development and makes recommendations for designing and conducting prevention research over the next decade, with the aim of reversing the insidious increase in social problems that confront children and adolescents in contemporary society. We show how research in prevention needs to cut across multiple problem domains and include both artistic and scientific components to promote a broad range of healthy behaviors for future generations of children and youth.

To the loves of our lives, Martha and Ben

The Art and Science of Prevention Research

Principles of Effective Programs

John G. Borkowski,
Carol E. Akai, and Leann E. Smith

George Albee (1991) once asked a provocative question: Who are more valuable to society, Albert Schweitzer and Mother Theresa or John Snow and Ignatz Semmelweiss? Although the former are widely admired humanitarians, the latter made important scientific discoveries that saved millions of lives. Snow figured out that cholera was a waterborne disease. He observed that the pattern of cholera infection was related to the origin of drinking water. By removing the handle from water pumps, he stopped the cholera epidemic. Semmelweiss, puzzled by the high rate of childhood fevers and deaths in women in the public wards of Budapest hospitals, eventually decided that somehow medical personnel and obstetrical trainees were spreading infections from the dissecting rooms of their anatomy labs to the women giving birth. His solution was simple: Order the staff to wash their hands for 10 minutes before delivering an infant. Suddenly, the rate of fever and death dropped to almost nothing. Albee's point was not to diminish the contributions of Albert Schweitzer or Mother Theresa, but rather to emphasize the importance of prevention research in solving human problems. The fore-stalling of human tragedy—at either the individual or group level—is the unique contribution that the science of prevention provides society at large.

Prevention research and its application in field settings are relatively new areas of interest among the social sciences. It is not surprising, then, that there is little in the way of standard practice with respect to the principles associated with research on the prevention of developmental problems. This book is about the thoughtful interweaving of innovative theory, carefully crafted methodologies, and best practice in conducting prevention research and applying those results in community settings. Effective prevention programs depend on the successful combination of the rigors of the scientific method with the art of workable, real-life practices.

A major challenge to maintaining a balance between art and science in developing prevention programs is the conflict between pressing social needs and the slow-moving demands of science. Part of the problem is society's quick-fix attitude, which often fails to assimilate the strenuous principles and characteristics of high-quality research into the demands of service delivery to those in need. In addition, society often fails to see the importance of providing prevention services until seemingly small problems develop into full-scale crises, sometimes at a national level. An important step for social science researchers, as well as for society at large, is to develop and apply a *culture of prevention,* wherein agencies and institutions recognize the necessity of intervening early, with high-quality programs, to halt the escalation of widespread social problems.

This book identifies a wide range of prevention programs that foster healthy development in infants, children, and adolescents. The domains covered include infancy and toddlerhood, early childhood developmental delays, maltreatment, risky sexual behavior, youth violence, negative consequences of marital conflict and divorce, and domestic violence. In each area, major intervention programs are described, suggestions are given for their effectiveness, a model program is created, and an example is presented to show how a specific child or adolescent would move through the model program. For all of the prevention programs reviewed, critical analyses of the major features or principles inherent in well-documented prevention programs were conducted. This initial chapter prepares the way for these critical analyses by showing how and why each of 15 principles is essential for prevention programs that produce strong and lasting effects on important problems facing society.

DESIGNING EFFECTIVE PREVENTION PROGRAMS: "GOOD SCIENCE MAKES GOOD ART"

Borkowski, Smith, and Akai (in press) identified the major principles associated with effective prevention research. The principles listed in Table 1.1 have been shown to lead to scientifically and clinically significant outcomes, meaning that

Table 1.1. Principles of effective prevention programs

Treatment principles	Procedural principles	Design and evaluation principles
Theory-driven	Sufficient dosage	Interpretative standards
Comprehensive	Appropriate timing	Outcome evaluation
Varied teaching methods	Well-trained staff	Internal validation
Positive relationships	Programmed generalization	Adequate effect size
Sociocultural relevance	Treatment fidelity	Clinical or social significance

these principles will likely promote successful outcomes if implemented systematically in field settings.

The 15 principles can be grouped into three overlapping categories: treatment principles, procedural principles, and design and evaluation principles. *Treatment principles* correspond to the specific curriculum and associated components of an intervention, *procedural principles* refer to how that intervention is implemented in the field, and *design and evaluation principles* relate to an appropriate and convincing assessment of program effectiveness. If endorsed in practice, these 15 principles will produce clear interpretations about the causal factors that produce meaningful outcomes following an intervention. In the sections that follow, the goal is to show how good science and artful practice go hand in hand to produce important, evidence-based, treatment-related outcomes for infants, young children, and adolescents who face a variety of potentially harmful life circumstances.

The creation of a list of effective principles rests heavily on the scholarship of Nation et al. (2003), who analyzed four areas of prevention research in an attempt to determine the most frequently occurring principles of effective programs: 1) substance abuse, 2) risky sexual behavior, 3) delinquency and violence, and 4) school failures. Across these four content areas, 35 well-designed studies were used for qualitative and quantitative analyses (Nation et al.). In the areas of substance abuse and risky sexual behaviors, the most important principles were the comprehensiveness of the intervention, varied methods of teaching, appropriate timing of the program with respect to the participants' age or stage of development, and sociocultural appropriateness and sensitivity of the program's contents. In the area of delinquency and violence, the building of positive relationships between participants and staff and the administration of sufficient treatment dosage also were important. All of the previously mentioned principles likewise appeared in successful programs designed to prevent school failures; in these instances, having a well-trained staff also was important for program effectiveness.

The thorough analysis of Nation et al. (2003), in combination with useful suggestions provided by Ramey and Ramey (1992), forms the conceptual and empirical foundation for the 15 principles listed in Table 1.1. The following sections describe these principles in greater detail, showing how each contributes to good prevention science and suggesting their importance for program implementation in field settings.

Treatment Principles

Treatment principles represent both the rigor of science and the art of everyday practice. These principles focus on how prevention programs can be carried out in a way that achieves scientific integrity when applied in complex, highly variable field settings. Perhaps the most important statements about the treatment under investigation are the following: Prevention curricula need to be driven by an established theoretical framework containing comprehensive modules that are relevant to the backgrounds and cultures of the participants. Positive relationships between the participants and the professionals (or paraprofessionals) delivering the intervention along with varied teaching methods make the curriculum more appealing and increase program participation. Adherence to the principles in the treatment category aids the success of prevention programs by accomplishing a difficult task: the artful implementation of scientifically sound principles that surround the development of a curriculum.

Theory-Driven Prevention research depends on innovative ideas to eradicate problems. A rich theoretical framework provides the conceptual foundation for testing these new programmatic ideas. Theories offer testable models that help explain how key concepts relate to one another and subsequently influence human behavior (Green & Piel, 2002; Miller, 2002). As its knowledge base expands, a theory-driven framework evolves and grows in scope, accuracy, and range of applications. Repeatedly testing a theoretical framework provides more information regarding the causes and correlates of an important behavioral outcome (e.g., antisocial behavior, preadolescent promiscuity) than not testing the theory or testing it only once. Theories aid prevention research by isolating the core components of a problem and by eradicating false tenets about the topic under study. More established theoretical frameworks attempt to guard against potentially ineffective or even detrimental prevention programs that might result from misconceptions and/or inaccurate information about a target problem. Theory-driven models provide both the explanation and the direction that prevention research requires.

Comprehensive Comprehensive programs use multiple intervention components to contend with all aspects of a target problem. Incorporating comprehensiveness into prevention curricula is important because deeply rooted problems are often multifaceted with numerous contributing factors. For instance, preventionists must consider the various influences on development such as individual, family, neighborhood, and cultural characteristics (Wachs, 2000). When the target problem has several domains, the number of components in a comprehensive program often corresponds with the number of domains presumed to be influential in promoting positive development. This thoroughness in prevention programming is especially important for populations with high levels of risk. Discovering which combination of components will be most effective in promoting healthy development is the initial task related to mounting prevention programs. Accordingly, comprehensive prevention programs address as many aspects of a specific problem as possible.

Varied Teaching Methods   The eventual success or failure of a prevention program relies on the participants' internalization of the contents of the treatment. The likelihood that vital components of the intervention will reach diverse groups with different backgrounds, abilities, and learning styles is determined by 1) the specific teaching approaches, 2) the circumstances surrounding the use of those teaching methods, and 3) the appropriateness of particular teaching tactics for the intended population. Because each individual has a unique constellation of learning needs, varying teaching methods ensures that all participants grasp the desired concepts and skills. Varied teaching methods not only respect unique learning styles, but they also keep learners engaged by making the materials and their presentation more interesting. The use of multiple techniques to present information increases learners' understanding of problem behaviors (creating a mental model that can guide future actions) as well as enhances the employment of specific skills (creating a new behavioral repertoire). Consequently, varied teaching methods produce good results by allowing participants to learn and apply content materials, ultimately achieving the goal of preventing negative behaviors from occurring.

Positive Relationships   Prevention programs that produce important results are those in which participants become invested in the intervention goals and are consequently committed to the treatment curricula. The outcome of treatment rests on the quality of the relationships between professionals and program recipients (Kohlenberg, Kanter, Bolling, Parker, & Tsai, 2002). Developing positive relationships is critical to creating a sense of connectedness that assures participants that the service delivery professionals are helping them to make gains in life skills, rather than trying to fix something that is wrong with them. Good relationships build support and encouragement for positive outcomes as well as create an accepting environment for possible setbacks. Furthermore, positive, mutually respective relationships between staff and families increase program attendance and reduce program attrition. Building rapport with intervention participants is essential to providing an affirming foundation on which the desired message is presented. In these ways, fostering positive relationships initiates the acceptance of, and adherence to, prevention curricula.

Sociocultural Relevance   The best prevention programs convey information in a manner that is both comfortable and nonoffensive to participants, allowing families to feel good about changing their current ways of thinking or behaving. Doing so requires curricula that have sociocultural relevance, meaning that the prevention program is tailored to the specific community and cultural norms of the participants. These programs concentrate on issues that are salient for a specific cultural group, and they mandate collaboration between practitioners and participants to establish program goals and determine the approaches that will be used to attain those goals. Prevention programs must consider local needs, respect cultural norms, and incorporate appropriate language use into their curricula. Socioculturally relevant programs also maintain close communication with target groups throughout the duration of the intervention. Continued interactions alert practitioners to unexpected problems and provide feedback for intervention components that are working well or those that are not producing the desired results. Accordingly, when practitioners and families work jointly to set goals for promoting healthy development by implementing prevention programs with sociocultural relevance, families deepen their investment in program objectives, making program success more likely.

Procedural Principles

Principles that fall into the procedural category help to integrate the elements of scientific accuracy with the artistic execution of the intervention. The smooth and effective administration of a prevention curriculum demands thorough attention to procedural details (e.g., determining exactly how much of the treatment will be given, assessing the best time for its administration, maintaining treatment fidelity). Likewise, high-quality staffing and programmed generalizations for the extension of acquired beliefs and behaviors are necessary for achieving both short- and long-term results. Principles within the procedural category serve to assure optimal program implementation, which in turn promotes intervention success.

Sufficient Dosage   Establishing a sufficient dosage involves determining which type of treatment should be presented, how long that treatment should be administered, and what will happen after the treatment is no longer provided. By manipulating the treatment dosage, researchers and practitioners can determine the amount of intervention required to produce the desired behavioral change(s). Nation et al. (2003) noted that a hallmark of effective prevention is an appropriate match between the intensity of the intervention and the needs of each individual in the program. Treatment dosage should correspond to participants' specific risks and needs. For instance, individuals with multiple risks typically require a greater treatment amount than participants with fewer risks to achieve positive and lasting effects (Nation et al.). Sufficient dosage typically occurs when the treatment amount adequately addresses the target problem without overwhelming or frustrating the clients by being too demanding. Program participants achieve their largest gains when each individual is administered the right amount and form of the treatment.

Appropriate Timing   To be successful, prevention programs should begin prior to the onset of problem behaviors and be tailored to the developmental needs of the individuals in the intervention; that is, effective programs utilize appropriate timing. Because the core of prevention is keeping problems from emerging, effective interventions promote positive behaviors and attitudes before problems commence to forestall potentially harmful trajectories from occurring. Appropriately timed interventions also must remain sensitive to the developmental needs of the participants. The developmental stage of the participants should be factored into curriculum development and its subsequent implementation. Information should not be presented in a way that overwhelms young participants or patronizes and bores older participants. Interventions that demonstrate long-term benefits for participants begin early enough to prevent the emergence of problem behaviors and utilize a developmentally appropriate curriculum and teaching strategy.

Well-Trained Staff   The effectiveness of prevention research relies heavily on the skills of the staff in implementing and executing the intervention. As such, it is critical for a prevention program to have well-trained staff members who are not only competent in program delivery, but who also are able to adapt as problems arise without departing from the core intervention goals and procedures. Successful programs establish a staff protocol that involves continuous checking over time to confirm that service delivery professionals have acquired, and are maintaining, the skills necessary for appropriately carrying out the intervention's components. This procedure begins prior to hiring, when potential staff members must demonstrate sufficient job-related skills (e.g., minimum levels of educational, occupational, and personal experiences necessary for the position). Once hired, supervisors or project managers should be responsible for ensuring that each staff member is appropriately trained as evidenced by the mastery of the intervention components; staff members should understand program goals and be competent in implementing strategies to achieve those goals. In many cases, a well-trained staff will demonstrate their mastery by becoming consistent or reliable with other interventionists (or the project manager) who represent the gold standard for service delivery. In other words, the prevention program will be implemented as intended and in exactly the same way across staff members to ensure that each participant receives high-quality programming. When staff training is viewed as a continuous process in professional development, prevention programs thrive because of reduced staff turnover and higher-quality supports for the participants themselves.

Programmed Generalization   A successful intervention must simultaneously tackle both the perpetuation of undesirable behaviors and the prevention of future problems. In this manner, effective programming offers a way for newly learned skills and positive behaviors to be maintained and generalized across settings and over time; such planned learning occasions are called programmed generalizations. Successful intervention programs are those that have built-in opportunities for participants to exercise their recently acquired skills via training sessions in multiple settings (e.g., home, school, after-school programs) as well as booster sessions, perhaps weeks or months after treatment has ceased. Follow-up contact with participants encourages the maintenance of positive behaviors and helps to prevent lapses into problematic behaviors by reminding participants of their goals and previous accomplishments. Employing a workable combination of intervention components across multiple domains, and over time, increases the likelihood of the development and continuation of positive behaviors. In short, programmed generalization is necessary to produce enduring treatment-related gains.

Treatment Fidelity   For prevention programs to ensure the greatest benefits for all individuals, it is imperative that each participant be given services of the highest quality possible. Assurance of first-rate treatment administration is shown through treatment fidelity, which is the documentation that each participant has received the intervention in the way that it was designed and represented in the curriculum. Prevention programs with good treatment fidelity continuously monitor various aspects of service delivery, carefully observing the precision of program implementation. Continuous supervision and feedback in the field between staff and program managers is essential to confirm that all clients are receiving the appropriate services. Not only does this process verify that each and every participant receives the correct amount of the treatment in the appropriate manner, but it also protects individual recipients from unintended biases during the intervention process. For example, a staff member may offer additional resources or supports to some participants and not to others based on his or her personal perceptions of familial needs. Establishing a clear protocol for when and how to provide additional resources eliminates the need for staff decisions based on personal judgments and priorities. By maintaining treatment fidelity, prevention programs ensure compliance to the curriculum during service delivery.

Design and Evaluation Principles

Principles belonging to the design and evaluation category rely on the interchange between science and art. Attention to scientific veracity is at the core of properly measuring a program's effectiveness and impact. For instance, appropriately evaluating outcomes, demonstrating an adequate effect size, and confirming internal validation all offer evidence of the success of a prevention program. Generating reasonable interpretive standards and verifying a program's clinical and/or social significance depend on the skillful work of practitioners and the insights of the entire research team. The principles associated with design and evaluation provide the means to interpret the causal factors associated with major changes following an intervention in an applied setting.

Interpretive Standards When evaluating a prevention program, researchers look for solid evidence that the prevention has worked. Verification that the prevention is effective depends on data that demonstrate clearly and convincingly that there is a statistically significant difference in major outcomes in favor of a treatment condition over an appropriately formed control condition. The failure to use randomized designs that employ active, rather than passive, control conditions may be the single greatest problem for prevention programs to meet the interpretive standards that reveal unequivocal treatment efficacy. Individuals in active control conditions receive attention (and sometimes information) that is similar to that received by those in the treatment condition(s). At times, several active control conditions are needed to isolate the impact of particular intervention components. Unfortunately, few prevention studies use active control groups that are suitable for clear comparisons with the treatment condition(s) and that allow for the decomposition of the overall treatment into its key causal components. Instead, research frequently includes passive control conditions, where participants are assessed in a pretest–posttest fashion, without the additional contact (or minimal information) that the active groups would receive. Sometimes solid methodological evaluation is compromised by a lack of random assignment, with the utilization of convenience samples acting as a barrier to forming true randomized designs. The inclusion of randomized, or at least quasi-randomized, designs is vital to meeting the interpretive standards associated with rigorous prevention research. Including active control conditions and using randomized designs ensures that differences between treatment and control groups can be attributed to the intervention curriculum and not to other factors, such as chance or frequent contact with staff. Appropriate interpretive standards demand the use of active control groups and permit unambiguous conclusions about the causal role of the treatment program in producing important behavioral changes.

Outcome Evaluation   In prevention research, program success is reflected by changes in the major outcomes, allowing the scientific community and the public to know what the prevention program has to offer. Programs must carefully select outcome variables for evaluation based on which constructs and processes are hypothesized to change as a result of the treatment. Frequently, the outcome variables will correspond with program goals. Good programs often have a wide range of outcome variables. Assessing gains in multiple domains is sometimes necessary to reveal the magnitude of a particular program's benefits as well as to identify specific areas for future improvements. Similarly, appropriate outcome evaluation involves measuring variables that are indicative of changes in causal processes, rather than static measures of behavior. By evaluating the achievement of process goals as well as performance goals, prevention programs demonstrate that the underlying core of the target problem has been addressed. Finally, the variables selected as major outcomes should reflect both short- and long-term changes; proof of lasting change provides the best evidence of the prevention program's effectiveness. Because practitioners hope to improve participants' lives following the delivery of an intervention, outcome evaluations provide confidence that the prevention program has been adequately tested and shown to be effective.

Internal Validation   The usefulness of a program in promoting healthy behaviors and preventing negative outcomes depends on the extent to which positive outcomes are due to behavioral changes resulting from the intervention; in research, this is called internal validation. Internal validation is the systematic attempt to show consistencies between the processes assumed responsible for change and the eventual outcome. Program evaluations are typically concerned with 1) whether the implementation results in major behavioral changes, 2) who changes, and 3) the extent of the change in relationship to underlying variability. However, whether the process itself has changed is sometimes more important than whether the targeted behavior has changed. That is, a visible behavioral change often requires great effort to produce a change in an underlying causal process, such as a belief or self-perception. Performance improvements sometimes follow related process changes only after a lengthy delay. Thus, significant correlations between changes in process measures and changes in outcome variables represent internal validation. Once underlying processes have been put in place or strengthened, important changes in performance should follow and, eventually, reflect statistically or socially significant results. This approach to data analysis ultimately helps to document when and where causal relationships occurred, thus lending support for attributing specific outcomes to the treatment-related process under investigation. In this sense, internal validation is a vital element for future prevention research.

Adequate Effect Size Establishing the quality and potential usefulness of prevention programming relies on demonstrating how much of the change in an outcome measure can be attributed to the treatment per se. In null hypothesis testing, the difference between means in the outcome (or dependent) variable in terms of the amount of error variance is called the effect size. One of the most popular measures of effect size, Cohen's d (1969), is expressed in its simplest form as $d = [\mu_1 - \mu_2] / \sigma$ (Howell, 2002). Including the effect size in evaluation research provides a valuable technique for standardizing the measures so that the importance of differences between the treatment and control conditions can be properly gauged. Scaling group differences in terms of standard errors provides a way to comprehend the magnitude and meaning of differences among groups when the number of units changes from measure to measure in different studies. For example, a difference of 100 points may constitute a small change on one measure, whereas a difference of only 10 units may represent a large change with another measure. Putting these differences in terms of their respective variances facilitates a clearer interpretation of treatment effectiveness (Howell, 2002). Cohen has suggested rules of thumb for interpreting the effect size, with d estimates of 0.20, 0.50, and 0.80 indicating small, medium, and large effect sizes, respectively (Howell, 2002). Establishing a reasonable effect size indicates the extent, in meaningful units, that the participants in the treatment condition have performed better than the participants in the control condition. Maxwell and Delaney (2004) have proposed that including the magnitude of an effect should regularly accompany hypothesis testing; effect size parameters are useful methods for accomplishing this end. In brief, expressing the degree that the null hypothesis is false using effect size helps to confirm the value and utility of a prevention curriculum.

Clinical or Social Significance Although effect size is one way to determine the magnitude of treatment effects, it is also important to remember that a good prevention program might result in a study with a small effect size but with important clinical or social significance. Clinical or social significance sometimes results from changes in several individuals that are dramatic enough to make the prevention effort worthwhile (e.g., completely altering a life-course trajectory) even if all participants do not exhibit the same benefits. For instance, a program would have significance if it prevented just one person from committing suicide or another from becoming a serial killer. Of course, positive changes in nearly all participants would be even better. The overall value of prevention research for society at large is established not only by meaningful changes in the treatment versus control group on the basis of statistical significance, but also by changes related to clinical or social significance.

CREATING EFFECTIVE PREVENTION PROGRAMS

When treatment, procedural, and design and evaluation principles are carefully considered in designing prevention research, the resulting program will likely display scientific integrity during the sensitive and artful implementation of its curriculum. By incorporating each of the 15 principles into prevention research, good science and good art overlap and intertwine to promote healthy development. For instance, a program with a varied and culturally sensitive curriculum administered with a sufficient dosage is likely to produce large, meaningful effects. Similarly, a comprehensive program that has appropriate developmental timing and that demonstrates good internal validation is likely to reflect the adequate interpretative standards necessary for matching the prevention of a major developmental problem with a given treatment. Evidence of the importance of each of the 15 principles will be demonstrated in a variety of ways in the book. All future prevention research should be designed and evaluated with these key principles in mind during each stage of the research formation and implementation process. This chapter acts as the foundation for the subsequent evaluation of prevention programs designed to advance the healthy development of infants, children, and adolescents.

The chapters that follow describe existing prevention programs within specific domains and critically analyze their current effectiveness as well as ways to enhance their potential impact. The 15 principles necessary for successful prevention programs serve as the criteria for the critical analyses contained in each chapter. Each chapter will show how and why the principles are necessary for promoting positive developmental outcomes. Each chapter also recommends the best approach to prevention, focusing on treatment, procedural, and design and evaluation principles. The model programs provided are generally modifications or extensions of existing prevention programs, although some are entirely new. In each case, the model programs are built around the combination of good art and science.

CASE STUDIES: THE PERSON IN THE PROGRAM

A unique feature of the review, analysis, and synthesis of prevention research in seven important domains is the development of a model program in each area and its application to the problems being encountered by a real-life family. This chapter concludes with three problem scenarios, one of which will be used at the end of each subsequent chapter to illustrate how the lives of children and adolescents can be enhanced through high-quality prevention research. These case studies give life to the model programs by focusing on how individual children and their families respond to and are affected by highly focused prevention programs.

❖

The Jackson Family: Steven's Problems at Home and School

Jason and Beth Jackson, a biracial couple, have been married for 8 years and have one 7-year-old son, Steven. Jason and Beth met in college and were married shortly after Jason's graduation from nursing school. Beth is a Spanish teacher at the local junior high school. Their combined income allows them to live comfortably, although they are certainly not wealthy by today's standards. Jason works 12-hour days on second shift, 3 days at a time, and then has 4 days off. Although it seems as though he has considerable free time, he usually takes that time to relax, catch up on his sleep, and spend time with Steven. Beth is supportive of Jason's career; however, she often finds herself feeling blue over their lack of time together. This has been a source of conflict for them, although neither feels that it is detrimental to their relationship. Occasionally, they disagree about who will take care of the household chores. Due to Jason's revolving schedule, they both have to keep track of who is doing what and when. More often, they argue over how to handle Steven, who was diagnosed with attention-deficit/hyperactivity disorder (ADHD) last year. Steven is now a third-grade student, and even though his social skills are minimal, he does have a few friends at school. Although Beth would like Steven to excel more in his studies, she knows that he is not failing any subject. Beth dealt with minor depression following Steven's birth and now finds his lack of attention and hyperactivity to be overwhelming at times. Jason is more concerned about Steven's progress in school than about how well he can play with his friends. Jason often scolds Steven for bringing home Cs and feels that his son just needs to concentrate more. The difference in their opinions about how to handle Steven's grade problems is probably the greatest source of conflict for Beth and Jason. Steven gets very upset when he hears his parents fighting, especially when they are arguing about him. He often thinks that it's his fault that they fight. Sometimes he feels like running out of his bedroom and yelling at them to stop fighting.

The Smith Family:
Family Violence and Keisha's Behavioral Adjustment Problems

Gary and Debra Smith are an African American couple with a 13-year-old daughter, Keisha. Gary and Debra divorced 2 months ago following a series of stressors including marital conflict and several instances of domestic violence. Keisha is disturbed by the violence between her parents and has ongoing talks with a teacher about how her parents always put her in the middle of their arguments. After hearing Keisha's story and noticing a bruise on her arm, the teacher made a report to the local child protective services agency, which has been monitoring the Smith family's situation since that time.

Although Gary and Debra thought that their divorce would solve their problems, they are still faced with ongoing difficulties. Keisha has been living with her mother since the divorce. Fearing Gary's violent behaviors, Debra obtained a restraining order against him, rendering him unable to have contact with either her or Keisha. Gary took Debra to court hoping to regain visitation with, or custody of, his daughter, but his request was denied because of his history of family violence. Because the Smiths have been living in poverty for several years, neither parent is able to afford adequate legal counsel. Gary is currently attending a support group for violent offenders in hopes of gaining the respect of his family and the courts.

Keisha, who was already having minor academic and behavioral difficulties prior to the divorce, has recently displayed increased problematic behavior. She is unhappy that she had to transfer to a different school when she and her mother moved away from the home that they shared with Gary, and she has expressed her discontent by acting out at her new school as well as at her new home. She has been talking back to her teachers, fighting with her classmates, breaking rules at home, and failing several classes. Keisha is angry at her father for not being involved in her life, but she is fearful that the violence she witnessed between her parents in the past might recur. She is angry with both parents because she feels that they always put her in the middle of their ongoing disagreements and conflict.

❖

The Taylor Family:
Intergenerational Teenage Parenting and Amy's Dilemma

Tom and Cassie Taylor, a European American couple, have been married for 11 years. They have two children together, Kevin (10) and Kathy (13). When Cassie was 16, she had a daughter, Allison, whom Tom adopted when they were married. Allison is now 17 and has a 6-month-old daughter, Amy. With the addition of another child to the household, Cassie finds that the family needs more money than Tom's income from his factory job. It was difficult for her to find a part-time job with only her GED, but Cassie finally found a janitorial position that allows her to be home when Kevin and Kathy get out of school.

Tension increased within the family after the birth of Amy. Cassie worried that Tom, a recovering alcoholic, might revert to drinking. When he drank regularly, problems in their relationship almost led to a separation; he also treated the children harshly. Tom has been sober for 5 years, but Cassie knows that she would be overwhelmed in their current situation if he had not joined Alcoholics Anonymous. Kevin and Kathy have had problems adjusting to the new infant in the house and the fact that Kathy must now share her bedroom with both Allison and Amy. Kathy has been falling asleep at school lately because Amy keeps her up at night. In addition, Kevin and Kathy have taken on more responsibility around the house since their mother went back to work, and they resent not having as much time with their friends. Although they love playing with Amy, they sometimes feel weighed down when they have to babysit for her, especially on weekends.

Allison is adjusting slowly, finding it hard living at home and having dual roles as a daughter and a mother in the same household. Amy's father is not involved with the family because he was incarcerated for drug possession shortly after Allison found that she was pregnant. Allison has not contacted him about the child because she is afraid he will not want to have anything to do with Amy. She remembers how it felt knowing that her biological father did not want to see her, and she would rather Amy not have to go through the same situation. Allison is tired of listening to her mom's advice about how to raise Amy, but she doesn't think she can afford to move out and raise Amy alone. In contrast to Cassie being overly involved, Tom has become less involved. He was very upset when he found out that Allison was pregnant and hasn't treated her the same since. Allison is sad that Tom is distancing himself from Amy and herself. She thought that being a mother would be easier, but much of the time she feels overwhelmed with the challenges and responsibilities that Amy brings.

APPLYING THE PRINCIPLES OF PREVENTION RESEARCH

The implementation of comprehensive intervention programs—guided by innovative theory—increases the likelihood that the challenging problems faced by the Jackson, Smith, and Taylor families can be prevented before they escalate to cause short-term developmental delays or lifelong damage. If targeted interventions are delivered in sufficient dosages by highly trained individuals who develop positive relationships with Steven, Keisha, and Amy and respect their ethnic, cultural, and racial backgrounds, then the model programs should produce large, meaningful changes in their lives.

REFERENCES

Albee, G.W. (1991). No more rock scrubbing. *The Scientist Practitioner, American Association of Applied and Preventive Psychology, 1,* 26–27.

Borkowski, J.G., Smith, L.E., & Akai, C.E. (in press). *Designing effective prevention programs: How good science makes good art.* Infants and Young Children.

Cohen, J. (1969). *Statistical power analysis for behavioral sciences.* Mahwah, NJ: Lawrence Erlbaum Associates.

Green, M., & Piel, J.A. (2002). *Theories of human development: A comparative approach.* Boston: Allyn & Bacon.

Howell, D. C. (2002). *Statistical methods for psychology.* Pacific Grove, CA: Duxbury.

Kohlenberg, R.H., Kanter, J.W., Bolling, M.Y., Parker, C., & Tsai, M. (2002). Enhancing cognitive therapy for depression with functional analytic psychotherapy: Treatment guidelines and empirical findings. *Cognitive and Behavioral Practice, 9,* 213–229.

Maxwell, S.E., & Delaney, H.D. (2004). *Designing experiments and analyzing data: A model comparison perspective* (2nd ed.). Mahwah, NJ: Lawrence Erlbaum Associates.

Miller, P.H. (2002). *Theories of developmental psychology* (4th ed.). New York: Worth Publishers.

Nation, M., Crusto, C., Wandersman, A., Kumpfer, K.L., Seybolt, D., Morrisey-Kane, E., et al. (2003). What works in prevention: Principles of effective prevention programs. *American Psychologist, 58,* 449–456.

Ramey, S.L., & Ramey, C.T. (1992). Early educational interventions with disadvantaged children—to what effect? *Applied and Preventive Psychology, 1,* 131–140.

Wachs, T.D. (2000). *Necessary but not sufficient: The respective roles of single and multiple influences on individual development.* Washington, DC: American Psychological Association.

2

PROMOTING INFANT
GROWTH AND DEVELOPMENT

Lane E. Volpe and Willow A. Wetherall

Infancy and early childhood represent a critical and particularly vulnerable stage of development, with implications for physiological health and safety as well as long-term developmental outcomes. Despite advances in medicine, reports on the status of infant health and mortality in the United States reveal surprisingly high rates of infant mortality and low immunization rates compared with other industrialized countries (Starfield, 2004). The overall U.S. infant mortality rate for 2002 was 7.0 infant deaths per 1,000 live births, translating into a total of 28,034 infant deaths for that year (Kochanek, Murphy, Anderson, & Scott, 2004).

Although the neonatal period, infancy, and early toddlerhood comprise a relatively small percentage of pre-adult development, this life stage is disproportionately important in setting the stage for optimal health and development across an individual's entire lifespan. Consequently, the physical growth and development that takes place in the first year of life directly influences children's subsequent health and nutritional status. It also fundamentally alters the trajectory of critical brain development and can even affect an individual's later risk of developing chronic diseases. Suboptimal health during this critical period is particularly detrimental because it occurs at a time when important milestones in physical growth and psychological development are achieved. Therefore, choices that parents make about how to create a healthy start for their children, including practices pertaining to feeding method- and sleep-related behaviors, can have long-term developmental consequences.

This chapter evaluates and critiques four exemplar programs designed to enhance healthy infant growth and development by 1) promoting breastfeeding (Infant Nutrition Study Community Health Intervention; Pugh, Milligan, Frick, Spatz, & Bronner, 2002), 2) reducing Sudden Infant Death Syndrome (SIDS; Back to Sleep Campaign; National Institute of Child Health and Human Development [NICHD], 2001), and 3) increasing the quality and regularity of early health care and improving parenting practices (My Baby U, Brown, Yando, & Rainforth, 2000; Healthy Steps for Young Children, Guyer et al., 2003a). These programs are presented in terms of their comprehensiveness, with the Healthy Steps for Young Children program being closest to what the authors advocate as a model program to promote early child health and development. The essential characteristics of these four programs are summarized in Table 2.1.

PROMOTING BREASTFEEDING INITIATION AND CONTINUATION

The parental choice to breastfeed or use infant formula has profound health implications for infants. The American Academy of Pediatrics (AAP; American Academy of Pediatrics; Work Group on Breastfeeding, 2005) affirmed that breast milk is the preferred form of nourishment for infants. The AAP currently recommends that all infants be breastfed exclusively for 6 months with continued breastfeeding to 1 year and for as long thereafter as mother and infant prefer. Breastfeeding is one of the most significant safeguards to infant health. Human milk provides infants with an optimal nutritional package and is especially important for the intensive brain development that takes place during infancy and early childhood. Because infants are born without a developed immune system, the antibodies present in breast milk offer the only available form of transferred immunity against a host of new pathogens that an infant will encounter outside the womb (Cunningham, 1995).

Research indicates that breastfeeding improves infant health and developmental outcomes in multiple areas. The incidence of postneonatal mortality in the United States is reduced by 21% overall for breastfed infants (Chen & Rogan, 2004). Breastfed infants experience significantly lower rates of numerous acute illnesses (Wolf, 2003), including diarrhea (Bhandari, Bahl, Mazumdar, Martines, Black, & Bhan, 2003), ear infections (Duncan, Ey, Holberg, Wright, Martinez, & Taussig, 1993), and respiratory illness (Lopez-Alarcon, Villalpando, & Fajardo, 1997). In addition, existing studies suggest that breastfed infants experience a decreased risk of chronic diseases such as leukemia and lymphoma (Bener, Denic, & Galadari, 2001), asthma (Oddy & Holt, 1999), and insulin-dependent and non–insulin-dependent diabetes (Kostraba et al., 1993; Pettit & Forman, 1997).

Although the mechanism of protection remains unclear, breastfeeding also has been associated with a decreased incidence of childhood obesity (Armstrong & Reilly, 2002). Breastfeeding has implications for improved cognitive and motor development (Bier, Oliver, Ferguson, & Vohr, 2002; Horwood, Darlow, & Mogridge, 2001) and has been associated with increased performance on IQ tests (Mortensen, Michaelsen, Sanders, & Reinisch, 2002).

The benefits of breastfeeding extend well beyond improved health outcomes for infants. Breastfeeding aids women in recovery following childbirth (Chua, Arulkumaran, Lim, Selamat, & Ratnam, 1994). In addition, women who choose to breastfeed experience postpartum weight loss (Dewey, Heinig, & Nommsen, 1993) and delayed return of ovulation, which naturally reduces the chance of subsequent pregnancies from occurring too soon after giving birth (Kennedy, Labbok, & Van Look, 1996). Women who breastfeed also may gain protection against later chronic illnesses, including osteoporosis (Lopez, Gonzalez, Reyes, Campino, & Diaz, 1996; Paton et al., 2003), breast cancer (Lee, Kim, Kim, Song, & Yoon, 2003; Newcomb et al., 1994), and ovarian cancer (Rosenblatt & Thomas, 1993). These health benefits for individual women and infants potentially yield significant advantages for society as well. Economic savings and environmental protection are frequently discussed as collective benefits. Other societal benefits from breastfeeding include lower rates of employee absenteeism (Cadwell, 2002), reduced insurance premiums, and decreased costs associated with public health care programs (Tuttle & Dewey, 1996).

The current rate of breastfeeding initiation in the United States is 70.9%, which approximates the national goal of 75%. However, at 1 week postpartum, only 68.9% of women are still breastfeeding, and only 62.5% are exclusively breastfeeding. By 3 months, rates of partial and exclusive breastfeeding have dropped to 50.2% and 41.1%, respectively (Centers for Disease Control and Prevention, 2003)—a time period that often corresponds with a mother's return to work or school (Li, Grummer-Strawn, Zhao, Barker, & Mokdad, 2003). This decline has significant health implications because many of the most important benefits for infants come from extended breastfeeding. Unfortunately, lack of information, preparedness, and support often lead to premature cessation of breastfeeding, and overcoming these obstacles to extended breastfeeding continues to pose significant challenges. Data from the 2002 National Immunization Survey revealed that continued breastfeeding fell short of the national goals at 6 and 12 months, with only 17.2% of mothers continuing to breastfeed at 1 year (Centers for Disease Control and Prevention). The Healthy People 2010 public health goals focus on breastfeeding as a national health priority and aim to increase the percentage of infants being breastfed to 75% percent postpartum, 50% at 6 months, and 25% up to 1 year (U.S. Department of Health and Human Services, 2000).

Table 2.1. Selected programs for promoting infant health and their defining characteristics

	INS Community Health Intervention	Back to Sleep Campaign	My Baby U	Healthy Steps*
Targets of intervention	Pregnant women, recruited prenatally	General U.S. population Entire population of pregnant women, parents, and child care providers Additional outreach efforts targeted at high-risk populations	Pregnant women Families of participants	Mothers of infants and young children Families of participants Pediatric practices and their staff
Content of intervention	Professional advice and support for lactation Peer support and role modeling Skill development and practical problem solving for managing breastfeeding	Population-wide health recommendation Recommendation to place infants in supine position for sleep Secondary program messages include avoiding the use of soft bedding in infant sleep environment and reducing infant exposure to cigarette smoke	Topics related to infant development including cognitive and motor skill development, infant temperament and behavior, developmental stages Common parenting concerns and experiences	Enhanced quality of preventive health care and developmental services Parental skill development Support services
Method of delivery	Direct daily contact with participants during postpartum hospitalization Home visits during first, second, and fourth weeks postpartum, and additionally as necessary	Blanket public health recommendations and public service announcements Direct advice given to parents and caregivers from health care practitioners	Eight videotapes mailed to participants' homes with supplementary reading materials, without accompanying instructions	Placed developmental specialists in existing pediatric practices to facilitate delivery of health care and developmental services for infants, young children, and families

	INS Community Health Intervention	Back to Sleep Campaign	My Baby U	Healthy Steps*
Method of delivery	Telephone support twice weekly through week 8, and weekly from week 8 to month 6 Additional contact and support as deemed necessary	Pamphlets, brochures, and other educational materials Creative outreach strategies for increasing awareness and compliance among high-risk populations	Videotapes feature topics related to infant development neonatally and at 1, 3, 5, 7, 10, and 12 months of age and distributed to parents when infants reach the corresponding age	Developmental specialists coordinated and facilitated telephone support, peer support groups, and parenting education and made home visits Specialists coordinated timing of appropriate services and tailored services to the needs of individual children and families
Outcomes of intervention	Increase in breastfeeding initiation, duration, and rates of exclusive breastfeeding After first week postpartum, more mothers in intervention group breastfeeding at all time points compared with control group Group differences not statistically significant due to small sample size	Widespread decrease in use of the prone infant sleep position Between 1992 (prior to campaign) and 1998, the proportion of infants placed to sleep in the prone position declined from 70% to 17% Significant decrease in rate of SIDS during the same time period Overall SIDS rate declined 40% from 1992 to 1998	Increase in maternal knowledge of infant development at 6 months Infants in intervention group experienced fewer serious illnesses during first year of life Intervention group required less medication, less medical care in the form of follow-up visits and referrals to specialists Mothers in intervention group were more likely to follow recommended vaccination schedules	Improvement in quality of care received at pediatric practices Intervention group more likely to follow recommended vaccination schedules and well-child visits Positive changes in parenting behavior Intervention children less likely to visit the emergency room with injuries

*This program is no longer in existence.

A variety of programs that promote breastfeeding initiation have been documented in the medical literature (Ryser, 2004; Volpe & Bear, 2000). However, programs that significantly increase the duration of breastfeeding using an active control condition are scarce. The few intervention studies that have been rigorously evaluated show promising results, but have been conducted on a relatively small scale (Pugh et al., 2002) or with low-risk populations (Dennis, Hodnett, Gallop, & Chalmers, 2002). One essential component that has been identified for increasing duration is the inclusion of peer support in the program design (Heinig & Farley, 2001). Lack of social support is a key risk factor for premature cessation of breastfeeding; however, programming that delivers peer support to mothers is able to overcome this barrier. In collaboration with Best Start, the Special Supplemental Nutrition Program for Women, Infants and Children (WIC) is currently implementing a nationwide initiative to provide peer support, in conjunction with other services, to its clients as part of the Loving Support Makes Breastfeeding Work campaign (McLaughlin, Burstein, Tao, & Fox, 2004).

Although peer support has been shown to be effective in increasing breastfeeding among high-risk groups (Milligan, Pugh, Bronner, Spatz, & Brown, 2000), peer support appears to benefit all women regardless of socioeconomic status or intention to breastfeed. Dennis and colleagues (2002) found that telephone-based peer support significantly increased breastfeeding duration for women who had already initiated breastfeeding, and two large-scale trials currently being conducted will likely provide new evidence-based strategies for promoting continuation of breastfeeding (K. Wambach, personal communication, July, 18, 2005; L. Pugh, personal communication, July 2005). The following section evaluates one small-scale program that produced promising results for increasing the duration of breastfeeding for women of low socioeconomic status.

Infant Nutrition Study Community Health Intervention

The Infant Nutrition Study (INS) is a hospital-based program that provides education, peer counseling, home visits, and clinical support for lactation to women of low socioeconomic status in the Mid-Atlantic region during postpartum hospitalization (Pugh et al., 2002). The goal of the INS is to increase breastfeeding initiation and continuation among women of low socioeconomic status and to develop cost-effective strategies for providing lactation support that decrease expenditures for formula purchase and health care. The INS model uses nurses and peer counselors to provide holistic professional and social support for breastfeeding. Community health nurses provide clinical and professional knowledge and educational support for women, whereas community-based peer counselors offer direct role modeling and emotional support.

Program Description Participants in the INS received daily visits from the community health nurse and peer counselor during hospitalization and three subsequent home visits during the first, second, and fourth week postpartum and additionally as necessary. Peer counselors also provided ongoing support via telephone twice weekly through the 8th week and weekly from the 8th week to 6 months, regardless of whether the mother was still breastfeeding (Pugh et al., 2002). The breastfeeding support team addressed common problems related to premature cessation of breastfeeding, including nipple discomfort, lack of social support, and physiological symptoms. Specific evidence-based breastfeeding advice and strategies were provided to participants, including use of cold compresses and other suggestions for decreasing breast discomfort (Pugh et al., 1996) and appropriate positioning for decreasing maternal fatigue (Milligan, Flenniken, & Pugh, 1996). The peer-counseling component served as a significant source of social support in line with the identified needs of women of low socioeconomic status (Milligan et al., 2000).

Program Evaluation Between 1999 and 2000, 41 women receiving financial and medical assistance were recruited at a large academic medical center to take part in the INS. Participants were randomly assigned to intervention or usual care conditions. Participants in the two groups did not differ on major demographic characteristics including age, ethnicity, education, marital status, and plans for infant feeding (Pugh et al., 2002). Women in the usual care group received standard hospital breastfeeding support services, including support from the nursing staff, assistance by telephone, and one visit from a lactation consultant if delivery happened to occur on a weekday. Mothers in the intervention group received this standard care plus all of the INS services. Intervention group mothers were contacted bimonthly for 6 months, and data were collected on each mother's occupation, employment or student status, the amount of time spent feeding (breast milk or formula), formula quantity used, health care provider, emergency room visits and reason for visits, and infant hospitalizations (Pugh et al.). Duration of breastfeeding measured in weeks was determined based on maternal self-report. Infant feeding was categorized as exclusive breastfeeding, partial breastfeeding, or exclusive formula feeding.

Results from the INS were promising. At 3 months, 45% of the intervention group was still exclusively breastfeeding compared with 25% of the usual care group. At 6 months, 30% of mothers receiving INS services and 15% of mothers receiving usual care were exclusively breastfeeding. Forty-five percent of intervention mothers were still partially breastfeeding at 6 months compared with 35% in the usual care group. Of the 12 chi-square analyses that were conducted to assess group differences in exclusive breastfeeding bimonthly from 1 to 24 weeks, none were statistically significant due to small sample size (Pugh et al.,

2002). However, these results were approaching significance and are suggestive of the potential impact of the INS program with a larger population.

Several important benefits were seen in terms of heath care among infants whose mothers participated in the INS program as compared with infants of mothers receiving usual care. Infants in the intervention group visited a health care provider less frequently, including checkups and visits due to illness, and used significantly fewer prescriptions (Pugh et al., 2002). Whereas these health outcomes may be a result of the protective effects of breastfeeding on infant health, it is also possible that home visits from the community health nurse may have replaced some doctor's office visits. Infants in the intervention group did have slightly fewer visits to the emergency room, although on average vaccinations and total hospitalizations did not differ between the two groups (Pugh et al.).

Critical Analysis of Treatment Characteristics   The INS was implemented in an effort to improve rates of breastfeeding among women of low socioeconomic status as a way to safeguard against many of the health issues faced by impoverished families (Pugh et al., 2002). The INS addressed gaps in previous efforts (e.g., education-only programs, limited postpartum hospital-based efforts) that only targeted breastfeeding initiation and used an extended intervention design to affect duration rates. The program was based on the concept that peer support is an essential component of programs formulated to increase the length of breastfeeding for individual women. The INS promoted the development of essential skills required for successful breastfeeding and included a focus on maternal and infant health. Positive relationships between intervention staff and program participants were a focal aspect of the INS program. The program's sociocultural relevance was reinforced by the peer counselor, who was not a medical authority but rather a support person who often shared the background and experiences of program participants.

The INS was designed for individual women and was not highly integrated into participants' social ecological systems. The program did not engage family members or other support people who may play a major role in a mother's decision to initiate and continue breastfeeding. Although the program design did include multiple home visits, a more systematic effort to target the individuals who comprise a woman's social support network may have further increased the success of the INS program. However, this expanded design would necessarily increase the cost of the intervention and may not be feasible given limited resources for intervention programs.

Critical Analysis of Procedural Characteristics   The INS program was appropriately timed, establishing contact with women prenatally and providing critical support during the postpartum period. Participants received the most contact and assistance during the early stage of breastfeeding when skills are still being adopted and refined and when breastfeeding problems, such as discomfort and fatigue, may pose the greatest risk for premature cessation. Telephone support occurred twice weekly through the 8th week and weekly through the 6th month. The intervention ended at 6 months, well after breastfeeding would have been established and any initial barriers to breastfeeding addressed.

The INS design relied on a highly trained staff, and the particular strength of the program was the collaboration between the community health nurse and the peer counselor. This team offered in-hospital and telephone support and conducted visits to participants' homes to promote, support, and maintain newly learned skills. Contact with participants was administered uniformly, but staff were able to provide additional support services to individuals at their discretion. This allowed for a more individualized approach to program delivery. However, because there was some variance in the amount of contact and support received by participants, it is difficult to evaluate the circumstances surrounding the need for additional support, as well as the minimum amount of support necessary to produce the desired outcome. The additional support given to mothers on an as-needed basis may well have contributed to the success of the program. However, this level of support may be difficult to replicate with a large-scale population, and may not be entirely necessary because some mothers may have been able to problem solve effectively without the additional support of the community health nurse or peer counselor. To establish a clearer relationship between specific levels of support and outcomes, a current large-scale breastfeeding intervention, built off the INS model, standardizes the amount of support received by each participant (K. Frick, personal communication, July 26, 2005).

Critical Analysis of Design Characteristics   The design strengths of the INS included use of a control group, clear goals and objectives for increasing breastfeeding initiation and duration, and systematic evaluation and documentation of results. In addition, the program surpassed many existing breastfeeding programs by focusing on increasing the length of breastfeeding and by working with mothers over a period of 6 months. This contrasts with many interventions that focus exclusively on breastfeeding initiation, often measuring breastfeeding only in the immediate postpartum period. However, the program did not provide long-term support for participants to encourage breastfeeding to 1 year and beyond, in line with AAP recommendations (American Academy of Pediatrics; Work Group on Breastfeeding, 2005). This may be one avenue for future refinement of the program design.

One of the major accomplishments of the INS was that it brought the breastfeeding rates of a high-risk group in line with those of more low-risk populations. The breastfeeding rates, especially exclusive breastfeeding, documented for women in the INS compared favorably with national rates at the same time points. This is particularly noteworthy because rates are substantially lower among women of low socioeconomic status than their middle- and upper-class counterparts (Ryser, 2004). This outcome, although not statistically significant, strongly suggests the potential to help narrow gaps in health status between women of low and high socioeconomic status and their children. Because the small sample size makes generalization of the findings across larger groups difficult, additional ongoing large-scale investigations may provide a more thorough assessment of the program's efficacy, especially with diverse and high-risk populations (L. Pugh, personal communication, July 2005). Such studies also may contribute to understanding the long-term protective effects of breastfeeding for women and children.

PREVENTING SUDDEN INFANT DEATH SYNDROME

SIDS continues to be the number one cause of postneonatal death for infants between the ages of 1 month and 1 year, claiming the lives of 2,295 infants in 2001 (Kochanek et al., 2004), and the incidence of SIDS has a marked peak between 2 and 4 months of age (Task Force on Infant Sleep Position and Sudden Infant Death Syndrome, 2000). Despite years of research and the proposal of numerous explanatory theories, the causes and mechanisms of SIDS remain unknown. A SIDS diagnosis is in essence a diagnosis of exclusion, defined as the sudden death of any infant or young child in which a postmortem examination fails to demonstrate an adequate cause of death (Willinger, James, & Catz, 1991). Of the numerous explanatory theories that have been proposed, few have translated into measurable protection for individual infants against SIDS. One of the only widespread policy changes resulting in a measurable decrease in SIDS deaths stemmed from the data on prone positioning. Studies conducted in Australia, New Zealand, and the United Kingdom demonstrated a highly significant relationship between the incidence of SIDS and prone infant sleep position (see Fleming, 1994). The public health campaigns that followed in these and other western European countries advocating the supine (lying on back with face upward) sleep position were associated with a dramatic reduction in SIDS rates. In 1992, the AAP issued a similar recommendation, advocating the use of supine or lateral sleep positions for healthy, full-term infants in the United States. Currently, part of the NICHD's strategic plan is to eradicate all SIDS deaths by emphasizing the importance of daily behavioral infant caregiving practices and by expanding research on the processes and mechanisms involved in SIDS (NICHD, 2001).

Back to Sleep Campaign

Based on the AAP's 1992 recommendation to place infants in the supine or lateral position for sleep, the NICHD initiated the Back to Sleep Campaign in 1994 in conjunction with a coalition of other agencies. This multidisciplinary, multi-level campaign serves as the primary program aimed at reducing the national rate of SIDS.

Program Description   The Back to Sleep Campaign aims to reduce SIDS rates by educating parents and other caregivers about the importance of placing infants in the supine position to sleep (NICHD, 2001). The campaign also includes secondary messages related to improving the safety of infant sleep environments, including use of firm mattresses and elimination of excess soft bedding and toys, thereby decreasing the risk for suffocation. In addition, the campaign promotes proper prenatal and infant medical care and advocates elimination of cigarette smoke from the infant's environment. The campaign message was further refined in 1996 to more specifically promote back rather than side sleeping for infants. The campaign also recognizes that to successfully reduce SIDS rates, efforts must be made to address related public health concerns—for example, women's health and prenatal care must be emphasized, and awareness of and sensitivity to cultural diversity in child-rearing practices must be incorporated into public health education materials (NICHD).

The Back to Sleep Campaign differs from other prevention programs in the scope of its efforts, operating as a public health campaign geared toward the national population rather than targeting a particular subgroup identified as specifically at risk for SIDS. This expanded approach is necessary because, by definition, SIDS deaths are sudden and unpredictable, and research conducted to date has failed to identify risk factors useful for predicting and preventing the risk of SIDS in individual infants. Therefore, all intervention components are intended for the entire population of infants and/or pregnant women.

Although changes in infant sleep position have been associated with a marked decline in the incidence of SIDS, African American, Alaskan Native, and Native American communities continue to be disproportionately affected by SIDS (NICHD, 2001). Beginning in September 1999, NICHD began collaborative work with the National SIDS Alliance, the National Black Child Development Institute (NBCDI), and a number of other national organizations to identify and implement strategies for delivering the Back to Sleep message to African American communities. After several meetings, these groups developed educational materials, including *Babies Sleep Safest on Their Backs: A Resource Kit for Reducing SIDS in African American Communities* (NICHD, NIH, DHHS, 2001), which contains culturally appropriate materials including fact sheets, brochures, magnets, videos, and leaders' guides for facilitating community discussions on reducing the risk of SIDS. Following the October 2000 launch of the resource kit, several organizations spearheaded efforts to train other leaders in the use of the resource kit, training approximately 10,000 regional chapter and affiliate members between 2001 and 2005.

These regional training efforts generated a multitude of strategies tailored to specific communities. For example, in Chicago, Illinois, campaign partners encouraged parents and expectant parents to gain access to local Walgreen's stores where pharmacists provided information and consultations on ways to reduce the risk of SIDS. In addition, efforts in the Detroit metropolitan area included *SIDS Sundays,* in which local church pastors were given SIDS risk-reduction materials and asked to share the information with their congregations and with the caregivers in their child care centers. In Mississippi, efforts were targeted at child care providers through a partnership with the Mississippi Head Start Association and the State Day Care Licensing division. The NICHD is beginning internal evaluations of the regional efforts to target African American communities that have been conducted thus far and is presently exploring strategies for reducing SIDS in Native American communities, particularly the Northwest and Northern Plains tribes, where SIDS rates are at the highest levels.

Program Evaluation   Although the Back to Sleep Campaign has never been formally evaluated, the campaign has demonstrated success in reducing the incidence of SIDS since its inception in 1994. The primary focus of the campaign is to reduce the incidence of SIDS by educating parents to place infants in the supine position when laying them down to sleep. NICHD employs two means of assessing success in meeting this goal. First, using data collected annually as part of the National Infant Sleep Position (NISP) study (see Willinger, Ko, Hoffman, Kessler, & Corwin [2000]), researchers are able to measure the number of infants placed in different sleeping positions. Since 1992, the NISP study has tracked behavioral changes in the U.S. population and has shown significant decreases in the use of the prone sleeping position following the Back to Sleep Campaign. Second, data from the National Center for Health Statistics examines changes in SIDS rates during the same time period. Although direct causality between changes in infant sleep position and declining rates of SIDS cannot be established, these two statistics enable researchers to examine the decline in SIDS relative to behavioral changes in placement of infants in the prone sleeping position during the same time period (Willinger et al., 1998).

The NISP study is a telephone survey conducted annually since 1992. The interview gathered information on sociodemographics; characteristics of the infant and the sleep environment, including infant sleep position; and sleep position recommendations from specific sources (Willinger, Ko, Hoffman, Kessler, & Corwin, 2003). The NISP study randomly sampled approximately 1,000 households in the 48 contiguous states with infants younger than 8 months. Beginning in 1993, households in which the mother of the infant did not complete high school were oversampled, adding approximately 35 infants each year to the national sample (Willinger et al., 2003). The median infant age in the survey sample, which did not vary significantly from year to year, was 136 days (Willinger et al., 2000). Interviews were completed with the primary nighttime caregiver, and 80% to 85% of participants interviewed were mothers. All analyses were based on the combination of the national sample and the oversample of mothers with less than a high school education.

In 1992, prior to the supine recommendation from the AAP, 70% of nighttime caregivers sampled by the NISP study *usually* placed their infants to sleep in the prone position, whereas the supine position was the typical choice for only 13% of caregivers (Willinger et al., 2000). Data from the 1994 NISP study, prior to the initiation of the Back to Sleep Campaign, revealed a rate of usual prone and usual supine placement for 43% and 27% of infants, respectively. The initiation of the Back to Sleep Campaign brought forth significant and rapid changes in infant sleep placement. Within just 1 year of the start of the campaign, the rate of supine placement among infants 8–15 weeks, who are at greatest risk for SIDS, doubled, rising from 17% to 35% (Willinger et al.). The use of the prone sleeping position declined for infants in all sleeping arrangements, although bedsharing infants were slightly less likely to be placed in a prone position. The prevalence of the usual prone sleeping position declined from the combined years 1993–1994 to the combined years 1999–2000, decreasing from 33.9% to 8.9% for infants who shared a bed and from 52.1% to 14.1% for infants who usually slept alone (Willinger et al., 2003).

The first 4 years following the initial recommendation by the AAP that infants be placed in nonprone sleeping positions saw a dramatic decrease in the number of infants dying of SIDS annually. Between 1992 and 1998, the proportion of infants placed on their stomachs to sleep declined significantly from approximately 70% to approximately 17% (NICHD, 2001). Although causality cannot be determined (Willinger et al., 2000), during the same years, the overall SIDS rate declined roughly 40% from 1.2 per 1,000 live births to 0.72 per 1,000 live births and continued falling to 0.53 per 1,000 live births in 2000 (Rasinski, Kuby, Bzdusek, Silvestri, & Weese-Mayer, 2003). The most significant decline in SIDS took place from 1993 to 1995, with a decline of 12% from 1993 to 1994 and 15.5% from 1994 to 1995. Although there may be more than one factor associated with this decline, such as decreasing rates of prenatal maternal cigarette smoking, the majority of the decline can be attributed to changes in infant sleep position (Willinger et al., 1998).

The message of the Back to Sleep Campaign has been largely successful in permeating the general population. Nighttime caregivers reported increasing exposure to recommendations from four primary sources (physicians, neonatal nurses, reading materials, and radio/television) favoring supine infant sleep position, and this exposure correlated temporally with the Back to Sleep Campaign

(Willinger et al., 2000). Recommendations of supine only or supine and lateral sleep positions from all sources more than doubled between 1994 and 1997/1998. By 1998, 95% of the national sample reported receiving a recommendation of back or side placement of infants for sleep (NICHD, 2001). Of all sources cited, nonprone recommendations from the infant's physician had the greatest influence on increasing probability of supine positioning. Receiving a nonprone recommendation from additional sources had an additive effect, with the highest probability of supine placement occurring among mothers who reported receiving a recommendation from all four sources (Willinger et al.).

Despite the overall success of the campaign, there appear to be ethnic and socioeconomic discrepancies in compliance with the Back to Sleep Campaign recommendations. For example, a study involving predominantly African Americans of low socioeconomic status found that recommendations from health care practitioners were less effective at influencing parents' choice of infant sleep position. Households with grandmothers had double the risk of prone placement. In addition, parents cited infant comfort and fear of vomiting and choking as reasons for continuing to place their infants prone (Willinger et al., 2000). The higher incidence of SIDS and the slower rate of decline seen among infants of African American mothers may be attributable to discrepancies in exposure to the campaign message and noncompliance with Back to Sleep Campaign recommendations (Rasinski et al., 2003). It also may reflect the influence of other risk factors, including higher rates of low birth weight, prematurity, and young maternal age (Willinger et al., 1998). Data from the NISP study reveal a higher rate of prone sleeping for infants of African American mothers compared with Caucasian mothers (Willinger et al., 1998). Between 1994 and 1998, prone placement decreased from 44% to 17% for infants of Caucasian mothers, but only from 53% to 32% for infants of African American mothers (Willinger et al., 2000). The disparate decline between these two subgroups resulted in an increase in the African American–Caucasian ratio for SIDS, which was 2.16 in 1992 prior to the Back to Sleep Campaign, but 2.52 in 1995 following the campaign (Willinger et al., 1998); this ratio has begun to decline with the 2000 statistics (Rasinski et al., 2003). Clearly, the central message of the Back to Sleep Campaign may not be reaching everyone, and it may not adequately address the motivations for a subgroup of mothers to place their infants in the prone position in spite of public health messages to the contrary.

Furthermore, the Back to Sleep Campaign may not be adequately educating child care providers, which is particularly problematic because 20% of SIDS deaths occur in child care settings (Moon & Oden, 2003). Despite the overall decline in SIDS and decrease in prone sleeping achieved by the Back to Sleep Campaign, the proportion of SIDS deaths that occur in child care settings has remained constant.

Most of these deaths are associated with prone positioning, which poses an even greater risk to infants who are not normally placed in that position to sleep. Use of the unaccustomed prone sleeping position may increase an infant's chances of succumbing to SIDS by as much as 18-fold (Moon & Oden, 2003).

Despite continuing challenges in reaching all subpopulations with the Back to Sleep Campaign message, this public health education campaign has achieved undeniable success in a relatively short period of time, causing significant changes in normative parenting behavior. It is important to note that the Back to Sleep Campaign has accomplished this success with a small budget of $750,000 per year, which has remained unchanged since the program's inception in 1994. Large-scale prevention efforts that are expensive and intensive may not be cost-effective because of the difficulties inherent in predicting SIDS risk for individual infants (NICHD, 2001). However, in communities where the rate of SIDS remains relatively high, more targeted and intensive efforts are warranted. To fund new initiatives for African American and Native American communities, the NICHD has sought additional contract dollars, bringing its annual budget to approximately $1.5 million in recent years. The ability of the Back to Sleep Campaign to achieve its success given its limited annual budget is due in part to the inexpensive nature of implementing the recommendations for individual parents. Adopting the supine infant sleep position does not require technical training for parents, nor does it necessarily involve the use of particular materials, specific furniture, or other medical or safety devices. Physicians and other health care practitioners can be encouraged in the knowledge that this simple and cost-free recommendation can produce possible lifesaving outcomes for their clients.

Critical Analysis of Treatment Characteristics The Back to Sleep Campaign incorporates several treatment characteristics, including a guiding theoretical framework and effective programming. The program message is based on empirical evidence that use of the supine infant sleep position is associated with lower rates of SIDS. This theoretical foundation, coupled with parents' innate desire to provide the best possible care for their infants, has contributed to improved outcomes associated with the Back to Sleep Campaign. The Back to Sleep Campaign addresses critical domains, including health care practitioners, parents, and expectant parents through educational efforts and repeated message exposure. However, increasing exposure to the Back to Sleep message among additional caregivers, such as grandparents and child care providers, could strengthen the campaign's efficacy. New approaches for targeted subpopulations emphasize the inclusion of multiple social systems such as family, faith institutions, community networks, and local businesses. These networks may prove instrumental in increasing exposure, support, and reinforcement of the behavioral changes in infant caregiving espoused by the Back to Sleep Campaign.

The success of the campaign is based on the simplicity of its central message. Therefore, the Back to Sleep Campaign does not employ widely diverse teaching methods, but instead focuses on consistency of its message and reaching the widest audience possible. This is done largely through the use of printed educational materials, public service announcements, and direct recommendations from health care professionals to their clients. This strategy supports positive outcomes because exposure to recommendations throughout infancy has been shown to strongly influence mothers' choice of sleep position for their infants (Willinger et al., 2000). Furthermore, the Back to Sleep message has permeated popular culture to such a degree that it has changed normative child care practices, even for those who are not directly exposed to the campaign message. For populations who have experienced less exposure to the campaign message and more barriers to compliance, the Back to Sleep Campaign has recently refined their educational materials to reflect greater cultural sensitivity. In addition, the campaign has initiated collaboration with local and national organizations that can lend valuable input to targeted program planning, delivery, and implementation.

Critical Analysis of Procedural Characteristics   Delivery of the Back to Sleep message is appropriately timed, with expectant parents and parents of young infants generally receiving recommendations on safe infant sleep positions from multiple sources, including health care providers, reading materials, and other media sources. The Back to Sleep Campaign incorporates a multilevel approach to maximize the likelihood that caregivers will be exposed to the recommendation from multiple sources and at multiple time points. However, this is not a carefully controlled aspect of the campaign strategy, and there is generally no systematic tracking or monitoring of individual families. The simplicity of the program message promotes ease of staff training and ease of implementation for most parents. One of the current challenges for the Back to Sleep Campaign is providing adequate training to address the varied factors that influence noncompliance, especially cultural norms about infant care that differ from contemporary recommendations. Continued efforts to engage communities where rates of SIDS remain disproportionately high will likely enhance strategies available to all health care practitioners and will advance efforts to further decrease the incidence of SIDS.

Critical Analysis of Design Characteristics   To date, no formal program evaluations have been conducted on the Back to Sleep Campaign. However, the campaign does have clearly defined goals and objectives and documents changes in infant sleep position among a national sample collected as part of the NISP study. The effects of this program are difficult to measure because the causal pathway between sleep position and risk of SIDS has not been clearly determined, and although the supine sleeping position is correlated with declining rates of SIDS, establishing causality has been elusive. It will be important to future evaluations to establish uniformity in death scene investigations, definitions, and postmortem procedures in order to collect more accurate statistics on the incidence of SIDS. More thorough documentation of the specific circumstances and conditions associated with a SIDS event will enhance the collective understanding of this phenomenon, improve the effectiveness of existing prevention programs, and refine ongoing research efforts (NICHD, 2001). Despite the fact that the Back to Sleep Campaign has not achieved its goal of complete eradication of SIDS (NICHD, 2001), the social significance of the Back to Sleep Campaign cannot be underestimated. It addresses a significant cause of infant mortality, and since the inception of the campaign, the lives of thousands of infants have surely been saved.

PROMOTING HEALTHY GROWTH AND DEVELOPMENT

On a number of key indicators, the health status of children in the United States lags behind other industrialized countries in terms of infant mortality, morbidity, and immunization rates (Starfield, 2004). Poor health outcomes for children are linked to economic disparities, barriers to gaining access to the health care system, and lack of parental information on child health and development (McLearn, Strobino, Minkovitz, et al., 2004). Children in families at or near the poverty level are less likely to have health insurance and "more likely to have unmet medical needs, delayed medical care, no usual place of health care, and high use of emergency room service than children and families who are not poor" (Dey, Schiller, & Tai, 2004, p. 5). Lack of access to the health care system keeps many children from receiving even the most basic medical care, including routine vaccinations to protect against preventable diseases. In the United States, poverty is the most significant factor associated with low vaccination rates (Rodewald & Santoli, 2001). However, research indicates that it is possible to overcome the challenges of poverty to provide needed immunizations to children (Vivier et al., 2001). Moreover, it is imperative that we overcome these challenges because poor health status in childhood compromises the health of future generations of adults (Starfield). Without a concerted and systematic effort to elevate the health status of children, national public health goals will remain unmet.

My Baby U

My Baby U is an educational program that was initiated in 1990 and is aimed at increasing parents' knowledge of infant development and caregiving practices (Brown et al., 2000). The program focuses on improving infant health outcomes by enhancing parents' skills in caring for their infant and increasing parental confidence. Using a series of eight videos and short books, the program covers important developmental milestones that occur during the first year of life. Topics covered include cognitive, emotional, and motor skill development; appropriate stimulation for skill acquisition; and intrinsic infant characteristics including individual temperament, skills, and needs.

Program Description   The My Baby U program employs a simple method of delivering its message to participants. Over the course of a year, eight hour-long videos are sent to parents' homes with an accompanying 50–70-page book that expands on the themes covered in the videos. The videos address topics in infant development at 1, 3, 5, 7, 10, and 12 months of age, and each video is sent to participants when their infants reach the corresponding age. The series of videos follows seven focal families as they learn about parenting and consult with experts on the challenges and experiences they encounter during their child's first year. The format of each video captures these families engaged in dialogue with each other and with a variety of experts on infancy. Each video also models various examples of parent–infant interactions. Participants in the My Baby U program were expectant mothers who were recruited through childbirth education classes at two medical centers in New England. The population was racially and socioeconomically heterogeneous and included families living in both rural and urban areas.

Program Evaluation   To assess the effectiveness of the My Baby U program, a sample of 200 participants was divided into a control group and an experimental group. The mean age of the mothers in the final sample, the majority of whom were first-time mothers, was 28.5 years; the average education level was some college without receiving a degree. The control group completed the regular series of prenatal education classes, and the intervention group additionally received the videos and books without any accompanying instructions. VCRs were available for participants who did not already have one at home; however, in this sample, all of the mothers reported having access to a VCR.

Participants in both groups completed questionnaires at three time points: prenatally and when infants were 6 months and 1 year. The data, combined with information from infant medical records, were used to evaluate how differences in maternal confidence and knowledge of infant development were related to maternal behavior and subsequent infant health outcomes. The My Baby U program was proven effective at increasing the mothers' knowledge of infant development, and the infants of intervention group mothers experienced fewer serious illnesses during the first year than infants of control group mothers. The mothers in the intervention group scored significantly higher on a measure of knowledge of infant development at the 6-month assessment and again at the 1-year assessment, and this difference remained after controlling for mothers' education levels. However, the intervention mothers did not differ significantly from the control group mothers on level of confidence as a parent (Brown et al., 2000).

Infants of mothers in both groups showed no significant differences at birth on a number of measures of physical well-being and were comparable in rates of physical growth over the course of a year. Both groups took their infants for a similar number of well-baby visits and contacted their infants' pediatricians by telephone at a similar rate. However, the intervention group mothers also took their infants for nonroutine visits significantly more often than mothers in the control group. Control group mothers were significantly more likely to receive telephone calls from pediatricians, including calls requesting that the mother bring her infant in for an office visit (Brown et al., 2000).

Although there were no group differences in the number of nonsevere illnesses, infants of mothers in the intervention group were significantly less severely ill than infants of mothers in the control group and required less medication and less medical care in the form of follow-up visits and referrals to specialists. My Baby U participants were significantly more likely to follow recommended vaccination schedules than control group mothers at 6 months, but this difference was not significant when infants were 1 year of age (Brown et al., 2000).

Critical Analysis of Treatment Characteristics   My Baby U is grounded in theory and uses Field's argument that increasing parents' knowledge about their infants also increases the likelihood that parents will engage in healthy interactions with their children (in Trotter, 1987). My Baby U follows a multimedia format to deliver its information on child development to parents. The program does not employ varied teaching methods and is limited to videos and printed materials reviewed independently in the homes of participants. However, the videos do offer variability in the teaching formats portrayed by following seven different families over the course of a year and incorporating dialogue between parents and varied experts. Similarly, My Baby U does not engage parents in direct relationship with each other or with experts on infant development. However, the videos do simulate and model such relationships and interactions and provide parents with a virtual peer group via the focal families.

My Baby U has clearly defined programmatic goals. Investigators developed the curriculum to "help parents learn to attune to their babies' individual learning abilities by providing an intimate, nonthreatening look at other parents going through a parallel experience" (Brown et al., 2000, p. 48). Part of the success of the My Baby U program may be attributed to the relevance of the program content to individual parents' lives. The program curriculum is delivered in the familiar context of the parents' own homes and presents information on infancy in a nonthreatening manner that reveals candid reflections of parents on their varied parenting experiences in the first year. However, one potential limitation of this method of delivery is that the degree to which parents can apply the material to their own lives may be affected by their perceptions of the featured families and whether they can relate to the experiences discussed on the videos. Furthermore, videos of this nature must be updated periodically so that the focal families continue to reflect a contemporary lifestyle.

Critical Analysis of Procedural Characteristics   The My Baby U curriculum had adequate dosage levels to produce desired change in maternal knowledge of infant development and infant health outcomes. However, increased exposure may potentially have produced even greater effects, especially in the long-term maintenance of these target behaviors past the first year of the infants' lives. The program content is appropriately timed and is delivered to mothers when their infants are entering the developmental and chronological stages that correspond to the topics covered in each video. Hospital staff notified researchers weekly of births that had occurred in order to maintain an exact protocol of scheduled mailings.

My Baby U did not provide participants with supplemental access to well-trained staff, although it did expose parents to child development experts featured on the videos. No booster sessions were provided to allow participants to refine and implement the skills learned from the videos, nor were peer groups created to allow participants to learn from each other's experiences. Although the lack of such follow-up opportunities may be perceived as a methodological or procedural limitation, it may have been a deliberate trade-off between maximum efficacy and practical cost considerations.

Critical Analysis of Design Characteristics   My Baby U has been scientifically evaluated using an active control group and was found to have a significant impact on maternal behavior and infant health outcomes. Differences in maternal knowledge of infant development between the control and intervention groups were explained by exposure to the My Baby U materials. The amount of time the intervention group mothers spent watching the My Baby U videos was significantly associated with total knowledge of infant development scores at the end of the year (Brown et al., 2000).

My Baby U is a cost-effective and easy-to-implement program that produces clinically significant results. Infants of intervention group mothers experienced fewer serious illnesses and experienced more frequent contact with health care practitioners during the first year of life. The fact that infants of intervention mothers adhered more closely to recommended vaccination schedules is of interest because the My Baby U videos did not contain any information regarding immunizations or other health care issues. Rather, the programming provided by My Baby U made mothers more aware of and attentive to their infants' needs and increased mothers' efficacy in managing their infants' medical care (Brown et al., 2000).

Healthy Steps for Young Children

Healthy Steps is a comprehensive, practice-based intervention program founded on a holistic model of health care that encompasses developmental and behavioral services. It emphasizes a preventive approach to child health care and provides parents with information and guidance on child care practices. The program promotes systemic change in pediatric care and aims to narrow the gap between recommended preventive health care services and the actual services that are received by children from birth to age 3. This disparity in recommended care is often particularly wide for families of low socioeconomic status who traditionally experience greater barriers to gaining access to needed health care services. Healthy Steps proved to be successful at improving care for these families at high risk. Since its initial implementation, Healthy Steps has been offered at more than 47 sites, and 15 of these participated in a program evaluation.

Program Description　　The Healthy Steps framework is based on the principle that high-quality health care and improved parenting behavior will necessarily have a positive impact on child health and developmental outcomes. Its model of improved care emphasizes a patient-centered approach, effective and efficient delivery of services, and increased parental satisfaction with services received. By creating a strong foundation in infancy and early childhood, Healthy Steps establishes a trajectory of positive parenting behavior with far-reaching implications for child health (Guyer et al., 2003a).

To improve the overall quality of infant and toddler care, Healthy Steps integrated child development specialists with training in nursing, child development, or social work into existing pediatric practices. These specialists assisted parents in addressing concerns about their child's development and behavior, facilitated the delivery of appropriate services, and made referrals as necessary. Healthy Steps specialists counseled parents on a variety of topical areas, including child development, nutrition, child health, injury prevention, family support, and maternal health. In addition, they staffed telephone hotlines, made home visits, provided parents with materials advocating preventive care and health promotion, administered developmental assessments, and organized parenting groups to facilitate learning and peer support. A key element of the Healthy Steps program was the strong relationship the specialists developed with families, enabling open communication and enhanced ties with the pediatric practice (Guyer et al., 2003b).

Program Evaluation　　Healthy Steps conducted a 15-site national evaluation. The sample included 5,565 children and their parents in both intervention and control groups (Guyer et al., 2003b). Newborns at six sites were randomly assigned to the intervention or control group. At the remaining nine sites, a quasi-experimental design was used, and a comparison location was selected. The practices included in this evaluation represented a range of settings, including community-based group practices, pediatric practices within academic medical settings, and staff model managed care organizations (Guyer et al., 2003a). The outcomes of the program spanned multiple domains and included improved quality of care, parenting practices, and child health outcomes.

Improvements in quality of care received at the pediatric practices occurred in the following areas: effectiveness, patient and family centeredness, timeliness, efficiency, and equity (Guyer et al., 2003b). For example, families in the intervention group were 20 times more likely to receive four or more of the Healthy Steps services than the control group and were twice as likely to report that someone in the practice went out of his or her way for them (Guyer et al., 2003a). Families receiving Healthy Steps services were more satisfied overall with the health care provided to them and were more likely to use the pediatric practice as a source of developmental information and guidance (Guyer et al., 2003a). Intervention families also were significantly more likely to follow recommended vaccination schedules and well-child visits and were significantly more likely to remain with the same practice until the child was at least 20 months of age (Guyer et al., 2003a). Significant gains were made in practices serving families with incomes below $20,000. Use of telephone information lines increased from 37% to 87% following the intervention; office visits that educated parents about child development increased from 39% to 88%; and the number of home visits more than tripled from 30% to 92% (McLearn, Strobino, Hughart et al., 2004).

Significant differences were found between intervention and control families in parenting practices related to infant health, safety, and development. Intervention mothers were less likely to place infants in the unsafe prone position for sleep and were less likely to give water or cereal to their 2- to 4-month-old infants (Guyer et al., 2003a). Parent–child interactions also were enhanced for intervention families, with mothers who received Healthy Steps services more likely to show picture books to and engage in playtime with their infants on a daily basis (Guyer et al., 2003a). The Healthy Steps program also decreased parents' use of harsh punishment (Guyer et al., 2003a) and increased the use of negotiations and time-out periods for managing their children's behavior (Guyer et al., 2003b).

Other aspects of maternal behavior revealed greater sensitivity to their children's cues during a teaching activity and greater awareness of their children's developmental levels. Interestingly, mothers who received Healthy Steps services were more likely to report behavioral problems in their children, including aggression and sleeping problems. Although this may indicate a higher incidence of behavioral problems among children of mothers in the intervention group, it is more likely that this finding reflects a difference in how mothers interpreted their children's behavior and their willingness to discuss behavioral issues with a member of the pediatric practice (Guyer et al., 2003b).

Although Healthy Steps produced a number of significant improvements in child health and development, the program did not affect other targeted outcomes. For example, factors related to constructing a safe home environment showed no effect, including use of safety latches and electrical outlet covers (Guyer et al., 2003a). Breastfeeding initiation and duration rates also were not affected by the Healthy Steps program (Guyer et al., 2003b), most likely because contact with mothers at pediatric practices generally occurred too late to influence breastfeeding behavior. Intervention children were less likely to visit the emergency room for injuries, but there were no significant differences in the overall number of hospitalizations between the control and intervention groups (Guyer et al., 2003a). This finding has implications for the overall cost-effectiveness of the program because reduction in number of emergency room visits could potentially offset the cost of the program (Guyer et al., 2003a). The estimated cost of implementing Healthy Steps ranges from $402 to $933 per family per year. Although this represents a considerable investment, Healthy Steps delivers important benefits at a far lower cost than programs such as Early Head Start and the Infant Health and Development Program, which average $4,500 to $10,000 per person per year, respectively (Minkovitz et al., 2003).

Critical Analysis of Treatment Characteristics   The Healthy Steps program increased parents' knowledge of child development and established a foundation of positive child care practices that launched children on a healthy developmental path. Healthy Steps also improved the overall quality of health care services received by children and their families by ensuring delivery of timely and appropriate services that enhance health outcomes for children. This comprehensive, multifaceted program expanded the scope of existing pediatric health care services, filling significant gaps in preventive care, parental education, and behavioral and developmental services. The program promoted change within individual families, strengthened relationships between families and health care providers, and restructured the way pediatric practices deliver services to their clients.

Healthy Steps did not rely on a one-size-fits-all approach to improving child health outcomes, but rather tailored its services to the specific needs of each child and family. In lieu of a standardized curriculum, the program emphasized flexibility in providing preventive health care and developmental services to children in the first 3 years of life. Healthy Steps relied on the skills and knowledge of highly trained professionals who employed a variety of teaching methods, including one-to-one counseling, home visits, written materials, telephone calls, and peer support groups. One of the cornerstones of the Healthy Steps program was the relationship that developed between the specialists and the families. This relationship ultimately strengthened the clients' connection with the pediatric practice and promoted continuity of care because intervention families remained with the same pediatric practice for a longer time period than control families.

To meet the needs of diverse client populations, intervention programs must be socioculturally relevant. Although Healthy Steps served more than 4,000 families of all ethnic backgrounds and socioeconomic status (Guyer et al., 2003a), it is difficult to assess the sociocultural relevance of Healthy Steps programming. Presumably, the degree of rapport that developed between Healthy Steps specialists and families would not have occurred in the absence of sensitive and culturally appropriate interactions. Furthermore, the intervention families indicated a high level of satisfaction with the services they received and felt that the staff went out of their way to help them (Guyer et al.). However, the development of specific socioculturally relevant guidelines and practices could become a more systematic part of the Healthy Steps program. Additional attention to and refinement of this treatment characteristic would likely increase the program's effectiveness.

Critical Analysis of Procedural Characteristics   One of the most important characteristics of the Healthy Steps program was the timing of implementation. Healthy Steps coincided with a critical period in child health and development, establishing a positive course of parenting behavior and well-child care during the first years of life. Healthy Steps was implemented by highly trained specialists who worked collaboratively with staff at pediatric practices and who enabled health care practitioners to deliver high-quality, comprehensive health care services (McLearn, Strobino, Hughart et al., 2004). However, given that the areas of expertise of each specialist may vary, it is important for practices considering implementing the Healthy Steps model to ensure consistency of programming.

The hallmark characteristic of the Healthy Steps program was its holistic approach to child health that involved assessing the needs of specific children and families and facilitating the delivery of the exact services that are required. Because the trajectory of development and the health care needs of each child are different, the flexible design of Healthy Steps was ideally suited to provide optimal and individualized care. The program was not designed to deliver specific and standardized dosage levels to all participants, but instead offered access to and coordination of health services as needed. Because implementation of program services was not uniform, treatment fidelity is not part of the program model. However, imposing standardization and precision of implementation would likely limit the program's effectiveness.

Critical Analysis of Design Characteristics   The Healthy Steps program was scientifically evaluated using active control groups and a quasi-experimental design. The goals of Healthy Steps are to promote improvements in the clinical capacity and effectiveness of pediatric primary care to better meet the needs of families with young children; the knowledge, skills, and confidence of mothers and fathers in their childrearing abilities; and the health and development of young children (Guyer et al., 2003b, p. 2).

The results of the program are well documented and include an analysis of numerous outcome measures. Healthy Steps potentially represents a more cost-effective strategy for improving child health and development than other more intensive programs (Minkovitz et al., 2003). By improving parental knowledge and skills, Healthy Steps established an infrastructure within the home that can perpetuate the benefits for children over time.

Although Healthy Steps produced significant benefits for children and families, it is difficult to measure the effect size of the program because of the potentially wide variation in the way the program was implemented and the types of services delivered. Healthy Steps specialists at different sites had various types of training, and families did not necessarily receive the same services even within a single pediatric practice. The benefits were achieved from improved communication, improved access to information, strengthened relationships, and better services and care delivered. It is difficult, therefore, to determine which program components or combination of services produced the results. However, the program did generate clinically significant results on a large scale. After implementation of Healthy Steps, the program was able to decrease disparities between high-risk and low-risk groups so that there were "no significant differences in the adjusted odds ratios for low- or middle-income families of an age-appropriate well-child visit at 1, 2, 4, 12, 18, and 24 months compared with high-income Healthy Steps intervention families" (McLearn, Strobino, Minkovitz et al., 2004, p. 563).

Healthy Steps achieved positive benefits in multiple domains for children and families, but it did not have a significant effect on other outcomes related to child health and development (Guyer et al., 2003b). In particular, Healthy Steps did not have an effect on breastfeeding behavior (Guyer et al., 2003a). Although breastfeeding initiation would likely have occurred prior to the initial contact with Healthy Steps specialists, one of the program's shortcomings is that breastfeeding duration was not increased for those mothers who had already established breastfeeding. As discussed previously, breastfeeding is one of the most significant safeguards for infant health and development, and an enhanced focus on breastfeeding promotion would further improve the overall impact of the Healthy Steps program. Another aspect of the program design that warrants refinement is the provision of booster sessions or continued support from developmental specialists for parents of children beyond the age of 3 years because the challenges inherent in each stage of child development change over time.

MODEL PROGRAM FOR PROMOTING GROWTH AND DEVELOPMENT AND PREVENTING CHILDHOOD INJURIES

A model program to promote a healthy start in early infancy must be comprehensive in its design and delivery. Successful programming must fully incorporate essential safeguards of early health and development, including optimal nutrition through breastfeeding, safe sleeping practices to reduce the risk of SIDS, and appropriate health and developmental care.

Characteristics of Successful Prevention Programs

The recommended components of a model prevention program in terms of the program focus, targeted participants, and delivery and implementation are found in Table 2.2. Successful programs must operate within a holistic paradigm, which is inclusive of women's health, parenting education, and caregiving skills. Healthy infancy begins with quality prenatal care and breastfeeding education and promotion and continues with access to high-quality and timely preventive health care services. Furthermore, the comprehensive program design should address all aspects of infant health and development, including medical care, immunizations, and developmental and behavioral services. Programs should assess the unique needs of each infant and assign appropriate care and services on an individualized basis.

Model programs must emphasize recruitment and retention of targeted participants, particularly among those families whose infants are at risk for poor health outcomes. Program success hinges on the ability to identify and engage those constituents who are most at need of prevention programming. In the United States, additional outreach efforts targeted at low-income and minority families are essential and require tailoring efforts to specific communities and developing culturally relevant approaches and materials. It is essential that program services be made easily accessible for women of low socioeconomic status who already experience greater barriers to gaining access to the health care system and social support services. WIC has been a central access point for multiple services relevant for low-income families, and securing partnership opportunities with WIC may be one avenue for targeted outreach. As noted in this chapter, existing public health campaigns have demonstrated additional creative approaches to reaching families from all socioeconomic and cultural backgrounds. For example, the Back to Sleep campaign distributed materials through local pharmacies and churches to increase exposure to SIDS prevention strategies within local communities (NICHD, 2001).

Highly trained staff ranging from medical professionals to lay support staff should deliver prevention curricula. Adequate training should include both updates on relevant medical information and a focus on interpersonal skills. The

Table 2.2. Components of a model program to promote infant health

Targets of intervention	Pregnant women
	Parents and caregivers
	Infants and children
	Hospitals, pediatric practices, and reproductive care practices
	Both general and high-risk U.S. populations
Content of intervention	Comprehensive approach to infant health that addresses breastfeeding, SIDS risk reduction, and promoting healthy growth and development
	Professional and peer support for breastfeeding
	Promotion of supine infant sleep positioning
	Educational materials related to infant care and development
	Enhance the quality of preventive health care and developmental services
Method of delivery	Professional and peer support prenatally and during postpartum hospitalization
	Public health campaign, distribution of educational materials, and professional advice about infant health and development
	Peer support groups
	Home visits
	Coordinated delivery of timely and appropriate health care services
	Creative approaches to reaching diverse and high-risk populations
Targeted outcomes of intervention	Increase breastfeeding initiation and duration
	Decrease incidence of SIDS
	Increase parental compliance with well-baby check-ups and vaccination schedules
	Enhance quality of health care and developmental services
	Promote continuity of care between reproductive, pediatric, and developmental care services
	Improve infant and maternal health

relationship between staff and participants is particularly important in programs designed to promote healthy infancy. Program staff must be able to build a strong rapport with diverse populations because trust and open dialogue facilitate the best possible care for mothers, infants, and families. Lay staff may be well positioned to enhance program delivery by offering social support and practical problem-solving skills. Previous research on breastfeeding programs has shown that women who have adequate peer support are most able to incorporate new practices into their parenting repertoire (Pugh et al., 2002). Social support is particularly critical to promoting breastfeeding initiation and duration because education-only campaigns are generally less effective (Turner-Maffei, 2002). Successful interventions occur where vicarious experience and modeling of new behaviors is a fundamental component of the program design.

Programs for promoting infant health should have a clear, simple message with information that is easily understood and assimilated by parents. The program message is best delivered to participants using multiple teaching formats, including educational media, authoritative medical and professional advice, group support, and interactive learning opportunities. Program curricula should support and facilitate dialogue between parents, medical professionals, and other service providers and should emphasize parents' roles in obtaining proper care for their infants.

Appropriate timing is a critical aspect of programs to promote infant health because prevention curricula must coincide with very specific developmental windows. For example, the efficacy of SIDS prevention efforts diminishes when programs are delivered after the peak ages for risk of SIDS, between 2 and 4 months. Similarly, there are physiological limits to the establishment of lactation, and all programs aimed at increasing breastfeeding must be delivered prenatally or in the immediate postpartum period. Prevention programs should ensure continuity of services between multiple health care practitioners, including obstetrical and pediatric providers. Ideally, prevention programs should be integrated with existing visits and procedures that occur in the first year of life such as well-baby visits and routine postpartum care.

In summary, a model program to promote infant health and development needs to effectively combine content related to SIDS, breastfeeding, and infant health and development. Within this holistic model, programming should be comprehensive, individually tailored, and delivered by sensitive and knowledgeable staff. Continuity of care between various service providers is essential to ensure that mothers, infants, and families receive appropriate and timely health care services. The following case study demonstrates the design and implementation of a model program for Allison Taylor, a 17-year-old expectant mother.

❖

A Program for Allison Taylor

Allison had a very difficult time breaking the news of her pregnancy to her parents because of her family's difficult history and the ongoing tension between her parents. In addition to her fears about how everyone would react and how the household would handle the addition of an infant, Allison is struggling with her own concerns about becoming a mother. She is scared that she won't be able to handle raising a child and that she won't get to do *normal* high school things such as going to parties and hanging out with her friends. At the same time, she is excited about having an infant to love. Allison is struggling to imagine what having an infant will really be like, but she knows that she wants to be a good mother and give her infant the best start in life. She has heard that breastfeeding is supposed to be the healthiest way to feed her infant, but she just can't imagine how embarrassed she would feel to do something like that in front of her friends or even in front of her parents and siblings. She is still leaning toward bottle feeding because it just seems easier, but she is paying close attention to the advice she has been given by her doctor and nurses about how to care for and keep her infant healthy. Some of the information she is getting is confusing because it is different from what her mom is telling her about how to be a good parent. After Allison's baby shower, she and her mom set up a new crib, and her mom told Allison that infants sleep better on their stomachs. Because her family is already worried about the infant keeping everyone up at night, Allison thinks that she should probably follow her mother's advice; after all, her mom raised three children and knows what it was like to be a teenage mother. Allison is worried, though, because the nurses at her doctor's office told her that infants should sleep only on their backs, and she is just not sure which advice to follow.

The case study shows that Allison is having mixed and complicated emotions about becoming a mother and being able to care for her infant. She has many perceived barriers to breastfeeding, such as embarrassment about breastfeeding in public. She also is uncertain about how to handle the conflict between the advice she receives from health care providers and from family members. It is important that Allison continue to receive quality prenatal care during the last trimester of her pregnancy as well as detailed information and support about how to keep her infant healthy during the first year of life. Allison must learn that although overseeing her child's health may cause short-term challenges for herself and her family, such as learning how to breastfeed and having disagreements with her mother about child care practices, the long-term challenges that would result from having an infant with health or developmental problems would be devastating for her family, emotionally and financially, and would only add to existing family stressors.

During one of Allison's early prenatal visits, her nurses talked about how her body was undergoing important changes to enable her to breastfeed her infant and how this process would continue throughout her pregnancy. This helped Allison understand why her breasts had changed so much, and she learned more about how breast milk was such a perfect food for infants. At each prenatal visit, the nurses continued to talk about her plans for feeding her infant, and they were able to discuss some common breastfeeding challenges that Allison might experience. Because Allison was still unsure about whether she would be able to handle it, the nurses encouraged her to go to a peer support group where teenage mothers talked about their experiences. At the meeting of this group, she met two other adolescent mothers who had breastfed their infants, and they shared a lot of information with her about what it felt like and how they managed to overcome feeling awkward when feeding their infants in front of family and friends. Talking to other mothers her age helped Allison decide that she would at least try breastfeeding to see how it worked for her. These women encouraged her to keep coming to the group, and one of them gave Allison her home telephone number if she ever had questions or was worried about breastfeeding.

During one of Allison's last prenatal visits, her nurses encouraged her to try breastfeeding. They gave her a video to take home, and she watched it that night with her mom and sister. The video described what newborn infants need and how to care for them in the first few weeks of life. It emphasized how dependent infants are on their parents for good care, safety, and nutrition. The video also showed parents putting infants to sleep on their backs and talked about how this was important for preventing SIDS. Allison and her mom talked about this advice after the video was over, and even though her mom was still worried that the infant wouldn't sleep well or that she might choke, they decided that it was most important to follow the advice of the doctors and nurses so that the infant would be safe and healthy.

As Allison's due date got closer, she felt anxious about the upcoming labor. When the time came, however, Allison's mom stayed with her the entire time, and the nurses were helpful and supportive. Although labor was difficult, she was overjoyed to finally meet her daughter Amy. The nurses helped Allison start breastfeeding her infant only 30 minutes after she was born. Allison enjoyed the close contact with her beautiful new daughter, but she could already tell that breastfeeding would be difficult and she felt that it was sometimes painful. She remembered from her earlier doctor's appointments that breastfeeding can be uncomfortable at first but that it shouldn't be painful. Although she was worried that she was already doing something wrong as a mother, she decided to ask the nurses for help because she knew from the video she had watched that many parents have problems with their newborn infants. The nurses arranged for a lactation consultant to come to her room, and the consultant taught Allison about different positions that would be more comfortable and how to make sure that Amy was latched correctly. Although Allison was still worried about breastfeeding when she went home, she decided that she would at least try to breastfeed for the rest of the week. The lactation consultant told her that she would call Allison at home the next day to see how things were going, and two people from the hospital planned to come visit Allison later that week. Allison took home another video about newborns that discussed what Amy could see and hear, why she cried, and how Allison could comfort and nurture her.

Three days after Allison arrived home, a nurse and a peer counselor came for a visit. They were very nice and kept telling Allison how beautiful Amy was. Because Allison was still having trouble with breastfeeding, they asked her to breastfeed Amy while they were visiting and suggested some practical solutions to make things easier. They knew the doctors and nurses at the pediatrician's office where Allison was planning to take Amy. They told Allison that the office was especially good because a woman who worked there helped parents make sure that their children were receiving quality health care.

At her first visit with the pediatrician, Allison received positive reinforcement that she had been successfully breastfeeding Amy. Christine, the specialist who was going to work with her, talked to Allison about how important vaccinations were for keeping Amy healthy, and she gave Allison a schedule of recommended well-baby visits and immunizations. Christine also talked to Allison about some of the things she had learned from the video, such as how her infant would grow and develop and what milestones she would reach at particular times. Christine told Allison that she would be receiving another video in the mail that dealt with Amy's needs at 1 month of age, and that she would be receiving videos at different times throughout Amy's first year. Christine also told Allison that there were many people available to help her. She gave Allison a telephone number to call if she had any parenting questions as well as information on a parenting support group that met twice a month. Allison found Christine to be immediately likeable. She felt that Christine was a good listener and seemed genuinely interested in her and Amy. She always took time in understanding and responding to Allison's questions. Allison looked forward to the times that Christine visited to see how Amy was growing.

Throughout the first year of Amy's life, Allison received a total of nine videos in the mail. The videos taught Allison about things such as schedules and routines, interactive playtime, how to comfort and sooth an infant, infant temperament, and infant physical and skill development. Allison breastfed Amy until the baby turned 6 months, and she was happy that her body was able to nourish Amy during that time. She took Amy for all of the recommended vaccination and well-baby visits and an additional time when Amy had an ear infection. Christine was always excited to see her when they came in for check-ups, and she kept encouraging Allison to read and play with Amy to help her develop new skills. Each time they spoke at the doctor's office or at Allison's house, Christine asked how Allison was doing. Allison liked this because everyone else seemed to focus mostly on Amy. Allison felt lucky that Amy was healthy and developing well.

❖

This example illustrates the positive outcomes resulting from a comprehensive program. Although Allison knows that protecting her infant's health will be a lifelong job, she feels good about giving her infant the best start in life. She knows that she has learned a lot about infants and what they need from their parents. Allison's success at breastfeeding, taking steps to prevent SIDS, and actively safeguarding her infant's health and development reinforces the idea that evidence-based prevention programs, combined with strong relationships between families and service providers, bring together the science and art of prevention programming to promote physical and psychological well-being for infants, mothers, and families.

FUTURE DIRECTIONS: IMPROVING PROGRAMS FOR PREVENTING INFANT ILLNESS AND INJURY

Significant advances have been made in efforts to promote healthy growth and psychological development in infancy, and progress has been made on a number of key health indicators. Although focused efforts related to particular aspects of infancy have had some impact on infant health and development, there remains a great need for more comprehensive, holistic programming. The challenge ahead will be to foster collaboration and cooperation among the multiple agencies and practitioners that directly affect infant health, and ensure continuity between medical services including women's health and reproductive care, infant medical and developmental services, parenting education initiatives, and large-scale public health campaigns. The model presented in this chapter represents an attempt to outline a cohesive and holistic program for promoting a healthy start for all infants.

Ongoing efforts to further develop and refine strategies to reach families most in need of these services will likely increase the potential impact of comprehensive programs aimed at promoting infant health. However, for prevention programming to be effective, the most important developments must occur in the collective approach to, and cultural attitudes about, infant health and development. Breastfeeding rates in the United States compare poorly with rates in other industrialized countries (Cadwell, 2002), and public perceptions of breastfeeding continue to undermine the efforts of individual programs attempting to increase its practice. Indeed, breastfeeding promotion efforts will accomplish only modest success until breastfeeding women are given adequate legal support and protection in the form of legislation. In addition to laws protecting women's right to breastfeed, policies that promote and protect breastfeeding for women in the work force, such as allowing short breaks and making private spaces available for pumping breast milk, are essential for increasing breastfeeding duration nationwide. More global public health campaigns that deliver information about appropriate developmental stimulation (e.g., reading to children) and that reinforce positive messages about breastfeeding and Back to Sleep recommendations are necessary. These campaigns will not only serve as reminders about appropriate parenting practices for individual parents, but will also help shift cultural norms in child care practices and remedy misconceptions about child health and development. This systemic change in the collective approach to infant care is critical to the future of prevention programs. Only in the context of these public health campaigns and national efforts will the art and science of prevention programming be realized.

REFERENCES

American Academy of Pediatrics; Work Group on Breastfeeding. (2005). Revised policy statement: Breastfeeding and the use of human milk. *Pediatrics, 115,* 496–506.

Armstrong, J., & Reilly, J.J. (2002). Breastfeeding and lowering the risk of childhood obesity. *Lancet, 359,* 2003–2004.

Bener, A., Denic, S., & Galadari, S. (2001). Longer breast-feeding and protection against childhood leukaemia and lymphomas. *European Journal of Cancer, 37,* 234–238.

Bhandari, N., Bahl, R., Mazumdar, S., Martines, J., Black, R.E., & Bhan, M.K. (2003). Effect of community-based promotion of exclusive breastfeeding on diarrhoeal illness and growth: A cluster randomised controlled trial. *Lancet, 361,* 1418–1423.

Bier, J.-A.B., Oliver, T., Ferguson, A.E., & Vohr, B.R. (2002). Human milk improves cognitive and motor development of premature infants during infancy. *Journal of Human Lactation, 18,* 361–367.

Brown, M., Yando, R., & Rainforth, M. (2000). Effects of an at-home video course on maternal learning, infant care and infant health. *Early Child Development and Care, 160,* 47–65.

Cadwell, K. (2002). Breastfeeding: A public health policy priority. In K. Cadwell, C. Turner-Maffei, A. Blair, L. Arnold, C. Cadwell, & K. Brimdyr (Eds.), *Reclaiming breastfeeding for the United States: Protection, promotion and support* (pp. 11–22). Boston: Jones and Bartlett Publishers.

Centers for Disease Control and Prevention. (2003). *Table 3: Any and exclusive breastfeeding rates by age.* Retrieved September 5, 2005, from http://www.cdc.gov/breastfeeding/data/NIS_data/age.htm

Chen, A., & Rogan, W.J. (2004). Breastfeeding and the risk of postneonatal death in the United States. *Pediatrics, 113,* e435–e439.

Chua, S., Arulkumaran, S., Lim, I., Selamat, N., & Ratnam, S.S. (1994). Influence of breastfeeding and nipple stimulation on postpartum uterine activity. *British Journal of Obstetrics and Gynaecology, 101,* 804–805.

Cunningham, A.S. (1995). Breastfeeding: Adaptive behavior for child health and longevity. In P. Stuart-Macadam & K.A. Dettwyler (Eds.), *Breastfeeding: Biocultural perspectives* (pp. 243–264). New York: Aldine De Gruyter.

Dennis, C.-L., Hodnett, E., Gallop, R., & Chalmers, B. (2002). The effect of peer support on breast-feeding duration among primiparous women: A randomized controlled trial. *Canadian Medical Association Journal, 166,* 21–29.

Dewey, K.G., Heinig, M.J., & Nommsen, L.A. (1993). Maternal weight-loss patterns during prolonged lactation. *The American Journal of Clinical Nutrition, 58,* 162–166.

Dey, A.N., Schiller, J.S., & Tai, D.A. (2004). Summary Health Statistics for U.S. Children: National Health Interview Survey, 2002. *National Center for Health Statistics, 10*(221).

Duncan, B., Ey, J., Holberg, C.J., Wright, A.L., Martinez, F.D., & Taussig, L.M. (1993). Exclusive breast-feeding for at least 4 months protects against otitis media. *Pediatrics, 91,* 867–872.

Fleming, P.J. (1994). Understanding and preventing sudden infant death syndrome. *Current Opinion in Pediatrics, 6,* 158–162.

Guyer, B., Barth, M., Bishai, D., Caughy, M., Clark, B., Burkom, D., et al. (2003a). *Healthy steps: The first three years.* Baltimore: Women's and Children's Health Policy Center, Department of Population and Family Health Sciences, Johns Hopkins Bloomberg School of Public Health.

Guyer, B., Barth, M., Bishai, D., Caughy, M., Clark, B., Burkom, D., et al. (2003b). *Healthy steps: The first three years. Executive summary.* Baltimore: Women's and Children's Health Policy Center, Department of Population and Family Health Sciences, Johns Hopkins Bloomberg School of Public Health.

Heinig, M.J., & Farley, K. (2001). Development of effective strategies to support breastfeeding. *Journal of Human Lactation, 17,* 293–294.

Horwood, L.J., Darlow, B.A., & Mogridge, N. (2001). Breast milk feeding and cognitive ability at 7–8 years. *Archives of Disease in Childhood, 84,* F23–F27.

Kennedy, K.I., Labbok, M.H., & Van Look, P.F. (1996). Lactational amenorrhea method for family planning. *International Journal of Gynaecology and Obstetrics, 54,* 55–57.

Kochanek, K.D., Murphy, S.L., Anderson, R.N., & Scott, C. (2004). Deaths: Final data for 2002. *National Vital Statistics Reports, 53,* 1–116.

Kostraba, J.N., Cruickshanks, K.J., Lawler-Heavner, J., Jobim, L.F., Rewers, M.J., Gay, E.C., et al. (1993). Early exposure to cow's milk and solid foods in infancy, genetic predisposition, and risk of IDDM. *Diabetes, 42,* 288–295.

Lee, S.Y., Kim, M.T., Kim, S.W., Song, M.S., & Yoon, S.J. (2003). Effect of lifetime lactation on breast cancer risk: A Korean women's cohort study. *International Journal of Cancer, 105,* 390–393.

Li, R., Grummer-Strawn, L., Zhao, Z., Barker, L., & Mokdad, A. (2003). Prevalence of breastfeeding in the United States: The 2001 National Immunization Survey. *Pediatrics, 111,* 1198–1201.

Lopez, J.M., Gonzalez, G., Reyes, V., Campino, C., & Diaz, S. (1996). Bone turnover and density in healthy women during breastfeeding and after meaning. *Osteoporosis International, 6,* 153–159.

Lopez-Alarcon, M., Villalpando, S., & Fajardo, A. (1997). Breast-feeding lowers the frequency and duration of acute respiratory infection and diarrhea in infants under six months of age. *Journal of Nutrition, 127,* 436–443.

McLaughlin, J.E., Burstein, N.R., Tao, F., & Fox, M.K. (2004, August). *Breastfeeding intervention design study: Final evaluation design and analysis plan.* Alexandria, VA: U.S. Department of Agriculture.

McLearn, K.T., Strobino, D.M., Hughart, N., Minkovitz, C.S., Scharfstein, D., Marks, E., et al. (2004). Developmental services in primary care for low-income children: Clinicians' perceptions of the Healthy Steps for Young Children Program. *Journal of Urban Health, 81,* 206–221.

McLearn, K.T., Strobino, D.M., Minkovitz, C.S., Marks, E., Bishai, D., & Hou, W. (2004). Narrowing the income gaps in preventive care for young children: Families in Healthy Steps. *Journal of Urban Health, 81,* 556–567.

Milligan, R.A., Flenniken, P.M., & Pugh, L.C. (1996). Positioning intervention to minimize fatigue in breastfeeding women. *Applied Nursing Research, 9,* 67–70.

Milligan, R.A., Pugh, L.C., Bronner, Y.L., Spatz, D.L., & Brown, L.P. (2000). Breastfeeding duration among low income women. *Journal of Midwifery & Women's Health, 45,* 246–252.

Minkovitz, C.S., Hughart, N., Strobino, D., Scharfstein, D., Grason, H., Hou, W., et al. (2003). A practice-based intervention to enhance quality of care in the first 3 years of life: The Healthy Steps for Young Children Program. *Journal of the American Medical Association, 290,* 3081–3091.

Moon, R.Y., & Oden, R.P. (2003). Back to sleep: Can we influence child care providers? *Pediatrics, 112,* 878–882.

Mortensen, E.L., Michaelsen, K.F., Sanders, S.A., & Reinisch, J.M. (2002). The association between duration of breastfeeding and adult intelligence. *Journal of the American Medical Association, 287,* 2365–2371.

National Institute of Child Health and Human Development (NICHD). (2001). *Targeting sudden infant death syndrome (SIDS): A strategic plan.* Retrieved September 5, 2005, from http://www.nichd.nih.gov/strategicplan/cells/SIDS_syndrome.pdf

National Institute of Child Health and Human Development (NICHD), NIH, DHHS. (2001). *Babies sleep safest on their backs: A resource kit for reducing SIDS in African American communities.* Washington, DC: U.S. Government Printing Office. Retrieved February 1, 2006, from http://www.nichd.nih.gov/sids/Entirekit.pdf

Newcomb, P.A., Storer, B.E., Longnecker, M.P., Mittendorf, R., Greenberg, E.R., Clapp, R.W., et al. (1994). Lactation and a reduced risk of premenopausal breast cancer. *New England Journal of Medicine, 330,* 81–87.

Oddy, W.H., & Holt, P.G. (1999). Association between breast feeding and asthma in 6 year old children: Findings of a prospective birth cohort study. *British Medical Journal, 319,* 815–819.

Paton, L.M., Alexander, J.L., Nowson, C.A., Margerison, C., Frame, M.G., Kaymakci, B., et al. (2003). Pregnancy and lactation have no long-term deleterious effect on measures of bone mineral in healthy women: A twin study. *American Journal of Clinical Nutrition, 77,* 707–714.

Pettit, D.J., & Forman, M.R. (1997). Breastfeeding and incidence of non–insulin-dependent diabetes mellitus in Pima Indians. *Lancet, 350,* 166–168.

Pugh, L.C., Buchko, B.L., Bishop, B.A., Cochran, J.F., Smith, L.R., & Lerew, D.J. (1996). A comparison of topical agents to relieve nipple pain and enhance breastfeeding. *Birth, 23,* 88–93.

Pugh, L.C., Milligan, R.A., Frick, K.D., Spatz, D., & Bronner, Y. (2002). Breastfeeding duration, costs, and benefits of a support program for low-income breastfeeding women. *Birth, 29,* 95–100.

Rasinski, K.A., Kuby, A., Bzdusek, S.A., Silvestri, J.M., & Weese-Mayer, D.E. (2003). Effect of a sudden infant death syndrome risk reduction education program on risk factor compliance and information sources in primarily black urban communities. *Pediatrics, 111,* e347–e354.

Rodewald, L.E., & Santoli, J.M. (2001). The challenge of vaccinating vulnerable children. *Journal of Pediatrics, 139,* 613–615.

Rosenblatt, K.A., & Thomas, D.B. (1993). Lactation and the risk of epithelial ovarian cancer. The WHO Collaborative Study of Neoplasia and Steroid Contraceptives. *International Journal of Epidemiology, 22,* 192–197.

Ryser, F.G. (2004). Breastfeeding attitudes, intention, and initiation in low-income women: The effect of the best start program. *Journal of Human Lactation, 20,* 300–305.

Starfield, B. (2004). U.S. child health: What's amiss, and what should be done about it? *Health Affairs, 23,* 165–170.

Task Force on Infant Sleep Position and Sudden Infant Death Syndrome. (2000). Changing concepts of sudden infant death syndrome: Implications for infant sleeping environment and sleep position. *Pediatrics, 105,* 650–656.

Trotter, R.J. (1987). The play's the thing. *Psychology Today, 21,* 26–34.

Turner-Maffei, C. (2002). Overcoming disparities in breastfeeding. In K. Cadwell & C. Turner-Maffei (Eds.), *Reclaiming breastfeeding for the United States: Protection, promotion and support* (pp. 105–123). Boston: Jones and Bartlett Publishers.

Tuttle, C.R., & Dewey, K.G. (1996). Potential cost savings for Medi-Cal, AFDC, food stamps, and WIC programs associated with increasing breast-feeding among low-income among women in California. *Journal of the American Dietetic Association, 96,* 885–890.

U.S. Department of Health and Human Services. (2000). *Healthy People 2010: Understanding and improving health* (2nd ed.). Washington, DC: U.S. Government Printing Office.

Vivier, P.M., Alario, A.J., Peter, G., Leddy, T., Simon, P., & Mor, V. (2001). An analysis of the immunization status of preschool children enrolled in a statewide Medicaid managed care program. *Journal of Pediatrics, 139,* 624–629.

Volpe, E.M., & Bear, M. (2000). Enhancing breastfeeding initiation in adolescent mothers through the Breastfeeding Educated and Supported Teen (BEST) Club. *Journal of Human Lactation, 16,* 196–200.

Willinger, M., Hoffman, H.J., Wu, K.T., Hou, J.-R., Kessler, R.C., Ward, S.L., et al. (1998). Factors associated with the transition to nonprone sleep positions of infants in the United States: The National Infant Sleep Position Study. *Journal of the American Medical Association, 280,* 329–335.

Willinger, M., James, L.S., & Catz, C. (1991). Defining the sudden infant death syndrome (SIDS): Deliberations of an expert panel convened by the National Institute of Child Health and Human Development. *Pediatric Pathology, 11,* 677–684.

Willinger, M., Ko, C.W., Hoffman, H.J., Kessler, R.C., & Corwin, M.J. (2000). Factors associated with caregivers' choice of infant sleep position, 1994–1998: The National Infant Sleep Position Study. *Journal of the American Medical Association, 283,* 2135–2142.

Willinger, M., Ko, C.W., Hoffman, H. J., Kessler, R.C., & Corwin, M.J. (2003). Trends in infant bed sharing in the United States, 1993–2000: The National Infant Sleep Position Study. *Archives of Pediatrics & Adolescent Medicine, 157,* 43–49.

Wolf, J.H. (2003). Low breastfeeding rates and public health in the United States. *American Journal of Public Health, 93,* 2000–2010.

3

PREVENTING EARLY
DEVELOPMENTAL DELAY

Leann E. Smith, Jody S. Nicholson, and Julie N. Schatz

According to the Individuals with Disabilities Education Improvement Act of 2004 (PL 108-446), a child is considered to have a developmental delay when he or she is diagnosed with problems in one or more of the following areas of development: physical, cognitive, communication, social or emotional, or adaptive. In 2000, special education services were provided for more than 6.5 million children diagnosed with developmental delays (U.S. Department of Education, 2002). Early delays have been shown to compromise later functioning and to have detrimental effects on child development. In the area of language and literacy, for instance, early delays have been associated with long-term reading difficulties (McGee, Prior, Williams, Smart, & Sanson, 2002; Scarborough & Dobrich, 1990) as well as problems in social, emotional, behavioral, and occupational areas during adulthood (Bennett, Brown, Boyle, Racine, & Offord, 2003; Maughan, 1995). Although the U.S. federal government has spent more than $321 billion (in 2002 dollars) since 1965 in attempts to enhance the educational achievement of disadvantaged children, 68% of fourth-grade students in 2000 could not read at grade level, with children living in poverty and minority children composing the majority of those with below-level reading proficiency (U.S. Department of Education, 2002). Given this societal problem, researchers and community leaders seek answers to help prevent adverse developmental outcomes for millions of America's children who live in poverty.

RATIONALE FOR PREVENTING
EARLY DEVELOPMENTAL DELAY

Current programs designed to prevent developmental delay have their roots in government programs initiated during the 1960s. In 1962, the Perry Preschool Project began as a preschool educational program and fostered long-term gains for children from disadvantaged economic backgrounds. Children in the treatment group of this project were provided with a half-day preschool experience for 2 years prior to school entry. In addition to attending preschool classes, treatment group families also received weekly home visits. The project compared three different classroom models: 1) direct instruction, 2) traditional nursery school with free play, and 3) High/Scope curriculum (Weikart, 1998). The High/Scope curriculum emphasized the child's role as an active learner; targeted areas such as social skills, art, math, reading, and science (Epstein, 2003; Schweinhart, 2003); and subsequently demonstrated the largest gains for participants in socioemotional, educational, and economic domains (Weikart). As such, the Perry Preschool Project laid a critical foundation on which later programs have been built by providing early empirical support for the possibility of preventing developmental delay.

With the dawn of President Johnson's War on Poverty in 1964, preventing developmental problems of children in poverty became a national priority. The Johnson administration spearheaded the formation of the Head Start program, which was based on the High/Scope curriculum of the Perry Preschool Project (Weikart, 1998). Subsequently, early educational services have been available for children in poverty for several decades (U.S. Department of Health and Human Services, 2004). Similarly, since the 1970s, legislation has paved the way for appropriate early education for children with disabilities. In 1975, Congress enacted the Education for All Handicapped Children Act of 1975, which provided support for the educational needs of infants, toddlers, children, and youth with disabilities in the form of early intervention, special education, and related services. In 1990, this act was renamed the Individuals with Disabilities Education Act (IDEA) of 1990, and renewed versions of the law have continued to delineate how educational supports should be made available to children with disabilities. According to the current IDEA law, it is mandatory for the state to provide intervention services for children with identified early delays. Specifically, before age 3, children are entitled to receive early intervention services such as occupational therapy, speech–language therapy, and family training. After age 3, children are similarly eligible for appropriate services to meet their educational needs, often within an inclusive classroom setting.

Early intervention services are also available for children who do not have identified delays but who are at risk for developmental problems. All children who meet a low-income criteria are eligible for enrollment in Head Start at age 3 or 4 depending on the state. For children aged birth to 3, Early Head Start (EHS), which will be discussed in subsequent sections, is also available in many areas. Given that children with identified delays and children at risk for delay due to economic disadvantage are eligible for early intervention services, current prevention research efforts focus on how programs can be improved to ensure the most optimal outcomes for these children.

Factors Associated with Risk for Developmental Delay

King, Logsdon, and Schroeder (1992) conceptualized risks for developmental delay as being either biological or environmental in nature. Biological risk factors such as premature birth or low birth weight are often related to developmental disabilities (Gallagher & Watkin, 1998; Hack et al., 2002; Wallace & McCarton, 1997). Working either independently or in conjunction with biological risks, environmental risk factors also have been connected with less than optimal child development. For instance, low-quality home environments (Bradley, Corwyn, Burchinal, McAdoo, & Garcia Coll, 2001; Harrington, Dubowitz, Black, & Binder, 1995; Liaw & Brooks-Gunn, 1993), child maltreatment (Masten & Wright, 1998), adolescent parenting (Levine, Pollack, & Comfort, 2001; Whitman, Borkowski, Keogh, & Weed, 2001), and maternal substance abuse (Moe & Smith, 2003; Weissman, Warner, Wickramaratne, & Kandel, 1999) have been identified in the literature as risk factors for child developmental delays and are often correlated with poverty.

Children in poverty are unfortunately doubly vulnerable to risk for developmental problems; economic disadvantage often entails a plethora of both biological and environmental risks (Guralnick, 1998). Poverty has been repeatedly related to problematic development in cognitive, academic, and socioemotional domains (e.g., Duncan & Brooks-Gunn, 1997; Pungello, Kupersmidt, Burchinal, & Patterson, 1996; Ramey & Ramey, 1999) and can be viewed as an overarching risk factor for developmental delay. Unfortunately, many children are exposed to the deleterious effects of simultaneously occurring biological and environmental risk. According to the U.S. Census Bureau (2003), 16.7% of children in the United States under age 18 were living in poverty in 2002. This figure, however, is for families below the federal poverty level ($18,850 for a family of four) and does not completely reflect the number of children with economic disadvantages. For instance, Bernstein, Brocht, and Spade-Aguilar (2000) demonstrated that families need to live at twice the federal poverty level to make ends meet. As such, low-income status is a more realistic estimate of the number of children at risk for developmental delay due to economic hardship. A staggering 38% of children in the United States live in families classified as having low incomes (Douglas-Hall

& Koball, 2005). In short, there remains a need to effectively intervene early in the lives of children who are at risk if major developmental delays and subsequent academic underachievement are to be prevented.

CURRENT PREVENTION PROGRAMS

Intervention programs have been shown to facilitate children's development in multiple domains (e.g., cognitive, social, emotional functioning [Guralnick, 1998; Ramey & Ramey, 1998; Reynolds, 1998]). Some programs address specific risk factors, whereas others aim to improve functioning for children with more global risks. Examples of targeted programs that documented success include the Infant Health and Development Program that was created for children with low birth weights (McCormick, McCarton, Brooks-Gunn, Belt, & Gross, 1998) and the Nurse Home Visitation Program (Olds et al., 1998) that was developed for children at risk for maltreatment. In contrast to these highly focused programs, the current review highlights three exemplar programs designed to prevent developmental delays for children with global risks because of their poverty status: 1) Chicago Longitudinal Study, 2) Abecedarian Program, and 3) Early Head Start (EHS). Table 3.1 provides a brief overview of each program. These programs have been selected because each contains unique characteristics that likely produced positive outcomes. The Chicago Longitudinal Study was exemplar in terms of its comprehensiveness, split treatment design, and active control group. The Abecedarian Program was included as a model program because of its theory-driven curriculum, comprehensiveness, and interpretable treatment design. EHS was notable because of its birth-to-3 focus and its unique design involving multiple formats (center-based, home-based, or combination).

The Chicago Longitudinal Study

The Chicago Longitudinal Study was a multisite, federally funded study of the Chicago Child–Parent Center (CPC) that began in 1967 and is still running today. Children were recruited for the initial study if they were not already attending another program and resided in a school neighborhood where at least 30% of the population was below the federal poverty level. Applicants who were deemed most at need due to economic and educational disadvantages were accepted into the program (Reynolds & Temple, 1998). Assessments were given each year of program participation and again at 13 and 21 years (Reynolds, Ou, & Topitzes, 2004).

The CPC aimed to increase competency in reading, math, and communication through diverse classroom and parent activities and field trips (Reynolds &

Table 3.1. Three prevention programs and their defining characteristics

	Chicago Longitudinal Study	Abecedarian Program	Early Head Start
Targets of Intervention	Male and female preschool children from economically disadvantaged backgrounds Parents	Male and female high-risk infants (e.g., low parent education, low income) Parents	Low-income families with infants or toddlers
Content of Intervention	Preschool education Parent education and resources Extensive referral system for families Continued involvement through third grade for extension group children	Early childhood education from infancy to age 5 Free formula and social work services School-age follow-up program Parent–teacher liaison	Three types of service delivery: 1. center-based programs 2. home-based programs 3. combination programs
Outcomes of Intervention	By third grade, program children had higher reading and math scores than controls At age 21, program children had higher graduation rates and lower juvenile arrest rates than controls	Higher cognitive scores, lower retention rates, and fewer special education placements for treatment children in comparison with controls By age 21, program children had higher levels of educational attainment and were more likely to be skilled employees than controls	At age 2 children in program group had higher cognitive and language test scores and lower levels of aggression than control group children EHS children in program group had more cognitively stimulating home environments and were more likely to be read to than controls
Costs and Duration	Preschool-only involvement: $6,730 per child ($7.10 return for dollar spent) 4–6-year involvement: $4,068 per child ($6.09 return for dollar spent)	Birth through kindergarten Birth through age 8 7:1 return rate for every invested dollar	Beginning as early as infancy and lasting through age 3

Temple, 1998; Reynolds, Temple, Robertson, & Mann, 2001). Specifically, the program focused on 1) providing comprehensive services, 2) increasing parent involvement in the children's educational experience, and 3) constructing a child-centered program concentrating on literacy/reading skills (Reynolds & Temple, 1998; Reynolds et al., 2001). The program was adopted under the philosophy that improving a child's early experiences will reduce the need for later remedial services and welfare programs by preventing school failure and social difficulties (Reynolds, 1998).

Beginning at four sites across Chicago, the Chicago Longitudinal Study followed the original sample consisting of 1,539 children: 989 children received the preschool intervention and 550 children were followed as the control group (Reynolds et al., 2001). Although all children in the intervention received both preschool and kindergarten components, 133 children exited the program after kindergarten, whereas 281 children continued through the second grade, and 155 children finished a third-grade component (Reynolds & Temple, 1998). Children in the control group were enrolled in non–CPC-government-funded programs such as Head Start, and the majority attended five randomly selected elementary schools in the Chicago area (Reynolds et al., 2004). The comprehensive services provided by the CPC study included four main components: 1) nutritional and health benefits through free breakfast and lunch services and health screening; 2) adult supervision provided by teachers, parent volunteers, school-community representatives, and teacher aides; 3) in-service trainings and supplemental instructional supplies for teachers; and 4) instruction in reading, mathematics, and language using a variety of teaching methods such as small-group activities, shared reading, and field trips (Reynolds & Temple, 1998).

Instructional activities within the Chicago EARLY (Early Assessment and Remediation Laboratory) project contained an assessment tool and curriculum component. The assessment tool was used to evaluate a child's strengths and weaknesses, whereas the curriculum component helped teachers remediate or advance developmental skills in the children as indicated by the assessment tool (Chicago Longitudinal Study, 2004). The curriculum in the Chicago EARLY was not used across all classrooms, but 66% of CPC teachers reported referencing it three times or more a week. The CPC program curriculum focused on learning activities that promoted language development as well as good social and psychosocial development through relatively structured classroom activities (Chicago Longitudinal Study, 2004). Learning activities addressed body image, gross motor and perceptual–motor skills, and language development. Body image and gross motor activities such as body-part recognition, balance, and body exercises were intended to increase body awareness and subsequently a child's self-concept. Perceptual–motor activities aimed at improving premathematic skills through

1) color and shape recognition, matching, and sorting and 2) fine motor and visual discrimination tasks. Language activities such as sound discrimination, sentence building, story comprehension, and verbal problem solving focused on developing both expressive and receptive communication skills (Chicago Longitudinal Study, 2004).

The program kept class sizes small with low teacher–child ratios (preschool: 1:8; kindergarten: 1:12) and coordinated a wide range of adult supervision in classrooms through parent volunteers under the leadership of a head teacher. With the small student–teacher ratios as well as the parent volunteers, the CPC intended to increase program effectiveness by fostering a child-centered environment that would help promote individual achievement in developmental tasks (Reynolds, 1998).

The head teacher was responsible for organizing in-service training and coordinating activities of the school-community representative, classroom teachers and aides, and the parent-resource teacher. The school–community representative provided outreach services to families by 1) conducting mandatory home visits; 2) referring families to community services such as employment training, mental health services, and welfare services; and 3) providing transportation services to families in need. A parent–resource teacher staffed a parent room that organized adult education classes and encouraged parent interaction to help create a social support system among participating families. There also was a strong parental component of the program: Eligible children were only accepted if their parents agreed to actively participate for at least half a day, 1 day a week in the classroom (Reynolds, 1998; Reynolds & Temple, 1998).

Program Evaluation   The resulting sample was composed entirely of minority children (93% African American, 7% Hispanic) with equal proportions of girls and boys. At age 8, children in the program were still considered to be high risk: 56.1% of the children's parents had not completed high school, 70.1% were single-parent households, and 69.4% of parents were unemployed (Reynolds et al., 2004). The CPC preschool had a significant positive impact on children's cognitive functioning, showing a 3-month performance gain in reading. Furthermore, children in the preschool treatment group had lower rates of special education (14% versus 25%) and lower grade retention rates when compared with the control group (23% versus 38%; Chicago Longitudinal Study, 2004). By third grade, children who had completed the extension beyond kindergarten were displaying significantly higher test scores than the comparison group of children who had completed only the kindergarten component. These children scored higher in reading (7.8 points higher) and math (4.5 points higher) with Cohen's d effect sizes of .48 and .35 respectively (Reynolds & Temple, 1998). By the seventh grade, children in the CPC follow-up program continued to have higher academic achievement than children who only received the preschool intervention. An 8.6 point advantage for the extended intervention group was found in reading achievement (d = .43). There was no significant difference between the extended group and the preschool-only group in math scores, although they were within the educationally important range (d = .28). In the treatment group in general, girls had the highest scores in reading and math at the seventh-grade level, as did children of high school graduates (Reynolds & Temple, 1998).

A monotonic relationship with school success was found for CPC participation; the longer the duration of the program, the greater the effects (Reynolds & Temple, 1998). At the final assessment, when the participants were 21 years old, higher reading and math scores and higher success scores on a life skills competency test were found for those who completed all 6 years of the program. In addition, reading achievement for treatment children was on average a full grade level above the control group, and 74% of the program group passed the life skills examination, a requirement for graduation from high school (Reynolds, 1998). Children who attended all components of the program through elementary school demonstrated the best school adjustment, supporting the notion that extended intervention programs are optimal (Reynolds). However, regardless of level of participation, all children who attended the CPC program had a 29% higher rate of high school graduation, a 33% lower rate of juvenile arrest, a 42% lower rate of arrests for violent offenses, a 41% reduction in special education placement, a 40% reduction in the rate of grade retention, and a 51% reduction in child maltreatment when compared with the control group (Reynolds et al., 2001). These findings suggest that any form of the intervention helped reduce the risk of adverse outcomes for these children.

Children who completed the extension program through the second or third grade also demonstrated higher achievement test scores in adolescence and lower rates of child maltreatment by age 17 as compared with the preschool-only participants (Reynolds et al., 2001). In contrast, children in the control group were twice as likely to be retained a grade (30.1% versus 15.3%) and more likely to be placed in special education (15.7% versus 10.0%) than those that completed all components of the study (Chicago Longitudinal Study, 2004). It is important to note, however, that differences in reading scores between the control and experimental group became nonsignificant (1.2 points instead of 4.0) when the mean was adjusted to account for cognitive readiness at kindergarten entry, parent education, and low family income (Reynolds & Temple, 1998).

The positive effects of the CPC study on child outcomes also had spill-over gains for the city of Chicago and society at large. The average cost for 1.5 years of program participation was $6,730 per child (1998 dollars), with a total return to society of $47,759 per participant—a $7.10 return per dollar spent. For the children who participated for 4–6 years, the return to society was $24,772 per participant, with an average cost of $4,068—a $6.09 return per dollar spent (Reynolds et al., 2001).

Critical Analysis of Treatment Characteristics Comprehensiveness was addressed in the CPC study by providing services at multiple time points and by encouraging parental involvement. Children received educational services beginning during preschool and lasting through elementary school. Parents were also highly engaged in the program; all parents were required to volunteer at least once a week in the classroom. In addition, the program provided parents with a resource room and continuing education classes. However, the program failed to target home environments, neighborhoods, or larger community contexts. If training components had been embedded in multiple arenas, then children might have been better prepared to generalize their skills across settings.

The mandatory parental involvement of the CPC, combined with low student–teacher ratios, potentially provided opportunities for positive relationships to be developed among both parents and teachers. The CPC study did not, however, use a uniform curriculum and did not cite a particular theoretical framework from which the program operated. Although the absence of a mandatory curriculum was a strength in that it allowed for individualization of treatment, there also were problems associated with this approach. For instance, it is unclear the extent to which the CPC utilized varied teaching methods because no uniform curriculum was espoused. The absence of theoretical grounding and curriculum specificity are significant limitations of the CPC program. Furthermore, the CPC also lacked sociocultural relevance. Although all of the children in the program were minorities, no mention was made of training teachers and staff in cultural sensitivity or implementing socioculturally relevant teaching practices. Lack of attention to community and cultural goals is a significant weakness of the CPC program. Effective programs must reach out to families so that their beliefs, values, and aims are not ignored or downplayed by intervention staff.

Critical Analysis of Procedural Characteristics The Chicago Longitudinal Study employed a research design that tested for the impact of dosage on development. The split treatment design (some children exited the program after kindergarten and others remained in the program through third grade) provided evidence for the benefits of intervention programs with a longer duration. This emphasis on determining appropriate dosage is a major strength and contribution of the CPC study. There were, however, limitations to the study's design, specifically in the absence of tests for timing effects. The CPC did not evaluate how treatment effectiveness might have been different based on age of entry into the program. As such, the treatment might have been more or less effective had children entered the program at different ages.

The CPC staff received regular in-service training and a master teacher was in charge of coordinating services and overseeing classroom teachers. Each classroom also had the added support of a teacher's aide and parent volunteers that ensured low student–teacher ratios. The presence of the master teacher, combined with the in-service training, provided the program with an avenue for promoting treatment fidelity, but the lack of a uniform curriculum made it impossible for all students to receive the same treatment. In addition, because there is no way to know if students received different amounts or forms of the treatment, change cannot be attributed to any specific program component. Furthermore, despite the multiple supports provided for teachers (training and low student–teacher ratios), without a specific curriculum for all teachers, it is difficult to determine if all children received high-quality classroom teaching.

Critical Analysis of Design Characteristics   The CPC program was strong in terms of interpretative standards. The split treatment group (3-year versus 6-year programs) allowed for a clear interpretation of the impact of duration on outcomes. The control group also was well designed as an active control group; children in the control group were enrolled in other government early education programs such as Head Start. The presence of the active control group makes the differences between the treatment and control groups more compelling. Because the control group received similar levels of contact and educational services, the significant positive changes exhibited by the treatment group indicated that the CPC curriculum, not just program involvement, was driving these developmental gains.

The program also had appropriate outcome evaluations with measures of various domains of functioning, thus allowing the program to demonstrate the breadth and depth of its effectiveness. Significant effect sizes also were reported, further documenting the successfulness of the treatment. Findings from the CPC project not only revealed statistically significant differences between the groups, but also socially significant differences. The lower incidences of crime in the treatment group, for example, lend support to this program's benefits to society at large. As such, gains for individual participants translated into community fiscal saving with a $7.10 return on every dollar (Reynolds et al., 2001). These strong design characteristics serve to demonstrate the multiple ways in which early prevention efforts can be effective.

The Abecedarian Project

The Abecedarian Project began in 1972 at the University of North Carolina. The program followed children from infancy (6 weeks) through age 8. Children were chosen for participation based on risk eligibility on a 13-item risk index, which included factors such as low parent education, low income, father absence, use of welfare services, poor maternal social support, and parents working at unskilled jobs (Ramey & Smith, 1977). The children in the project were assessed every year during the program (birth to 5 years) and then again at 12, 15, and 21 years (Campbell, Ramey, Pungello, Sparling, & Miller-Johnson, 2002).

The Abecedarian Project was developed to address two primary questions: 1) how malleable is cognitive development among children who are at risk when they are given early environmental support and enrichment, and 2) to what degree can their school performance be enhanced when provided with preschool and primary school services (Campbell et al., 2002)? The program was based on General Systems Theory (Ramey, MacPhee, & Yeates, 1982) and the Ecological Systems Theory (Bronfenbrenner, 1977), both of which acknowledge the effects of multiple environments (i.e., home, school) and relationships (i.e., parents, siblings, peers, child care) on the growing child and encourage intervention in early development for improving long-term outcomes.

Children were recruited and matched on high-risk index scores and then randomly assigned to either the control group (n = 54; 57% girls) or experimental group (n = 57; 49% girls). Supportive social services were made available to both the treatment and control groups when needed (Campbell et al., 2002). The children in the treatment group were further divided into two groups during the primary school years, with 25 children receiving preschool and school-age intervention (a total of 8 years of treatment) and the remaining 24 children receiving preschool-only intervention (a total of 5 years of treatment). The control group also was further divided into two groups when the children were 5 years old: One received a school-age intervention program (n = 21; a total of 3 years of treatment), whereas the other remained a strict control group. The control group received pediatric follow-up services on a schedule recommended by the American Academy of Pediatrics, were provided with unlimited iron-fortified formula, and received social work services and home visits. They were not provided with early childhood education, but many of the children attended other child care facilities with age-of-entry ranging from infancy to preschool age (Ramey & Ramey, 1998).

Although a rigid curriculum was not enforced, *Partners for Learning* was implemented at each treatment site. This program targets 31 skill areas in four broad themes: cognitive and fine motor, social and self, motor, and language development (see Sparling & Lewis, 1991). Game-like learning activities were tailored to these skill areas and cycled through in about 2-week intervals to keep the activities interesting and novel while allowing enough time for mastery (Ramey & Ramey, 1998; Sparling & Lewis, 1991). Similar to the Chicago Child–Parent study, the Abecedarian Project focused its curriculum on cognitive outcomes, specifically conversational language development.

Teachers were required to have formal training and professional experience and demonstrate skills for working with young children. Ongoing training updated teachers' knowledge, including a course covering language development and a technical assistance program. Furthermore, child–teacher ratios were kept low, with three children to every adult during infancy and four children to every adult for children between 1 and 3 years of age (Ramey & Smith, 1977).

The program was partially modeled after the Ecological System's Theory (Bronfenbrenner, 1977), so home-based resource teachers, parents, and social services were used to target areas of influence in the child's life outside classrooms. Parents of children in the preschool intervention were encouraged to be involved with their children's development; parents received a curriculum aimed at enhancing the environmental conditions that their children experienced at home. Parents also were given the opportunity to be involved in a parent group and received home visits by CPC staff. In addition, parents whose children participated in the school-age component of the treatment group were assigned to a home-based resource teacher. The purpose of this liaison between the program and the home was to increase parental involvement in the children's progress in the school-age component through individualized curriculum packets. Parents were encouraged to work with their child for 15 minutes a day on key skills provided in the curriculum packets throughout the 3 years (Ramey & Ramey, 1998).

Program Evaluation   Ninety-eight percent of the 111 participants recruited were African American, with the typical mother being young (M = 20 years) and unmarried, having less than a high school education (M = 10 years), living in a multigenerational household, and reporting no earned income (Ramey & Campbell, 1984). At 18 months, differences between the experimental and control groups emerged as the treated children had significantly higher scores on intellectual measures (Ramey & Campbell, 1984). Reading and mathematics scores increased as a linear function of the number of years in the program's treatment group; larger effect sizes in reading and mathematics scores were found for the preschool-only group when compared with the elementary education-only group at ages 8, 12, 15, and 21. Effect sizes ranged from small to medium for the preschool-only group; effect sizes were in the small range for the elementary education-only group (Ramey et al., 2000). These results indicate that the intervention seemed to be more effective in improving reading abilities, and results were better if the children received the intervention at an earlier age. Children in the preschool treatment group also showed reduced academic retention rates and lower rates of placement in special education at ages 12 and 15 in comparison with controls. A difference in IQ scores between the treatment and control groups persisted through age 15, although treatment effect sizes were largest during the preschool years and diminished over time (Campbell et al., 2002).

The final assessment for the Abecedarian Project was given when the children were 21 years old. Cognitive scores were significantly higher for the children in the preschool-only group as compared with those in the control group in terms of IQ scores and reading achievement (Campbell et al., 2002), indicating that the program was successful in fostering the children's cognitive development. Interesting differences were found when cognitive scores were investigated for males and females separately. Cognitive scores for women in the preschool treatment group approached statistically significant levels; they had IQ scores 8 points higher than women in the control group, but no difference was found for men. Although these findings only approached statistical significance, they suggest that girls may have benefited more from the program than boys.

In terms of educational attainment at age 21, individuals who were in the preschool treatment group completed more years of school, were more likely to be in school, and were three times as likely to have attended a 4-year college than individuals who were in the control condition (Campbell et al., 2002). Women in the treatment group earned 1.2 more years of education than women in the control group, whereas men in the treatment and control group did not differ in level of educational attainment. Overall, adults who were in the preschool treatment group were more likely to be skilled employees (47% versus 27%) and were less likely to use marijuana (18% versus 39%) or smoke (39% versus 55%) than adults in the control group (Campbell et al., 2002). However, there were no differences between the groups for violent behaviors or weapon-carrying (Campbell et al., 2002).

The Abecedarian Project also resulted in benefits for families of children in the treatment group. Mothers of children involved in the treatment program had higher educational attainment and better paying jobs at the 5-year assessment than mothers whose children were in the control condition (Campbell & Ramey, 1994). Furthermore, adolescent mothers of children in the preschool-only experimental group appeared to benefit the most from participation: By the 15-year assessment, their employment rate was 92% as compared with 66% for teenage moms whose children were in the control group (Ramey et al., 2000). Not only did children and their families gain from involvement in the early childhood program, but benefits also were passed on to society in areas such as participant earnings, maternal earnings, educational attainment, and health status; a projected net benefit to society for each individual who participated in the program was estimated to be around $75,000. With the program cost per individual estimated at $35,000, the net benefit totaled $40,000 by the 2002 dollar standard (Massey & Barnett, 2002). In sum, the program passed benefits on to society by decreasing participants' dependency on social services and helping them make their own contributions to the economy.

Critical Analysis of Treatment Characteristics   The Abecedarian Project is an exemplar early childhood program displaying both the art and science of prevention. First, the curriculum and design of the project was theory driven, using both General Systems Theory (Ramey et al., 1982) and Ecological Systems Theory (Bronfenbrenner, 1977) as the foundation for program development. The program also was comprehensive in nature, with both treatment and control groups receiving medical and social services. Children in the 8-year treatment group received not only full-day intervention for the first 5 years of life, but also tutoring upon school entry. This allowed for skills that were already acquired to be maintained and for difficulties with a particular subject area to be addressed prior to the development of large problems. In terms of teaching methods, multiple learning activities were provided as part of the curriculum, thus providing teachers with options for variety and flexibility.

Although the Abecedarian Project was successful in addressing important treatment characteristics such as being theory driven and comprehensive, the program was found lacking in terms of attention given to cultural sensitivity. If teachers and program staff were not trained to recognize the community norms and cultural values of program families, then some parents may have felt their concerns and goals were not addressed and subsequently participation and attendance may have decreased. Similarly, no reference was made to specific attempts to develop and maintain positive relationships as part of the program involvement. Again, without an emphasis on positive relationships, program staff may have inadvertently distanced some families by failing to create a friendly environment.

Critical Analysis of Procedural Characteristics   The Abecedarian Project also was noteworthy because of the emphasis placed on determining appropriate dosage. By having a research design consisting of groups receiving different levels of treatment, the project was able to assess the benefits of smaller and larger dosages. Similarly, the design allowed for testing timing effects by providing that some participants received only the treatment during elementary school. This attention to procedural characteristics provided a means for testing when and how much intervention is necessary to prevent developmental delays in an at-risk group.

The project ensured quality staffing by hiring staff with both formal education and experience with children. Staffers also received ongoing training that provided for treatment fidelity. In this way, there was documentation that all students received the same level and quality of services, a necessary step in attributing change to treatment components. Furthermore, through the elementary school tutoring program and the academic summer camp, children in the treatment group received opportunities to maintain and generalize skills.

Critical Analysis of Design Characteristics   The Abecedarian Project was strong on several design characteristics. The study displayed strong interpretative standards, with the control group receiving medical services, free formula, and home visits from social workers. There also was a middle-class comparison group. The presence of multiple, active control groups allowed for changes in treatment participants to be attributed to the intervention curricula and not simply to interaction with staff or better access to other social services.

The program also was successful in terms of outcome evaluation. Evaluations were conducted regularly throughout childhood as well as at 12, 15, and 21 years of age. The assessment scheme was broad, measuring academic, cognitive, and behavioral domains. Penal system involvement, drug use, and employment history also were measured. By incorporating measures of multiple aspects of development over time, comparisons could be made between treatment and controls that demonstrated the numerous gains possible from participating in the program. The program also reported large effect sizes early on, particularly for participants who received the 8-year treatment package. This further verified that substantial changes in participant behavior and functioning could be attributed to the treatment.

Early Head Start

The Head Start Reauthorization Act of 1994 expanded the preschool program to include services to low-income families with infants and toddlers (Raikes & Love, 2002). An initial research phase called the Early Head Start Research and Evaluation Project (EHSREP) was designed to include 3,000 children at 17 sites nationwide. The locations and participants for the study were chosen to represent diversity in factors such as geographic region, racial–ethnic status, urban-rural settings, and program auspice (Early Head Start National Resource Center, 2005). Early Head Start (EHS) was designed to provide intensive services prenatally through the first 3 years not only to help improve the child's development, but also to aid the family in child rearing and to encourage staff and community development (Paulsell, Kisker, Love, & Raikes, 2002).

Using an ecological perspective, EHS staff identified the needs, resources, and aspirations of families and devised individualized service agreements based on the program's established principles (Mann, 2002). These goals were drawn from empirical findings to form the requirements of the program; their implementation is notably interconnected. First, through careful documentation and revision of services, EHS aimed to uphold a high-quality program to prevent developmental delays and promote positive developmental outcomes. Central to achieving these goals were positive relationships and continuity across services, direct parent involvement, and sensitivity to cultural differences. As a result of EHS's commitment to comprehensive, flexible, responsive, and intense learning environments, the program was able to include children regardless of developmental difficulties. In addition, the program aimed to ease the children's stresses associated with transitions such as changes from school to home and from EHS to future educational settings. Finally, program staff connected participants with other community resources not provided via program involvement (Early Head Start National Resource Center, 2005).

The children in the EHS treatment group were involved in one of the 17 initial programs. Due to an emphasis on adherence to general principles, rather than specific techniques, each site was allowed to individualize a program to service their community's unique needs. As a result, not all programs were identical and included 1) a center-based option, 2) a home-based option, 3) a combination option in which families received a prescribed number of home visits and center-based experiences, and 4) locally designed options based on the resources available at each site (Fenichel & Mann, 2001). For example, at EHS sites in Vermont, the center-based option addressed EHS goals through a full-day, year-round, comprehensive child care environment (Central Vermont Community Action Council, 2005). For the home-based option, staff visited families in their homes three times a week to help assist the parents in providing educational experiences in the home environment. Parents also are given the opportunity to attend bimonthly meetings called *socializations* that provide group activities for families and children in the program. The combination option offered half-day child care three times a week, as well as a monthly home visit (Central Vermont Community Action Council, 2005).

EHS defined *curriculum* as a written plan based on sound child development principles about how children grow and learn (Fenichel & Mann, 2001). The different sites formed personal agendas that were to achieve these developmental and learning goals by formulating meaningful experiences for children, devising appropriate roles for parents and teachers, and collecting suitable materials. EHS stressed the importance of flexibility in designing curriculum so that the program accommodated each site's unique needs (Fenichel & Mann, 2001). Specifically, an EHS Manualized Assessment of Progress (MAP) system documented the progress of children and their families and the developmental, educational, and community services they received in order to be sensitive to the individual needs and unique characteristics of each child (Dickstein, Seifer, Eguia, Kuersten-Hogan, & Magee, 2002). In addition, federal and local staff monitors implemented a Program Review Instrument of Systems Monitoring (PRISM) to keep individual sites up to nationally set Program Performance Standards. This process aimed to help individual programs uphold the standards of the program at large while maintaining unique characteristics that best served their children (Fenichel & Mann, 2001).

Teachers in EHS classrooms were required to have a Child Development Associate credential or equivalency. EHS also provided training for staff on infant and toddler development and communication skills for effectively interacting with the children in the program and their parents. Staff–child ratios were kept strictly at 1:4 with a maximum group size of eight, unless more stringent requirements were stipulated by the state in which the program resided (Fenichel & Mann, 2001).

Program Evaluation The 3,000 children who participated in the research and evaluation phase were randomly assigned to the control and experimental groups. The control group was free to receive other services from the community. Evaluations occurred at 6, 15, and 26 months after entering the program and again at completion. The children and their families were also assessed at 14, 24, and 36 months of age. The programs sites were critiqued two times, in the fall of 1997 and again in 1999. Overall, the results from the 17 EHS sites showed that children profited in many areas of development from being a part of the program. Four of the 17 programs adopted a full-day, full-year, center-based child development program. These programs had a higher quality of care for their infants and toddlers as compared with nationwide center-based programs, especially for children from low-income homes. The children in these programs were found to show enhanced developmental outcomes, specifically in language and cognitive development, with no evidence of lower child well-being or higher rates of aggressive behavior being associated with spending more time in the center-based program (Early Head Start National Resource Center, 2005).

Children in EHS at 2 years of age scored higher on a standardized assessment of infant cognitive development (90.1 versus 88.1 on the Bayley Mental Development Index), had larger vocabularies (56.3 versus 53.9 on the MacArthur CDI), and used more grammatically complex sentences (CDI scores of 8.6 versus 7.7) than children in the control group. EHS seemed to be reducing overall risk of cognitive delay; children in the treatment group were less likely to score in the at-risk range of developmental functioning than controls (33.6% versus 40.2% scoring below 85; Raikes & Love, 2002). These gains were maintained at 3 years of age; children in the treatment group continued to perform better on the Bayley than controls (M = 91.4 versus M = 89.9). In addition, a smaller percentage of EHS children were in an at-risk range in comparison with control group children (27.3% versus 32.0%; Love et al., 2002). Children in EHS also displayed better socioemotional outcomes than children in the control group (Fenichel & Mann, 2001). At 3 years of age, children in the treatment group were shown to engage with their parents more and have less negativity during interactions with their parents than children in the control group. Children in the treatment group also were more attentive during play and displayed fewer aggressive behaviors (Early Head Start National Resource Center, 2005).

Both parental competency and children's home environments also were evaluated, with families in the treatment group displaying greater gains in these areas than those in the control group. Using the Home Observation for Measurement of the Environment (HOME) scale, children in the treatment group were more likely to live in homes that were cognitively stimulating in reference to language and literacy development; parents of children in the treatment group were more likely to read to their children daily (57% versus 52%) and at bedtime (34% versus 27%) than control participants (Raikes & Love, 2002). Mothers of children in EHS were shown to be more sensitive, supportive, and likely to extend play to stimulate cognitive growth while simultaneously being less likely to be detached or report spanking in the previous week in comparison with mothers in the control group. In fact, discipline techniques of mothers in the treatment group were milder and more prevention-oriented than controls (Raikes & Love, 2002), and children in EHS were found to be less aggressive at both 24 and 36 months than children in the control group (Love et al., 2003). Effect sizes were in the modest range, 10%–15%, although larger in some subgroup analyses. As a result of late implementation, some programs did not report results as positive as others, and the programs whose implementation was on schedule showed greater effect sizes ranging from 15% to 25% (Raikes & Love, 2002).

Critical Analysis of Treatment Characteristics   The EHS program utilized an ecological perspective and drew from empirical research to develop its core principles. Principles included comprehensive learning environments, positive relationships, and cultural sensitivity. Unfortunately, it is difficult to know how and to what extent these principles were translated into practice at each individual program site. Furthermore, it is challenging to evaluate the program in terms of comprehensiveness and variety in teaching methods because of the diversity of program forms (home-based, center-based, and combined programs). Because the specific components of the intervention were governed by each site, the degree to which EHS was comprehensive and used varied teaching methods cannot be determined.

Critical Analysis of Procedural Characteristics   The EHS program did not specifically design a way to evaluate appropriate dosage or timing of the intervention. Records were kept, however, regarding attendance and age of child at program entry, which provided a way to measure the impact of treatment level on outcomes. Two specific systems were designed by EHS to operate as a check of treatment fidelity. The MAP provides systematic documentation of services families receive, whereas the PRISM serves to evaluate each program's adherence to EHS subscribed principles. These systems fail, however, to provide specific evidence of treatment fidelity because no uniform curriculum was established across sites, only a unified set of principles. As such, it is unclear to what extent all children received high-quality services. In addition, no mention was made regarding any programmed generalizations of the treatment, probably because it is assumed that upon turning age 3, children would become eligible for Head Start or other preexisting programs. The lack of structured transition for leaving EHS could have resulted in some children not consistently attending Head Start and subsequently not maintaining gains developed during the program.

Critical Analysis of Design Characteristics   Although control group participants in the EHS program were allowed to use other preexisting community services, questions regarding actual utilization of such services on a regular basis kept EHS from having a true active control. Documentation of an active control group is critical for making judgments regarding treatment effectiveness. For instance, without an active control group, it is unclear if gains for participants are due to the intervention or just to interactions with service professionals. The study did benefit, however, from the clustering of treatment programs into three basic types (center-based, home-based, and combined). This provided an avenue for testing which form of service provision might be most effective for certain families. In terms of outcome evaluation, EHS had assessments scheduled at multiple time points. These assessments were broad in scope and included evaluations of cognitive and language development, behavioral characteristics, the home environment, and parenting. The study did not identify any specific process variables, however, which makes internal validation difficult to evaluate.

Because EHS is a relatively young program, evaluations are not complete. A full critique of EHS is somewhat challenging given that there is, as of yet, no data on school and adult functioning. In turn, the clinical or social significance also is difficult to place in context. Effect sizes for EHS have been small, although specific program sites sometimes have displayed greater gains than others. Site differences bring to light the importance of fully implementing programs, adequate staff training, and attention to treatment fidelity. Overall, however, the small differences between groups in standardized scores of child functioning, although statistically significant, bring to question the clinical meaning of the findings. It will be important for EHS to continue to follow and assess the children over time to see a more complete picture of the impact of the early intervention program.

MODEL PROGRAM FOR THE PREVENTION OF DEVELOPMENTAL DELAY

The aforementioned programs—CPC, Abecedarian, and EHS—have brought prevention planning for children's developmental delays to a new level. Each project has made individual contributions to the understanding of what works in promoting the positive outcomes for children including a program's timing and length, specific participant targets, and risks to be addressed. Exemplary programs must begin early, address multiple risk factors, and incorporate interagency collaboration. In addition, programs should include components to support the child as well as the parent(s) with an emphasis on fostering positive dynamics within the family system. Dimensions of the model program can be found in Table 3.2 and include recommendations for the targets of intervention, curriculum content, outcome goals, and program duration.

A model program to prevent developmental delay should target the child and parent(s) and utilize multifaceted components administered in both the home and child care setting. In the home, a program caseworker can discuss curriculum topics such as teaching new skills to the child and handling misbehavior in an environment where the majority of these issues occur. In addition, by bridging to the child care center, the same key components can be further reinforced by child care teachers that have received special supportive training. Providing high-quality child care with well-qualified teachers exposes the child to a controlled environment while allowing overtaxed parents to work without worrying about their children's safety and/or causing a financial burden. Also, the time spent in a child care setting affords children direct educational instruction by well-trained child care providers. By incorporating the two most important contexts of the child's immediate caregiving environment into the prevention program, continuity in teaching can be accomplished and multisetting translation of effects can be seen more clearly.

Appropriate timing and duration of service delivery also is essential in the model program. For optimal success, the model program should begin in infancy before problems have become long-standing and resistant to change. Delivering

Table 3.2. Components of a model developmental disabilities prevention program

Targets of Intervention	High-risk families with infants and toddlers
Content of Intervention	Parent training and home visits High-quality child care programming Community referrals Tutoring and parent resources provided through elementary school
Outcomes of Intervention	Lower rates of child maltreatment Higher parental educational attainment Higher cognitive and language test scores for program children Fewer child behavioral problems
Costs and Duration	Infancy through age 5 with continued supports through grade 5

services through the children's 5th birthday also would ensure that a critical period of development is being supported, which is particularly important for families facing multiple risks including poverty or having a single head of house. Moreover, providing booster sessions and additional supports once the intensive services have ended can strengthen program effects and ensure maintenance over time.

To summarize, the model program must start in infancy and continue through the first 5 years of life, employing a multifaceted approach to remedying potential problems that place children at risk for developmental delay. In addition, components must address parent and child concerns in both the home and child care environment. To put the model program into action, the case study of Allison Taylor and her daughter Amy is used to illustrate how the model prevention program works.

❖

Allison and Amy

Allison Taylor wasn't sure about being a mother. At age 17, she was trying to finish high school, deal with her boyfriend's incarceration, and fulfill her role as a daughter in a struggling family. But when her little girl was born, Allison couldn't bear to give her up for adoption. Allison's parents, Tom and Cassie, agreed to help out and allowed their daughter and the infant, Amy, to stay with them. Money was tight, and making matters worse was the constant bickering between her parents.

Allison loved her daughter, but she was beginning to feel that she had no control over her life. She felt that she was responsible for her parents' increased worries and fighting. Adding to her stress were the responsibilities involved in being a new parent. At 6 months, Amy still got up at least once in the middle of the night and was beginning to crawl. Allison felt like she could never rest. She lived with her family, but because they were busy with their own lives, most of the responsibility of caring for Amy fell to Allison.

However, Allison was thankful for the help she was receiving. In particular, the food supplement she got from the Women, Infants and Children (WIC) program helped reduce her grocery bills and ensured that she got all the nutrition she needed to breastfeed her infant. She enjoyed the WIC appointments because she got a chance to talk about Amy and ask questions about the right way to care for her. It was at one of these appointments that Allison first heard about a parenting program that was looking for families like hers. Although somewhat unsure about the program, Allison thought that she would try it (they told her she could quit at any time).

Allison had been nervous about her first home visit, but the first time she met Rachel, her home visitor, she was struck by how easy it was to talk with her. Rachel had prepared extensively for her meeting with Allison, as she did before meeting all participants in the program. She was hired because of her experience working with children and her easy manner. She had had several months' training on specific parenting techniques and ideas, as well as on how to interact with the mothers, and she had been made aware of the many issues young mothers face, particularly single mothers, and how to handle such issues sensitively. When she met with Allison, Rachel asked many questions about topics Allison hadn't thought about before. During the first session, Rachel suggested that Allison respond to Amy's cooing and noises. Allison was amazed—she had never thought that Amy was actually trying to communicate with her! Allison was even more amazed when Rachel told her that Amy could go to a free quality child care center for up to 50 hours a week. That meant that Allison could finish school and not worry about Amy.

As the weeks passed, Allison kept thinking that she and Rachel couldn't possibly talk about anything more, but every week she learned something new. She began to feel less frustrated with the things Amy did, realizing that the behaviors were common to all children. Moreover, Allison was beginning to feel competent in her parenting skills; she had learned new ways to teach her child and felt great when Amy mastered a new task.

Amy had settled well into her new school. At first, Allison had a hard time dropping her off because Amy would cry and cling to her, but all the teachers assured Allison that this was normal. With their extensive training and continued education, the teachers were able to suggest things that Allison could do to help Amy make the transition into the new child care center (e.g., be consistent with drop-off and pick-up times). There were four teachers in a classroom of 12 children, and Allison believed that Amy was being well cared for. She knew that the children received a lot of individual attention yet still had time to interact with one another. Even more, once a week Allison got a chance to volunteer in Amy's classroom and see the variety of activities the children participated in each day.

Over the course of the next 4 years, the lives of Allison and Amy continued to change. Amy grew to love school. It seemed to Allison that her daughter's vocabulary increased every day. Amy described the fun games she played at school and counted for the whole family all the way up to 80! Allison appreciated the way Amy had grown both in her newfound abilities and emotionally, evidenced by the large number of friends she had at school. Allison was proud of her daughter and thankful that she could finish her own education while Amy was at school. Appreciating Rachel's impact on her life, Allison decided to become a social worker. Now nearing the end of her studies, she eagerly awaits her graduation after which she and Amy will move into their own place. Even though finances are still tight and she sometimes worries about the future, Allison is hopeful about the direction her life is taking.

Almost 5 now, Amy is thriving. She sings constantly and is not shy about sharing her ideas with whoever is around. She is confident about the things she has learned and can't wait to go to kindergarten and be a *big girl*. She also can't wait to be an astronaut when she grows up and touch the stars someday. Sometimes Allison watches Amy play and thinks about how far they've come. Starting out with the odds stacked against them, Allison and Amy are well on their way to a bright future.

The positive experiences and continued growth of Allison and Amy are clear markers of the success of a program targeted at preventing developmental delays. Beginning early, the curriculum was able to address problematic issues before they had a significant negative impact on Amy. In addition, Amy's positive, enriching child care situation provided her with new learning opportunities. It also allowed Allison to have the crucial worry-free time necessary to better herself and to foster an opportunity for success for mother and child. Prevention programming works toward this goal, which is manifested by each child's triumph.

FUTURE DIRECTION

In closing, three key areas are highlighted that will need to be addressed by future programs designed to prevent developmental delays: 1) programmed generalizations, 2) treatment fidelity, and 3) sociocultural relevance. As the Abecedarian Project documented, starting an intervention during the early years of life and then continuing to provide supports to children during elementary school is critical for developing and maintaining strengths in academic domains. Future prevention programs should similarly be mindful of the need to provide opportunities for programmed generalizations such as tutoring and regular parent meetings. Booster sessions also are necessary during transitions times such as preschool to kindergarten. Providing additional supports after the completion of the program help children stay on track for future success.

Prevention programs need to incorporate indicators of treatment fidelity into the implementation of the curriculum. To demonstrate effectiveness there must be documentation that all children received the same high-quality services so that gains are attributable to the specific curriculum components and are not the spurious result of the extra attention provided by program participation. Programs cannot exhibit strong treatment fidelity when it is unclear what the treatment is, in fact, all about. The lack of clearly delineated intervention curricula plagues this area of research. Programs may be theoretically grounded and comprehensive and incorporate innovative teaching methods, but without a structured curriculum, it is impossible to know if all children are receiving the same level and quality of services. At the same time, however, programs must pay special attention to individualizing programming. Effective programs balance the art of responding to the unique needs of individual participants with the science of maintaining treatment fidelity.

Finally, future programs designed to prevent developmental delay must seek to ensure sociocultural relevance. This is especially important because many children receiving prevention services are from ethnic or racial minority groups. Researchers should collaborate with community leaders to best understand the needs, goals, and cultural values of participants. For instance, in a qualitative study of parenting, teaching children about racial themes was found to be highly valued and practiced among African Americans of low socioeconomic status (Coard, Wallace, Stevenson, & Brotman, 2004). In light of their findings, Coard et al. suggested that intervention programs should include racial socialization in parent training programs. This is just one example of successful collaboration between intervention designers and community members. Community partnerships enable science and art to come together to promote the optimal development of children who are at risk through their participation in prevention programs.

REFERENCES

Administration for Children and Families. (2005). *What is Early Head Start?* Retrieved August 22, 2005, from http://www.ehsnrc.org/AboutUs/ehs.htm#principles

Bennett, K.J., Brown, K.S., Boyle, M., Racine, Y., & Offord, D. (2003). Does low reading achievement at school entry cause conduct problems? *Social Science & Medicine, 56,* 2443–2448.

Bernstein, J., Brocht, C., & Spade-Aguilar, M. (2000). *How much is enough? Basic family budgets for working families.* Washington, DC: Economic Policy Institute.

Bowe, F.G. (1995). Population estimates: Birth-to-5 children with disabilities. *The Journal of Special Education, 20,* 461–471.

Bradley, R.H., Corwyn, R.F., Burchinal, M., McAdoo, H.P., & Garcia Coll, C. (2001). The home environments of children in the Unites States Part II: Relations with behavior development through age thirteen. *Child Development, 72,* 1868–1886.

Bronfenbrenner, U. (1977). Toward an experimental ecology of human development. *American Psychologist, 32,* 513–531.

Campbell, F.A., & Ramey, C.T. (1994). Effects of early intervention on intellectual and academic achievement: A follow-up study of children from low-income families. *Child Development, 65,* 684–689.

Campbell, F.A., Ramey, C.T., Pungello, E., Sparling, J., & Miller-Johnson, S. (2002). Early childhood education: Young adult outcomes from the Abecedarian Project. *Applied Developmental Science, 6,* 42–57.

Central Vermont Community Action Council, Inc. (2005). *Head Start and Early Head Start.* Retrieved September 3, 2005, from http://www.cvcac.org/Services/headstart.htm

Chicago Longitudinal Study. (2004). *Chicago Longitudinal Study.* Retrieved August 28, 2005, from http://www.waisman.wisc.edu/cls/index.htmlx

Coard, S.I., Wallace, S.A., Stevenson, H.C., Jr., & Brotman, L.M. (2004). Towards culturally relevant preventive interventions: The consideration of racial socialization in parent training with African American families. *Journal of Child and Family Studies, 13,* 277–293.

Dickstein, S., Seifer, R., Eguia, M., Kuersten-Hogan, R., & Magee, K.D. (2002). Early Head Start MAP: Manualized Assessment of Progress. *Infant Mental Health Journal, 23,* 231–249.

Douglas-Hall, A., & Koball, H. (2005). *Basic facts about low-income children in the United States.* Retrieved June 23, 2005, from http://www.nccp.org/pub_lic05.html#2

Duncan, G.J., & Brooks-Gunn, J. (1997). *Consequences of growing up poor.* New York: Russell Sage Foundation.

Early Head Start National Resource Center. (2005). *Early Head Start benefits children and families.* Retrieved August 28, 2005, from http://www.ehsnrc.org

Education for All Handicapped Children Act of 1975, PL 94-142, 20 U.S.C. §§ 1400 *et seq.*

Epstein, A.S. (2003). Early math: The next big thing. *High/Scope ReSource: A magazine for educators.* Ypsilanti, MI: High/Scope Press.

Fenichel, E., & Mann, T.L. (2001). Early Head Start for low-income families with infants and toddlers. *Future of Children, 11,* 135–141.

Gallagher, T.M., & Watkin, K.L. (1998). Prematurity and language developmental risk: Too young or too small? *Topics in Language Disorders, 18,* 15–25.

Guralnick, M.J. (1998). Effectiveness of early intervention for vulnerable children: A developmental perspective. *American Journal on Mental Retardation, 102,* 319–345.

Hack, M.B., Flannery, D.J., Schluchter, M., Cartar, L., Borawski, E., & Klein, N. (2002). Outcomes in young adulthood for very-low-birth-weight infants. *New England Journal of Medicine, 346,* 149–157.

Harrington, D., Dubowitz, H., Black, M.M., & Binder, A. (1995). Maternal substance use and neglectful parenting: Relations with children's development. *Journal of Clinical Child Psychology, 24,* 258–263.

Head Start Reauthorization Act of 1994, PL 103-252, 42 U.S.C. §§ 9831 *et seq.*

Individuals with Disabilities Education Act (IDEA) of 1990, PL 101-476, 20 U.S.C. §§ 1400 *et seq.*

Individuals with Disabilities Education Improvement Act of 2004, PL 108-446, 20 U.S.C. §§ 1400 *et seq.*

King, E.H., Logsdon, D.A., & Schroeder, S.R. (1992). Risk factors for developmental delay among infants and toddlers. *Children's Health Care, 21,* 39–52.

Levine, J.A., Pollack, H., & Comfort, M.E. (2001). Academic and behavioral outcomes among the children of young mothers. *Journal of Marriage and Family, 63,* 355–369.

Liaw, F., & Brooks-Gunn, J. (1993). Patterns of low-birth-weight children's cognitive development. *Developmental Psychology, 29,* 1024–1035.

Love, J.M., Harrison, L., Sagi-Schwartz, A., van IJzendoorn, M.H., Ross, C., Ungerer, J.A., et al. (2003). Child care quality matters: How conclusions may vary with context. *Child Development, 74,* 1021–1033.

Love, J.M., Kisker, E.E., Ross, C.M., Schochet, P.Z., Brooks-Gunn, J., Paulsell, D., et al. (2002). *Making a difference in the lives of infants and toddlers and their families: The impacts of Early Head Start. Executive summary.* Retrieved August 22, 2005, from http://www.acf.hhs.gov/programs/opre/ehs/ehs_resrch/reports/impacts_exesum/impacts_execsum.pdf

Mann, T.L. (2002). The role of training and technical assistance in supporting the delivery of high quality services in early head start. *Infant Mental Health Journal, 23,* 36–47.

Massey, L.N., & Barnett, W.S. (2002). *A benefit cost analysis of the Abecedarian Early Childhood Intervention.* Retrieved August 29, 2005, from http://nieer.org/resources/research/AbecedarianStudy.pdf

Masten, A.S., & Wright, M.O. (1998). Cumulative risk and protection models of child maltreatment. *Journal of Aggression, Maltreatment & Trauma, 2,* 7–30.

Maughan, B. (1995). Long-term outcomes of developmental reading problems. *Journal of Child Psychology and Psychiatry and Allied Disciplines, 36,* 357–371.

McCormick, M.C., McCarton, C., Brooks-Gunn, J., Belt, P., & Gross, R.T. (1998). The Infant Health and Development Program: Interim summary. *Journal of Developmental and Behavioral Pediatrics, 19,* 359–370.

McGee, R., Prior, M., Williams, S., Smart, P., & Sanson, A. (2002). The long-term significance of teacher-rated hyperactivity and reading ability in childhood: Findings from two longitudinal studies. *Journal of Child Psychology and Psychiatry, 43,* 1004–1017.

Moe, V., & Smith, L. (2003). The relation of prenatal substance exposure and infant recognition memory to later cognitive competence. *Infant Behavior & Development, 26,* 87–99.

Olds, D., Henderson, C.R., Jr., Cole, R., Eckenrode, J., Kitzman, H., Luckey, D., et al. (1998). Long-term effects of nurse home visitation on children's criminal and antisocial behavior: 15-year follow-up of a randomized controlled trial. *Journal of the American Medical Association, 280,* 1238–1244.

Paulsell, D., Kisker, E.E., Love, J.M., & Raikes, H.H. (2002). Understanding implementation in Early Head Start programs: Implications for policy and practice. *Infant Mental Health Journal, 23,* 14–35.

Pungello, E.P., Kupersmidt, J.B., Burchinal, M.R., & Patterson, C.J. (1996). Environmental risk factors and children's achievement from middle childhood to early adolescence. *Developmental Psychology, 32,* 755–767.

Raikes, H.H., & Love, J.M. (2002). Early Head Start: A dynamic new program for infants and toddlers and their families. *Infant Mental Health Journal, 23,* 1–13.

Ramey, C.T., & Campbell, F.A. (1984). Preventive education for high-risk children: Cognitive consequences of the Carolina ABC. *American Journal of Mental Deficiency, 88,* 515–523.

Ramey, C.T., Campbell, F.A., Burchinal, M., Skinner, M.L., Gardner, D.M., & Ramey, S.L. (2000). Persistent effects of early childhood education on high-risk children and their mothers. *Applied Developmental Science, 4,* 2–14.

Ramey, C.T., MacPhee, D., & Yeates, K.O. (1982). Preventing developmental retardation: A general systems model. In L.A. Bond & J.M. Joffe (Eds.), *Facilitating infant and early childhood development* (pp. 343–401). Hanover, NH: University Press of New England.

Ramey, C.T., & Ramey, S.L. (1998). Prevention of intellectual disabilities: Early interventions to improve cognitive development. *Preventive Medicine, 27,* 224–232.

Ramey, C.T., & Ramey, S.L. (1999). Early experience and early intervention for children "at risk" for developmental delay and mental retardation. *Mental Retardation and Developmental Disabilities Research Review, 5,* 1–10.

Ramey, C.T., & Smith, B. (1977). Assessing the intellectual consequences of early intervention with high-risk infants. *American Journal of Mental Deficiency, 81,* 318–324.

Reynolds, A.J. (1998). Developing early childhood programs for children and families at risk: Research-based principles to promote long-term effectiveness. *Children and Youth Services Review, 20,* 503–523.

Reynolds, A.J., Ou, S.R., & Topitzes, J.W. (2004). Paths of effects of early childhood intervention on educational attainment and delinquency: A confirmatory analysis of the Chicago Child–Parent Centers. *Child Development, 75,* 1299–1328.

Reynolds, A.J., & Temple, J.A. (1998) Extended early childhood intervention and school achievement: Age thirteen findings from the Chicago Longitudinal Study. *Child Development, 69,* 231–246.

Reynolds, A.J., Temple, J.A., Robertson, D.L., & Mann, I.A. (2001). Long-term effects of an early childhood intervention on educational achievement and juvenile arrest: A 15-year follow-up of low income children in public schools. *Journal of American Medical Association, 285,* 2339–2346.

Scarborough, H.S., & Dobrich, W. (1990). Development of children with early language delay. *Journal of Speech and Hearing Research, 33,* 70–83.

Schweinhart, L.J. (2003, April). *Benefits, costs, and explanation of the High/Scope Perry Preschool Program.* Paper presented at the meeting of the Society for Research in Child Development, Tampa, FL.

Sparling, J., & Lewis, I. (1991). Partners: A curriculum to help premature, low birth weight infants get off to a good start. *Topics in early Childhood Special Education, 11,* 36–47.

U.S. Census Bureau. (2003, September 26). *United States Department of Commerce News.* Retrieved January 3, 2004, from http://www.census.gov/Press-Release/www/2003/cb03-153.html

U.S. Department of Education. (2002). *Why "No Child Left Behind" is important to America.* Retrieved January 6, 2004, from http://www.ed.gov/nclb/overview/importance/edlite-index.html

U.S. Department of Health and Human Services. (2004, March 22). *Administration for Children and Families questions and answers support.* Retrieved December 20, 2004, from http://faw.acf.hhs.gov

Wallace, I.F., & McCarton, C.M. (1997). Neurodevelopmental outcomes of the premature, small-for-gestational-age infant through age 6. *Clinical Obstetrics and Gynecology, 40,* 843–852.

Weikart, D.P. (1998). Changing early childhood development through educational intervention. *Preventive Medicine, 27,* 233–237.

Weissman, M.M., Warner, V., Wickramaratne, P.J., & Kandel, D.B. (1999). Maternal smoking during pregnancy and psychopathology in offspring followed to adulthood. *Journal of the American Academy of Child and Adolescent Psychiatry, 38,* 892–900.

Whitman, T.L., Borkowski, J.G., Keogh, D.A., & Weed, K. (2001). *Interwoven lives: Adolescent mothers and their children.* Mahwah, NJ: Lawrence Erlbaum Associates.

4

PREVENTING CHILD MALTREATMENT

Julie N. Schatz

Since the Battered Child Syndrome was first recognized (Kempe, Silverman, Steele, Droegemueller, & Silver, 1962), awareness of child abuse and neglect and its devastating repercussions has become part of the public consciousness. Media coverage of stories of children who have been victimized has fueled a deeper understanding of child maltreatment and has put faces on the often elusive victims. The country learned about the devastating experiences of five children from a Florida family who had been intentionally tortured by their parents. Not only were these children denied food and severely malnourished, there also was evidence that the parents had pulled the young children's toenails out with pliers (CNN News, 2005). Although an extreme case, this example of child abuse is not an isolated occurrence.

In 2002, nearly 1 million U.S. children were substantiated victims of maltreatment (U.S. Department of Health and Human Services Children's Bureau [USDHHS], 2004). The majority (60%) were victims of neglect, another 20% were physically abused, 10% were sexually abused, and 7% experienced emotional maltreatment. Yet, the most alarming statistic is the fatality rate: In one year alone, nearly 1,400 children in the United States were killed as a consequence of maltreatment (USDHHS). Of those children, 75% were from 0 to 4 years old, suggesting that younger children may be at the greatest risk for suffering the most serious physical consequences. Findings such as these have led the U.S. Advisory Board on Child Abuse and Neglect (1990) to issue a warning—child abuse and neglect in the United States now represent a national crisis.

Although the tragic stories continue to mount, considerable progress has been made in identifying families at risk for maltreatment as well as in designing programs aimed at reducing that risk. More important, many prevention programs have shown substantial effects in both ameliorating maltreatment and reducing instances where it has already occurred. This chapter provides 1) discussion of relevant literature and issues central to the prevention of child maltreatment, 2) specific design and implementation concerns for maltreatment prevention programs, 3) presentation and evaluation of three successful prevention programs, and 4) recommendations for a model child maltreatment prevention program.

WHEN POOR PARENTING BECOMES CHILD MALTREATMENT

A long-standing conundrum central to both identification and prevention of child maltreatment has been defining exactly what behaviors constitute child endangerment (Hutchison, 1990). Acceptable parenting behaviors vary from culture to culture, family to family, and even from parent to parent within the same family. For example, Cia Gao, or coin rubbing, is a type of folk medicine practiced in different cultures in which a coin is dipped in heated oil and then rubbed on the chest or back, and it can leave painful-looking marks (Gellis & Feingold, 1976; Johnson, 1996). This cultural attempt at helping the child can be mistakenly viewed as intentional abuse (Johnson).

Aside from cultural differences, a wide continuum of parenting exists, and specific threshold cutoffs of acceptable, unacceptable, and outright dangerous parenting practices are not easily determined. Further complicating the matter is that the same parenting actions may have different ramifications at various times in a child's development. For example, slapping an adolescent may not leave a bruise, but applying the same force behind the slap on a toddler may cause injury. This type of scenario lends itself to the ongoing definitional confusion and creates difficulties for child protective agencies and public policy makers in discerning child maltreatment. It can then be seen that a clear, generalizable conceptualization of abusive and neglectful parenting has been elusive, but it is very much the foundation for understanding how to prevent it.

Because of the complications in defining child maltreatment, the government has attempted to provide a framework to guide the professionals working with child maltreatment victims. Legislature's attempt to promote unification of what is considered negligent and harmful caregiving has been the Child Abuse and Prevention Treatment Act (CAPTA) of 1974 (PL 93-247). CAPTA has been updated on occasion until as recently as 2003, to set forth specific definitions that would foster identifying maltreatment and promote protection of children. At minimum, according to CAPTA,

Abuse and neglect is any recent act or failure to act on the part a parent or care-taker that results in death, serious physical or emotional harm, sexual abuse or exploitation; or an act or failure to act that presents an imminent risk of harm.

Sexual abuse is the employment, use, persuasion, inducement, enticement, or coercion of any child to engage in, or assist any other person to engage in, any sexually explicit conduct or simulation of such conduct for the purpose of pro-ducing a visual depiction of such conduct.

Although these minimal guidelines provide a base for discerning reportable parenting behaviors, each state is allowed to delineate their conceptualizations of legal maltreatment. Clearly these variations in reportable specifics can create prob-lems. Foremost, what can be considered child maltreatment in one state may not constitute child maltreatment in another regional area. For instance, Michigan and Indiana share a border, but different levels of evidence are required to substantiate a maltreatment occurrence (USDHHS, 2004). Because of discrepancies and sub-sequent difficulties in verifying maltreatment instances, substantiated cases may actually be largely underreported (Pelton, 1994).

Consequences of Child Maltreatment

All forms of maltreatment can lead to serious pathology in multiple domains of the child's life, including cognitive, adaptive, and behavioral development. Cognitive functioning (e.g., school-related outcomes, intelligence) is often signif-icantly impaired. Compared with children who are not maltreated, maltreated children perform lower on math and reading tests and are more likely to repeat a grade (Eckenrode, Laird, & Doris, 1993). Adaptive skills also are influenced; mal-treated children score significantly lower on indices of home, school, and peer adjustment than non-maltreated peers (Wodarski, Kurtz, Gaudin, & Howing, 1990). Victimized children have problems with socioemotional well-being as evi-denced by withdrawn behaviors, low self-esteem, and antisocial behaviors (Kaufman & Cicchetti, 1989; Lewis, 1992).

Research also has advanced understanding of the physical repercussions of maltreatment beyond the immediate broken bone or burn. Evidence suggests that maltreatment may impact a child's biological make-up through altering the lim-bic system, neural structure, and even the functioning of the developing brain itself (Teicher, 2002). The limbic system, which serves to regulate memory and emotion, shows overexcitation in children who are abused (Teicher). Structural changes in the brain have also been identified within a group of maltreated chil-dren that had been admitted to a hospital for psychiatric evaluation (Teicher et al., 2004). Teicher and colleagues examined magnetic resonance imaging scans of the victimized children and found that their total corpus callosum area was 17% smaller than in comparison children who had not been maltreated. This emerg-ing area of research alludes to a possible physiological mediator of child maltreatment's effects on later socioemotional well-being in addition to highlighting the strong direct effects of maltreatment on children's biological development.

Maltreatment also places individuals at an increased risk for serious and chronic illnesses throughout their life, including asthma, ischemic heart disease, and cancer (Kendall-Tackett & Edwards, 2004). The cost of maltreatment for the child is extensive and apparent, but additional effects are experienced by many others including siblings, the nonperpetrating parent, and society as a whole. For example, siblings who are not victimized must worry not only for their own safety, but also for the safety of their maltreated brother or sister. Teachers must deal with an unfocused child and classmates may experience compromised instruction.

The financial repercussions felt by society further underscore the far-reaching effects of maltreatment. In one year alone, it is estimated that $6 billion will be spent on hospitalizations for children who are victimized, and an additional $2 billion will be needed for the care of their chronic medical problems (Fromm, 2001). Judicial costs are estimated to be near $350 million, and juvenile delinquency incarcerations of children who are maltreated are expected to cost $9 billion (Fromm).

Causes and Correlates of Child Maltreatment

The consequences of maltreatment are long lasting and extensive; the importance of early intervention and, ideally, prevention, becomes obvious. To identify families at risk for child abuse or neglect, researchers have investigated potential factors thought to be related to maltreatment with a particular focus on the mother and the immediate environment of the family. Statistics show that the majority of perpetrators of child maltreatment are the immediate caregivers of the child. In fact, 80% of the perpetrators are parents of the victim (USDHHS, 2004). Of this percentage, nearly 50% involve mothers acting alone. Fathers acting alone account for only 19%, with both parents acting together accounting for an additional 18% of cases.

Among the most consistently cited sources of risk are parenting orientations (e.g., unrealistic expectations, rigidity toward children's behaviors) and age of parent. Parenting orientations, particularly a lack of knowledge about children's typical development and behaviors, have been consistently associated with child maltreatment (Twentyman & Plotkin, 1982). It has been suggested that when developmentally inappropriate behaviors are expected, the child's failure to meet such standards can result in parental frustration and subsequent child maltreatment. Furthermore, because young parents often hold unrealistic expectations for their children (Whitman, Borkowski, Keogh, & Weed, 2001), it is not surprising that teenage parents evidence higher rates of maltreatment than older parents (Bolton, 1990).

Risks are also found beyond the immediate characteristics of the parent and include low socioeconomic status, single parenthood, and a lack of social support. A family's meager financial resources may cultivate a neglectful environment for the child. For instance, Sedlak and Broadhurst (1996) reported that families with annual incomes of less than $15,000 were more likely to be identified as neglectful than families with annual incomes above $30,000. Family structure and functioning also have been linked to child maltreatment. Connell-Carrick's (2003) review associated single-parent homes with incidences of child neglect and proposed that father involvement in children's lives was a key process variable for child maltreatment. Beyond the influence of the father, other social supports may play a role in maltreatment occurrences (Belsky, 1993). For example, an overburdened mother with no friend to turn to may vent frustrations on her child.

PREVENTION PROGRAMS: DESIGN AND IMPLEMENTATION ISSUES

The aforementioned risks are often interrelated and difficult to disentangle. Understanding these risks, however, is fundamental in designing effective and efficient prevention programs for several reasons. First, risks serve as a guide for selection of participants. Each program utilizes these risks to form their eligibility requirements. Second, the curriculum for the programs is built around ameliorating these risks and providing supports for change. Third, the change in these risks over time often becomes the outcome criterion to which the program is evaluated in terms of success. For these reasons, a thorough understanding of sources of risk for child maltreatment is key to understanding prevention programming.

Programs for preventing child maltreatment must also take into account several additional essential dimensions, besides identifying those at risk for maltreatment, for optimal impact. Particularly important in the design and implementation of these programs are 1) the comprehensiveness of the program and its components, 2) location of service delivery, 3) timing and length of service delivery, and 4) delineating the outcome(s) to be evaluated and related—the evaluative standards used to measure the success of the program.

Programs must be comprehensive because the emergence of child maltreatment is multiply determined (Belsky, 1993). Targeting only discipline practices is likely too simple an approach; rather, additional domains of family functioning must also be addressed by the program's curriculum. Programs that have used a comprehensive approach to preventing maltreatment and that have included in their curriculum components to foster social supports, refer families to appropriate social services agencies, and strengthen the parent–child bond have shown successful outcomes (Olds, 1997).

Prevention programs must consider where to deliver their services, and utilizing the home environment is important for two reasons. First, young children are not yet in school and therefore spend the majority of their time in the home. In addition, practical utility makes the home an optimal place for visitation, particularly for high-risk participants who can be difficult to contact and who can have high attrition rates with research programs. Utilizing home visitation takes away the participants' responsibility to make appointments at a different location. Moreover, caseworkers spending time with families in their homes are able to make continuous observations about the home environment and its changes, as well as to subsequently tailor the program treatments and goals accordingly. For these reasons, it has been concluded that home visitation is an essential dimension of all successful child maltreatment prevention programs (Lutzker & Bigelow, 2002; U.S. Advisory Board on Child Abuse and Neglect, 1991).

Timing of services as well as their length of delivery also are important aspects of prevention programming. Beginning while the mother is pregnant is ideal. Initiating services before parenting patterns are well-established can lead to detection and subsequent alteration of potential problems before the official parenting process has begun. In addition, the majority of maltreatment fatality cases involve a child under the age of 4; it is clear that waiting too long is not only impractical but also irresponsible. Moreover, the program must continue for an extended period of time. Although short-term service delivery may be less costly and time-consuming, little support for success has been found for abbreviated programming. Rather, child maltreatment prevention programs should last years rather than a few weeks. In their meta-analytic review of 56 programs designed to prevent maltreatment, MacLeod and Nelson (2000) found the lowest effect sizes for home visitation programs that had 12 or fewer visits and that lasted less than 6 months.

Finally, it should be noted that the scientific rigor by which researchers design prevention programs can contribute to not only assessing the components' impact but also in furthering knowledge about what works best in the program, including types of staff employed, setting of services, and methods of service delivery. Control groups, different treatment levels, and randomization into groups are important aspects of a prevention program in order to empirically evaluate its components as well as its effects. Furthermore, determining at the outset which variables of interest will be indicators of the program's success is essential. Recidivism rates can be skewed as discussed earlier by inconsistent definitions of child maltreatment behaviors; for this reason, it is important to incorporate other measures of positive effects of the program, including the health and well-being of the child in addition to clear indicators of the parent–child relationship (e.g., attachment, child report measures of parenting).

PREVENTION PROGRAMS AND THEIR EVALUATIONS

Each of the aforementioned design and implementation issues plays a role in understanding the utility of current child maltreatment prevention programs. Although the goal of many programs is to prevent child maltreatment, three programs stand out because they consider many of the characteristics necessary for optimal success. This chapter evaluates and discusses three exemplar child maltreatment prevention programs: 1) Nurse Home Visitation Program (NHVP; Olds, Henderson, Chamberlin, & Tatelbaum, 1986), 2) Project SafeCare (PS; Lutzker, Bigelow, Doctor, & Kessler, 1998), and 3) Healthy Families America (HFA; Daro & Harding, 1999). A brief overview of each program's characteristics is provided in Table 4.1. The NHVP employs empirically rigorous methodology and a longitudinal assessment scheme; PS delivers a multicomponent curriculum and utilizes continuous assessments to adequately determine individual needs; and HFA provides a long-lasting, multidimensional, high-intensity program.

The Elmira Nurse Home Visitation Program

The Nurse Home Visitation Program (NHVP) was specifically designed to prevent child maltreatment through supporting families who are at risk. The NHVP started in 1977 in Elmira, New York, and set the example for creating a scientifically rigorous prevention program in both design and evaluation. Thoroughly grounded in well-supported theories, this program employed professional nurses as home visitors and attempted to improve 1) outcomes of pregnancy, 2) parental caregiving, and 3) mothers' life-course development (Olds, 1997). Multiple evaluations of the NHVP have shown significant long-lasting positive effects on both mothers and children that received the full services from the nurses.

The NHVP was an intensive program that delivered a variety of services to mothers beginning during the prenatal period and continuing through the children's second birthday. Mothers were recruited for the NHVP if the target child was the mother's first live birth and the mothers were 1) young in age (less than 19 years at registration time), 2) single parents, or 3) low in socioeconomic status (Olds, Henderson, Chamberlin, & Tatelbaum, 1986). Eligible mothers were randomly assigned into four groups—two treatment and two control groups—with all groups receiving developmental screening for their infants at 1 and 2 years of age (Olds, Henderson, Chamberlin, & Tatelbaum). Treatment group 1 (T1) re-

Table 4.1. Three child maltreatment prevention programs and their defining characteristics

	Nurse Home Visitation Program	Project SafeCare	Healthy Families America
Targets of intervention	Primiparious mothers and their children, as well as their family and friends (Families at high risk recruited but program open to all)	Mothers, fathers, and their children (Recruited from Child Protective Services for confirmed abuse or neglect or request involvement)	Mothers, fathers, and their children (Recruited from several agencies including prenatal clinics and Planned Parenthood, with a focus on families who are at high risk)
Content of intervention	Nurse home visitors provided: 1. Fetal and child development 2. Strengthening supports (family/friend) 3. Referrals to community supports	Multiple services delivered with a focus on: 1. Home safety 2. Health training 3. Parenting Role playing Video supplements	Home visitation and some parent groups (dependent on site) focus on three components: 1. Promoting positive parenting 2. Enhancing child development 3. Preventing child abuse and neglect
Outcomes of intervention	Extensive evaluations (prenatal and when children were 0–4 years, 15, 19, and soon to be 27 years) Low rate of maltreatment Treatment mothers had improved maternal life course outcomes (e.g., drank less, had fewer subsequent births) Children of mothers in full treatment group had better emotional and behavioral outcomes	Reduced recidivism rates Case studies revealed 1. Parents used more positive parenting behaviors (e.g., less scolding, more leveling) after treatment 2. Videotapes were useful in promoting positive parenting	Low rate of maltreatment Promoted family and child health Promoted positive parenting Promoted school readiness
Costs and duration	Lasts from mid-pregnancy (30th week) through children's 2nd year	24 weeks but varied (contingent on each family's needs)	Lasts from birth through child's 5th year Average cost per family is $2,764

ceived the screening, transportation, and prenatal home visits that were given once every 2 weeks. Treatment group 2 (T2) received the aforementioned services but visitation was extended to include postnatal visits lasting until the child was 2 years of age. Control group 1 (C1) was provided only with the screening, whereas Control group 2 (C2) also was provided with transportation to the screenings.

Trained nurses delivered multiple components to the participants in their homes, with each visit involving three major activities: 1) educating the parent regarding fetal and child development, 2) involving friends and extended family to support the mother and her child, and 3) connecting the mother to appropriate service supports with an emphasis on strengthening families' relationships to medical resources (Olds, Henderson, Chamberlin, & Tatelbaum, 1986). A curriculum was used to guide the activities; however, the nurses were able to tailor the content of the visits to meet the individual needs of each family (Olds, Henderson, Chamberlin, & Tatelbaum).

The number of visits varied depending on the age of the child. During pregnancy, visits were scheduled once every other week. For the period of the first 6 weeks postpartum, the visits increased to once every week and gradually were diminished until the children reached the age of 2. Nurse visitors averaged nine completed visits for mothers receiving visits during their pregnancy and 23 visits from the time of birth until the child was 2 years of age.

Program Evaluation   Although the NHVP lasted only 2 years, both mother and child effects were found during the prevention program as well as several years later. Assessments were conducted continuously from the prenatal period until the children were 4 years of age, then again when the children were 15 and 19 years old. Multiple forms of information were gathered from different sources including medical records, interviews, and assessments of the mother–child dyads, as well as records of substantiated child abuse and neglect creating a multimodal understanding of effects. Because multiple evaluations were conducted, only key findings highlighting the program's effects on maternal life course, parenting, maltreatment instances, and children's adolescent development will be discussed. It should be noted that due to nonsignificant differences in evaluations after pregnancy and birth, C1 and C2 were collapsed into one comparison group (Olds, Henderson, Chamberlin, & Tatelbaum, 1986). T1 findings also were of nonstatistical significance and, subsequently, T1 was not utilized in several analyses unless specifically specified (Olds, Henderson, Chamberlin, & Tatelbaum).

During pregnancy, women who were visited by a nurse (T1 and T2) improved the quality of their diets and by the end of pregnancy, had better health outcomes, experienced greater informal social support, and made better use of formal community services (all $p < .05$) than comparison mothers (Olds, Henderson, Tatelbaum, & Chamberlin, 1986). By the end of pregnancy, among women who smoked, nurse-visited mothers had 25% fewer cigarettes and 75% fewer preterm deliveries than their counterparts in the comparison group (Olds, Henderson, Chamberlin, & Tatelbaum, 1986). Among the 14–16-year-old mothers, those visited by nurses had infants who were 395g heavier than their counterparts in the control group (Olds, Henderson, Tatelbaum, & Chamberlin, 1986).

Parenting behaviors between the comparison group and the full treatment groups were also significantly different (Olds, Henderson, Chamberlin, & Tatelbaum, 1986). High-risk mothers (i.e., poor, unmarried teenagers) who were visited by a nurse were more positive in their interactions with their children at both 10 and 22 months in comparison with control mothers. The high-risk treatment mothers also provided more appropriate play materials than their control counterparts.

Of central importance, the program served to reduce the number of substantiated child maltreatment instances among families at highest risk (Olds, Henderson, Chamberlin, & Tatelbaum, 1986). Among the high-risk mothers in the comparison group, 19% had abused or neglected their children in the first 2 years of life. In comparison, only 4% of high-risk mothers who had nurse-visits maltreated their children during this time.

In a 15-year follow-up study, for children who were maltreated and came from full-treatment families, the program served to buffer the developmental effects typically associated with child abuse and neglect. Eckenrode and colleagues (2001) examined the relationship between child maltreatment and the early onset of behavioral problems. Early onset of behavior problems was determined by children's early initiation of problematic behaviors including use of cigarettes (at or before 12 years), drugs or excessive alcohol (at or before 15 years), sex (at or before 13 years), and involvement with the law (at or before 15 years). For participants who were in the full-treatment condition, a moderational effect of the prevention program was found such that for the children of these mothers, maltreatment did not have a significant relationship with the onset of problematic behaviors. The researchers attributed this finding to the program reducing maltreatment occurrences in addition to delaying the timing of incidences (Eckenrode et al., 2001).

Positive program effects also were found 15 years later for mothers who were single and had a low socioeconomic status at the time of the initial visit. The high-risk mothers in the full treatment group had a lower number of subsequent pregnancies, received Aid to Families with Dependent Children (AFDC) benefits for fewer months, and used alcohol and drugs less frequently than their counterparts in the control groups (Olds et al., 1997). Their adolescent children also showed program benefits evidenced by fewer instances of running away, fewer arrests, and fewer convictions and violations of probation than their counterparts in the comparison groups (Olds et al., 1998). Moreover, these adolescents had fewer sexual partners and smoked and drank less frequently than their counterparts in the comparison group (Olds et al., 1998).

Replications of the NHVP have been conducted in both Memphis, Tennessee, and Denver, Colorado, with both of these programs employing a more diverse sample of mothers to remedy the lack of cultural variability in the original program. Positive outcomes have been found at these sites, with mothers who were visited by a nurse having fewer subsequent pregnancies, longer birth intervals, and fewer months of using food stamps in contrast to comparison mothers (Olds et al., 2004). The children in the treatment group also showed benefits, with higher intellectual functioning and fewer behavior problems than their counterparts in the control group (Olds et al.).

Although the NHVP was one of the first longitudinal prevention studies directed at ameliorating child maltreatment and its repercussions, strong evaluative evidence suggests that it accomplished its goal, particularly among mothers at highest risk. This already well-evaluated prevention program is still assessing the impact it had on children's functioning even as they become adults—outcome data will be measured again when the children turn 27 (J. Eckenrode, personal communication, January 11, 2005).

Critical Analysis of Treatment Characteristics   The NHVP incorporated several essential treatment characteristics into its programming including a theoretical grounding and building of positive relationships. The design and composition of the NHVP were well-conceived with ecological, self-efficacy, and attachment theories serving as guiding frameworks (Olds, 1997). The overall program foundation rests on the tenets of ecological theory, stressing the importance of understanding the dynamic relationship between the parent–child dyad and further placing this relationship into perspective among the broader social context, such as friends and community agencies (Bronfenbrenner, 1979). In addition, this theory emphasizes the concept of process including program processes, parental processes, and parental interaction processes (Olds).

Self-efficacy and attachment theories also guided the design. Self-efficacy theory played a role through the project's emphasis on aiding the participants to set minimal, achievable goals that would support their confidence for the possibility of change (Olds, 1997). For example, a mother's goal could be to contact a vocational training agency as one step of several to eventually procure a job. Attachment theory was evident in the design of the home visits. Three components of the visits addressed attachment issues: 1) visitors developing a positive relationship with the mother and her family social supports, 2) mothers and caregivers reviewing their past childhood histories, and 3) program components emphasizing positive caregiving (sensitive and responsive) in early child development (Olds). Clearly, the program rested on well-evaluated theories.

The building of positive relationships was another strong treatment characteristic of the NHVP. Because of the emphasis on attachment theory, positive relationships were cultivated not only with the mother and her child, but also with the home visitor and the mother, as well as the mother, child, and extended family. The nurses fostered positive relationships to serve as sources for continued program success, particularly by encouraging members of the family to participate in the visits, thus creating additional supports to ensure the maintenance of treatment effects.

Critical Analysis of Procedural Characteristics   The NHVP was appropriately timed and employed a well-trained staff. Because of the qualifications necessary for the home visitors, a high level of key training in nutritional, physical, and safety needs of children was already ensured. Nurses also received 3 months of training regarding the program's protocol. With program implementation during the prenatal period, the well-trained home visitors could target potential difficulties (e.g., a lack of knowledge about appropriate child development) before the official parenting process had begun. As discussed earlier, by altering potential parenting problems before they become habitual practices, changes may be made more easily. Thus, implementation of programming during this period had been recommended for the most promising results (Daro, 1996).

Because children under 4 are the most vulnerable to maltreatment's physical repercussions, the NHVP's program falls short in program duration and sufficient dosage domains. Effects were apparent in multiple domains over time for mothers and children; however, lengthening service delivery or utilizing booster sessions may have further contributed to program impact. Limited duration may be one reason that 4% of families in the full treatment group still had documented cases of child maltreatment (Olds, Henderson, Chamberlin, & Tatelbaum, 1986).

Critical Analysis of Design Characteristics   The NHVP, in comparison to other programs, is clearly among the best in methodology and design characteristics. Randomization of participants was carried out in a complex manner to ensure adequate sample size and subsequent statistical power needed to detect treatment effects. Participants were randomly assigned to one of the four treatment groups already discussed through a process that began with participant stratification by marital status, race, and seven geographic regions within the county (Olds, Henderson, Chamberlin, & Tatelbaum, 1986). Decks of cards were used to assign mothers, and the deck was reconstituted periodically to over-represent the groups with smaller numbers of participants (Olds, Henderson,

Chamberlin, & Tatelbaum). This random assignment to groups is a rare but important component of child maltreatment prevention programming.

Furthermore, the multiple follow-up assessments of both mother and child outcomes were essential design components that strengthened the conclusions about the success of the program. The follow-up studies were able to reveal additional information regarding the program's impact on mothers' life course and multiple domains of children's development. By not simply utilizing substantiated child maltreatment instances as the criterion for success, a much broader picture of the program impact was gained. In addition, the social significance of reduced maltreatment instances coupled with maternal and child gains several years after the program services ended is apparent.

Project SafeCare

Project SafeCare (PS) was a theoretically driven ecobehavioral approach to both prevent child maltreatment and reduce and ameliorate its occurrence where it had already appeared (Lutzker et al., 1998). PS was based on the earlier program Project 12-Ways. This program consisted of 12 components that included parent–child training, stress reduction, self-control training for parents, basic skills training for children, activity planning, relationship counseling, alcoholism referral, job finding, money management, health and safety training, multiple-setting behavior management, and prevention (Lutzker, 1984). Although the program was comprehensive, it was not as effective as the researchers had planned. Therefore, the creators sought to create a streamlined, efficient systematic replication of Project 12-Ways that would be applicable for multiple populations. Initially carried out in urban Southern California with a large proportion of Latinos and Latinas from Mexico, PS consisted of only three of its predecessors' 12 components and was an in-home program.

Participants for PS consisted of two different types of families. The first group was referred by the child protective services for child abuse and/or neglect. The second group was referred by a social worker at the hospital for meeting certain risk requirements—for example, being young, single, or low in socioeconomic status (Lutzker & Bigelow, 2002).

Most of the home visitors (family counselors) for PS were graduate students at the doctoral level, although some possessed a master's degree. All counselors were required to have experience working with at-risk families. In addition, individuals involved in any aspect of the project (e.g., counselor, management) received extensive training.

Counselors delivered the following three components to families in their homes: bonding, safety, and health. The parenting component, also termed PAT

(Planned Activities Training), was designed to increase positive interactions between the parent and child with the goal of increasing bonding between the two (Lutzker et al., 1998). PAT encouraged parents to employ positive interaction skills and use everyday moments for teaching (incidental teaching). An additional focus was to help parents learn to prevent discipline situations from arising through positive and proactive parenting. Parents also were given cards that depicted an activity appropriate for practicing the targeted parenting skills.

The home safety training component was designed to reduce the risk of children's accidental death or injury due to unsafe home environments (Lutzker et al., 1998). This component addressed hazards that may have been present in the home and attempted to identify and remove potential problems for the children. For example, parents were asked where they kept household cleaners, and if they reported an unsafe location, steps were taken to ensure the children's safety (Lutzker & Bigelow, 2002). Parents also were given safety equipment including outlet plug covers and drawer latches (Lutzker et al.).

The health component was created with the goal of teaching parents to identify symptoms of common childhood illnesses and provide appropriate care to their children (Lutzker et al., 1998). Parents were given two texts: a health manual containing information on a variety of health topics (e.g., prevention of illnesses, home treatments) and the A–Z Symptom and Illness Guide. Families were also given basic health supplies including a thermometer, a medicine dropper, and antibiotic ointment (Lutzker & Bigelow, 2002).

A protocol was utilized for the order of components as well as the administration of the curriculum; however, variations were allowed. The entire training was designed for administration over a period of approximately 24 weeks, but actual length of the program involvement varied for each family depending on the progress observed (Lutzker & Bigelow, 2002). The three components were generally administered in the following order: health training, home safety (and cleanliness), and parenting, with the goal of every family completing each of these components in four or five sessions per component (Lutzker & Bigelow). Individual tailoring for each family was allowed so that families with few safety concerns or with more knowledge about health issues were allowed to spend less time on a particular component. At the close of each session, parents were encouraged to give feedback on whether they felt that they had successfully completed the activities of the session and their feelings about the family counselor.

Each session followed seven steps: 1) Describe target behavior or skills, 2) Explain rationale for behavior, 3) Model behavior, 4) Ask parent to practice behavior; observe with checklist, 5) Provide positive feedback, 6) Provide constructive feedback, and 7) Review parent's performance and set goals for upcoming week (Lutzker & Bigelow, 2002).

These steps could vary slightly according to the component being administered but generally adhered to the full seven procedures.

Program Evaluation   Although not as rigorously tested as the NHVP, PS has been evaluated several times. Investigations into the program's effects, components, and procedures have been conducted with evidence generally supporting positive results.

Recidivism data were evaluated to assess the program's success in stopping maltreatment. Survival analyses revealed a large discrepancy between PS participants and a similar comparison group. Two years after program completion, 85% of the PS families had survived without an additional report to the child protective agency, whereas in the comparison group, only 54% of families were without a report (Gershater-Molko, Lutzker, & Wesch, 2002).

Several case studies were conducted with findings suggesting positive program effects. For instance, a two-family case study was carried out to assess a video teaching method and its utility in promoting positive parenting. Parenting behaviors, including leveling, touching, verbalizing, and instructing, were assessed before the viewing and then compared with measures obtained after the video (Bigelow & Lutzker, 1998). Five video segments were watched in the participants' homes and described the targeted parenting skills and modeled appropriate activities and interactions. In comparison to the baseline scores, the scores after viewing the video were higher for positive touching and verbalizations. Moreover, in follow-up information, the two families had no additional reports to the child protective agency 1½ years later (Bigelow & Lutzker, 1998).

Evaluations by the participating families and service agencies also were conducted to assess service quality. Surveys were left with the family or agency to fill out after a visit and addressed several issues including the appropriateness of the set goals, the practicality of the intervention delivered, and the professionalism shown by the counselor (O'Brien, Lutzker, & Campbell, 1993). Overall, the feedback received suggested that the services of PS were satisfactory with only one exception: staff knowledge about legal issues pertinent to the consumers (O'Brien et al., 1993). This feedback was utilized to remedy the problem, and training was provided to improve the deficit. Additional investigations found further support for the methods employed, materials used, and measurement validity (cf. Lutzker & Bigelow, 2002).

The findings, however, must be considered with caution. Although 206 families consented to be in the project, only 41 families completed all three training components. Due to the 90% attrition rate, the statistical validity of the findings warrants concern.

Critical Analysis of Treatment Characteristics   PS met many critical treatment characteristics, including being theory driven, varying teaching methods, and having sociocultural relevance. Grounded in a socioecological framework, the program utilized multidimensional components to target parenting and create a safe environment for the child (Lutzker et al., 1998). These components were delivered through varied and creative teaching methods utilizing scenarios and role playing so that the families could have a chance to apply their newfound knowledge. These characteristics of the program created a multimodal method of delivering services to the families. By employing such methods, learning and retention of the key information is likely to be significantly improved.

This project also demonstrated sociocultural relevance through its tailoring of services to meet the needs of many Spanish-speaking participants. Program components and curriculum were in both English and Spanish, and the study employed fluent Spanish-speaking caseworkers to ensure that the participants felt comfortable (Lutzker & Bigelow, 2002). Of great importance in all prevention studies is their likely generalizability to other populations. This program demonstrated that components resting on ecology theory were in fact influential in altering repeat child maltreatment cases in a largely Hispanic population.

An additional positive treatment characteristic demonstrated by PS was the building of positive relationships. In fact, strengthening relationships was a core dimension of PS and was emphasized by the home visitor showing great sensitivity to each family's individual needs (Lutzker & Bigelow, 2002). Telephone calls were made to the participants before the visit to ensure an appropriate time to visit the family. In addition, each visit started with a warm-up time in which greetings were to be exchanged. These strategies fostered rapport and trust between the home visitor and the family.

Critical Analysis of Procedural Characteristics   Overall, PS demonstrated several key procedural characteristics: A well-trained staff and treatment fidelity are among the most salient. All of those involved with administering each of the components of PS had a thorough background in working with at-risk families. Staff training was conducted through the employment of several modalities, including role playing, simulations, direct observation, and videotapes (Lutzker & Bigelow, 2002). Training checks also were administered to measure trainees' skills and abilities to administer the protocol; quizzes and a training checklist were filled out by a supervisor to assess where each potential family worker was in terms of skill development (Lutzker & Bigelow). This well-articulated training plan ensures a staff capable of providing program protocol in the manner it was intended to be delivered.

With regard to timing and dosage levels, PS was not sufficient. Created as a secondary prevention program to aid families already reported for maltreatment, the program must not only support and teach the curriculum but also defeat problematic parenting patterns that have already been well established. However,

PS's biggest problem is the dosage level of the program. Designed to last 6 months or less, depending on the individual family's needs, PS programming falls short of a long-lasting intervention and lacks the time necessary to ensure that sufficient dosage levels of the curriculum have been delivered. In fact, according to MacLeod and Nelson's (2000) review, because of the short duration, program effect sizes are likely to be quite low.

Critical Analysis of Design Characteristics   PS evaluated its service delivery methods as well as several outcomes. The program's multidimensional delivery of services (e.g., instruction, role playing, video instruction) allowed for individual components to be assessed in terms of their utility. It was discovered that the innovative approach of using video technology proved useful with participants and promoted positive parenting (Bigelow & Lutzker, 1998). In addition, the outcome evaluations of recidivism data and parenting have shown the program to be internally valid.

However, several key design limitations deserve attention. PS lacks a longitudinal assessment scheme with well-defined outcomes, which include multiple indicators of family and child functioning. Although case studies provide valuable clinical information, the generalizability of the findings is questionable. Following up with families over an extended period of time to examine maternal life course and children's emotional and behavioral well-being would have contributed to understanding the program's full utility in helping at-risk families.

Healthy Families America

Healthy Families America (HFA) is a 5-year, multicomponent, home visitation-centered program. HFA is loosely based on the Healthy Start Program (HSP) that has been implemented across the state of Hawaii for more than 3 decades. HSP is a long-lasting, comprehensive program that utilizes community supports to strengthen the families it serves. Beginning at birth and lasting through the child's fifth birthday, this home visiting program aims to prevent child maltreatment, support child development, and promote positive parent–child relationships (Duggan et al., 1999). HSP screens mothers at the hospital to assess potential sources of risk for the family, including single parenthood, substance abuse, and social isolation. The HFA program developers incorporated many of the elements of the HSP program, including a similar risk assessment scheme and providing services for 5 years, but did not create an exact replication.

In 1992, HFA was begun in the mainland United States and now has sites in more than 450 communities in the United States and Canada (Prevent Child Abuse America, 2002b). Prevent Child Abuse America is HFA's national headquarters and assumes responsibility for ensuring that sites adhere to the core tenets of the program. The program has three goals: 1) promote positive parenting, 2) enhance child development and health, and 3) prevent child abuse and neglect (Prevent Child Abuse America).

The program begins with a systematic assessment of all families in an intended population within a community; this is an important dimension of HFA. More universal in its approach than other programs, 90% of all HFA programs reach out to either all new parents or all first-time parents within a particular community. Families at greater risk of potential parenting difficulties are encouraged to participate in the home visiting that begins with weekly visits that are reduced over time as the families meet goals with success (Prevent Child Abuse America, 2001a).

Using a strength-based model versus a medical model, family support workers (FSWs) help parents to maximize their current strengths and minimize stressors. The FSWs attempt to educate parents about children's abilities at different ages as well as how to use discipline in a positive manner. In addition, the program serves to create a community support system by linking the families with pertinent agencies and providing support for other needs including referrals for employment and housing and aiding in their decisions to seek counseling for substance abuse or family violence (Prevent Child Abuse America, 2001a).

Twelve critical elements clustered around the topics of service initiation, service content, and staff characteristics provide guidance for each HFA program but allow for flexibility depending on the community's needs:

1. Initiate service delivery prenatally or at birth
2. Utilize a standardized assessment tool to systematically identify families most in need of services
3. Offer services voluntarily and foster family trust
4. Offer services intensively with well-defined criteria for adjusting services over time
5. Ensure that services are culturally competent, and that staff understand, acknowledge, and respect cultural differences among participants—program materials should reflect the diversity of the population served
6. Focus services on supporting the parents, the parent–child interaction, and child development
7. Link families to appropriate services with an emphasis on supporting families' utilization of medical resources
8. Limit staff caseloads
9. Involve personal characteristics in the selection of FSWs
10. Ensure that FSWs have training and experience in handling typical at-risk families
11. Ensure that service providers receive training specific to their role

12. Ensure that service providers receive ongoing supervision to guarantee that they are effective with their families (Prevent Child Abuse America, 2001a)

HFA protocol requires adherence to the onset of program initiation as well as an ability to screen for participants. According to these requirements, services must begin prenatally or, at the latest, at the time of the child's birth. Moreover, screening for participants must be done by employing a standardized assessment tool to assess each family's potential risks. Screening is carried out at multiple sites including Planned Parenthood, prenatal clinics, and hospitals by reviewing maternal medical records or interviewing the family to assess risk for maltreatment in 10 domains—for example, an individual's past child maltreatment experiences, social isolation, single parenthood, and expectations about a child's development and behaviors. The Kempe Family Stress Checklist is used to screen participants for risk, with families scoring at or above 25 usually offered services. Standardized scoring is employed; however, each site is allowed to place the bar higher depending on their budget and the individual needs of the population their program targets. However, services are usually instantly offered if a family has any of these specific risks: a single parent, a mom who had no prenatal care or delayed care, or a mom who wanted an abortion but didn't follow through (C. Wessel, personal communication, August 10, 2005). Utilization of the standardized screening process allows for systematic identification and keeps consistency in defining *at risk* across sites (Prevent Child Abuse America, 2001a).

Once potential participants have been deemed eligible, services should be discussed in a positive manner, with emphasis placed on voluntary participation (Prevent Child Abuse America, 2001a). By offering the program as an option rather than compulsory, services can seem like a positive choice. In addition, promoting the program in this positive manner allows trust to begin to be forged between the family and the program. For those who choose to enter the program, HFA protocol requires services to be offered intensively, at least once a week, with well-defined criteria for adjusting these visits over time (Prevent Child Abuse America, 2001a).

HFA's respect for culture within their foundational elements is especially noteworthy. This critical tenet holds all staff responsible for being understanding of and respecting cultural differences among participants. Moreover, the materials employed in each individual program site should reflect the multidimensional nature of culture, including accounting for the linguistic, racial, and geographical variations of the people served (Prevent Child Abuse America, 2001a).

Service delivery requirements must be met (Prevent Child Abuse America, 2001a). For instance, services must be comprehensive, rather than simply focusing on the parents. The parent–child relationship and the child's well-being also must be targeted. Social services agencies must be utilized; at minimum, families should be put in touch with a medical provider with additional resources employed for families with other needs. In addition, the home visitors must have limited caseloads to ensure adequate capabilities to meet each family's individual needs and to allow adjustments in intensity level to be met.

The critical elements also address the characteristics necessary to be a caseworker. According to HFA protocol, home visitors should be selected for their personal characteristics (rather than strictly educational experience), which show the skills necessary to do the job; the home visitor should be an empathetic, nonjudgmental source of support for the family. Also important, providers should have a framework, based on education, or experience in handling the variety of situations they may encounter when working with at-risk families. For this reason, service providers receive extensive training. Specifically, service providers receive training specific to the essential components of family assessment (for Family Assessment Workers) or home visitation for FSWs that ensures consistency in program delivery (Prevent Child Abuse America, 2001a). HFA requires 1 week of preservice training and 1 day of continuing training quarterly (C. Wessel, personal communication, August 10, 2005). Moreover, an additional 80 hours of training during the first 6 months of service is recommended by Prevent Child Abuse America (2001b). Supervision is provided in an ongoing manner to aid caseworkers in establishing realistic and effective plans that strengthen the family's functioning.

Program Evaluation   Multiple evaluations have been conducted on many of the individual sites of HFA programs. These findings suggest that HFA promotes positive effects for the families in a variety of domains. The results from the states' year-end reports are too numerous to be detailed here (cf. Daro & Harding, 1999); however, an overview of key findings regarding program effects on participants' health, parenting, and child maltreatment instances will be highlighted.

Notably, HFA promotes family health. For instance, in Arizona, parent and child health effects were apparent across 23 sites that serve a culturally diverse sample of mothers—Hispanic, Caucasian, Native American, African American, Asian American. Among parents who have been in the program longer than 18 months, 80% reported that they had a primary care physician (LeCroy & Milligan Associates, Inc., 2004). In addition, although the immunization rate for 2-year-olds in Arizona is 77%, HFA families had 94% of their toddlers fully immunized. In Virginia, HFA families again exceeded state percentages with 82% of HFA children receiving the full amount of vaccinations, whereas the statewide percentage was 74.6% (Galano & Huntington, 2004).

The HFA program also was found to foster positive parenting. According to the Arizona report, participating families had a reduction in parenting stress. On six of the subscales of the Parenting Stress Index, scores improved such that from the baseline to 6-month assessment, increased competence and attachments and decreased feelings of depression, isolation, negative mood, and feelings of restricted role as a parent were noted (all $p < .05$; LeCroy & Milligan Associates, Inc., 2004). The 12-month assessment echoed this finding again with each of the subscales maintaining a significantly improved score from the baseline assessment.

Most important, HFA families had low numbers of substantiated maltreatment instances. In Virginia, the rate of substantiated cases of child maltreatment was 1.1% for 2,272 families (Galano & Huntington, 2004). Other state findings place the range of substantiated instances of maltreatment among HFA families from less than 2% to 12% (Jacobs, Easterbrooks, Brady, & Mistry, 2005; LeCroy & Milligan Associates, Inc., 2004).

Critical Analysis of Treatment Characteristics   The HFA program rests on strong treatment characteristics. At the heart of HFA is its focus on building positive relationships between the home visitor and the family, the family and support agencies, and the individual family members, with an emphasis on the relationship between the parent and child. To foster these relationships, home visitors employ an empathetic, nonjudgmental listening style and help families address crises and strengthen positive supports.

The HFA program also is among the most comprehensive in child maltreatment prevention programming. In its attempt to promote family well-being, the HFA program targets multiple sources of potential risk, including parental mental health, home safety, and child developmental issues. Because the FSW is deeply involved with individual families, appropriate referrals can be made to address the needs as the FSW becomes aware of problematic areas.

Sociocultural relevance is exemplified by the HFA program with cultural sensitivity as one of the program's 12 critical elements (Daro & Harding, 1999). According to HFA protocol, culture must be respected and taken into account in all interactions between the FSW and the families. In addition, materials utilized for the program must account for cultural differences (Daro & Harding, 1999). Clearly, HFA's sensitivity to culture is of key import in dealing with populations at risk that are comprised of all ethnicities and the multiple program sites across the nation.

Critical Analysis of Procedural Characteristics   HFA is particularly strong in procedural characteristics with notable dosage, timing, training, and treatment fidelity criteria. Clear guidelines are in place for consistency across sites in training, dosage administration, and treatment fidelity. Training updates, 1-day quarterly training, and an additional 80 hours of training during the first 6 months of service experience support program delivery that adheres to the HFA curriculum (Prevent Child Abuse America, 2001b). Home visitors are regularly supervised by professionals with advanced training and experience who are employed by HFA. In addition, HFA managers and supervisors from each site meet regularly with personnel from other sites to coordinate and compare program developments. The fidelity checks foster an optimal, consistent delivery of services.

The continuation of services for families through the children's fifth year is a strength of HFA programming that puts it head and shoulders above other programs in terms of duration. By supporting parents through their children's critical developmental years, optimal outcomes can be fostered at a time when the children are most vulnerable. HFA places great emphasis on being sensitive to each family's individual needs, and tailoring the visits accordingly serves to foster family retention over time.

Critical Analysis of Design Characteristics   The HFA program meets many of the essential design characteristics, including outcome evaluation, internal validation, and social significance. Each site is free to set their own goals and evaluate them accordingly, with many reports supporting a wide-range of positive program effects and the internal validity of the overall HFA curriculum. Because of its multiple sites and universal delivery approach, the social significance of the HFA program is substantial.

Particularly important for HFA as it continues to grow across the nation, however, will be incorporating systematic evaluations of its components and effects into the design scheme. Many individual sites have conducted year-end reviews of their projects with similar outcomes; however, implementing a nationwide outcome criterion may serve to make programs targeting different populations that are at risk in various geographical locations more comparable in terms of determining levels of success. Although several HFA implementations are beginning to use randomization and incorporate a more rigorous methodology in designing their programs, consistent use of active control groups could strengthen the empirical support for the utility of HFA. Because each of the sites is able to utilize a curriculum of their choosing (as long as it adheres to HFA goals) and is able to define their target population, considerable variations exist. Using control groups within these sites could provide valuable information about which curriculum works best for which at-risk population.

MODEL PROGRAM FOR THE PREVENTION OF CHILD MALTREATMENT

Programs such as the NHVP, PS, and HFA have shown impressive results and provided solid footing for building future prevention programs. A model child maltreatment prevention program would incorporate exemplary characteristics from each of these programs and add innovative components that recent investigations have shown lend themselves to positive results. A complete description of the model program components can be found in Table 4.2, including specifics about the targeted participants, content of the intervention, evaluative outcomes, and duration of services.

A model program must begin prenatally, providing at-risk families with a solid foundation on which to build relationships, ameliorate risks, and strengthen parenting skills before parenting behaviors become established. In addition, delivering services through the first 5 years of the children's lives will ensure optimal support during critical years of development. Through employing home visitors that are well-trained and sensitive to individual needs, family retention will be fostered for the duration of the program.

The model program design should include multiple treatment levels, random assignment of subjects to groups, a core curriculum that is multifaceted in remedying risks, and a longitudinal assessment scheme. Within this design, home

Table 4.2. Components of a model child maltreatment prevention program

Targets of intervention	Families who are at risk (child in utero)
	Extended family and friends who are present in child's life
Content of intervention	Parenting skill building
	Education about children's development
	Multimodal teaching techniques (e.g., face-to-face visits, telephone calls, videotapes)
	High-quality child care
	Community agency collaborations
	Individualization of services
Targeted outcomes of intervention	Prevent child maltreatment
	Increase positive parenting interactions
	Reduce problematic parenting behaviors (e.g., punitive language directed toward child, physical punishment)
	Support parental well-being and life course development (e.g., career and education referrals, counseling for depression)
	Improve family relations
	Foster a positive growing environment for the child
	Promote optimal child development
Duration	Prenatal through 5 years with intensive service delivery through the first 4 years, slowly decreasing in intensity until the 5th year; booster sessions begin at age 8 and continue every 2 years subsequently

visitors would be able to tailor the dosage to the specific needs of the individual family. The longitudinal scheme would allow for multiple evaluations to determine program impact over time.

Because of the prominent role that many outside agencies play for at-risk families, their inclusion in the model program is vital for success. The services fulfill many needs (e.g., low-cost housing, WIC food supplements, reduced-fee clinics) and are essential referrals for the majority of at-risk families that child maltreatment prevention programs target. Agencies can serve as valuable resources for prevention efforts, both as sources for referral and for providing individualized knowledge. For example, having a contact with a child welfare agency aids in understanding which specific parenting behaviors are necessary to report. By taking advantage of resources in the community, free expertise and services can be used to foster the overall goals of the prevention program and maximize cost efficiency. For these reasons, the model program will build interagency collaborations within the community.

Drawing from other prevention areas, two important dimensions seem particularly important for a model child maltreatment prevention program, but were lacking in each of the exemplar reviewed programs: a child care component and booster sessions. Although many programs to prevent developmental delays have used first-rate child care settings to supplement their interventions (e.g., the Abecedarian Project), this potentially enriched environment has yet to be fully employed in child maltreatment prevention programs. Yet, child care providers can offer additional supports including monitoring children's development and giving attention to their unmet needs (Thompson, 1995). The child care staff also can support parents through providing parenting groups, fielding child-related questions, and giving overburdened parents a chance to fulfill educational and occupational needs with worry-free care for their children (Thompson). In addition, provision of booster sessions to foster maintenance of program effects has yet to be utilized but seems particularly applicable to child maltreatment prevention. Middle childhood and teenage years pose important challenges for all parents, including dealing with increased autonomy and peer issues, and providing occasional supports could foster continued positive parenting and parent–child relations.

In short, the model program must 1) begin prenatally and continue for 5 years, 2) use a comprehensive curriculum that targets multiple risks, 3) be scientifically rigorous, 4) ensure that staff is well-trained in curriculum and sensitive to the individual needs of at-risk families, 5) specify at the outset clear evaluative standards that assess multiple domains of child and family functioning, and 6) foster interagency bridges.

A case study of Debra Smith and her family is provided below to illustrate the model program and its specific components.

❖

A Child Maltreatment Prevention Program
for Debra Smith and Her New Baby

Debra Smith felt that she was finally getting her life back on track. After several difficult months of divorce proceedings and telephone calls from school about her teenage daughter Keisha, Debra felt confident that things were turning around. Keisha's father was no longer involved in their lives, and Debra believed that her exhaustion and worry would finally abate. It was after dinner that she got a telephone call that changed everything: The test results from her annual check-up were in and she was pregnant! She had thought that stress was causing her physical symptoms.

Debra felt as though her world had been turned upside down. She worried about one more mouth to feed and child care costs. How was she going to handle this new life by herself? After several days of thinking things through, Debra decided to keep the baby. At one of her prenatal doctor visits, a nurse talked to Debra about a program that offered help to mothers like her (single and having a hard time making ends meet). It sounded interesting to Debra and she decided to call the number the nurse gave her for more information.

It was near her last trimester of pregnancy that Debra met Kristin, a social worker who had been extensively trained in all components of the program. Despite Debra's initial uncertainty about starting something new, she enjoyed Kristin's company. During their weekly visits, Debra learned about child behaviors and developmental milestones. She was given a chance to voice her concerns and add her thoughts about each of the topics. The two women talked about everything from home safety to Debra's financial worries. Kristin taught Debra techniques for handling stress and referred her to an employment agency that found her the perfect job.

Debra went into labor just 2 weeks after starting her new job at the local library. She was glad that she had worked out her maternity leave with her employer as soon as she was hired and that Kristin had provided information about the program's child care facility. All she needed to do for the next few weeks was spend uninterrupted time with her new baby boy, whom she named Jackson, and "bond" with him, as Kristin liked to put it.

Although Debra was anxious about leaving Jackson at the program's child care center while she went to work, she felt better after visiting the center, where she was able to watch the teachers and witness their apparent love for teaching and for the children. Even though she knew that the teachers had rigorous training on child development and management issues in addition to having a degree in child education, Debra was surprised at the genuine care they showed for each child. While on maternity leave, Debra began to believe that her family would succeed. She even looked forward to going back to work despite the added stress she knew that would bring (e.g., having to rush and drop off Keisha at school and Jackson at child care). But the techniques she learned from Kristin about how to deal with stress, as well as her continual conversations with Kristin, helped her remain optimistic about the future.

As Jackson continued to grow, Debra continued to appreciate Kristin's support. She couldn't believe the interesting things they did during their visits. One week, Kristin brought music over and practiced *dancing* with Jackson. As Keisha, Debra, and Kristin laughed at their little dance party, Jackson was soothed to sleep with his mom's rocking motions. Now Debra or Keisha *dance* Jackson to sleep almost every night. Although initially Keisha thought the visits her mom received would be boring, watching the things that her mom and Kristin did began to interest her. The dancing thing was really fun! During one visit, Keisha got involved in the meeting and talked about her thoughts on being Jackson's big sister and her worries about not having a dad around all the time. She also got to watch a videotape on how to teach her infant brother new things. Every day after school Keisha held Jackson and put toys just a little out of his reach. Keisha cheered the day Jackson was finally able to pull his bear close to his body!

At Jackson's child care facility, Debra had become a regular at the monthly parenting group. She enjoyed talking with the parents of other children who were dealing with similar problems and voicing her thoughts on how to handle teething or talking back. When she shared her insights, she felt a sense of pride and self-efficacy at her own skills as a mom.

Since Jackson's birth, Debra has really enjoyed the program's sessions. Now that he's 2, she can't believe all the new things she's learned from Kristin, despite already having parented one child, and how her life is changing. With the free child care and a few scholarships, she's been able to afford to reduce her hours at work and take classes at the local college. She can't wait until the day she becomes a teacher and gets to make a difference in the lives of children. Debra also knows that she's setting a good example for both of her children, especially Keisha. Just the other day, when they were at the table studying together, Keisha said, "I'm so proud of you!" and talked about where she wanted to go to college.

As the lives of Debra and her children continue to unfold, it's clear that they have an optimal start. Most salient is the positive relationship that Debra has with both of her children and the bond that is growing between brother and sister. The program provided support in multiple areas through a variety of means, but in the end, the most important contribution was the betterment of one family and the unending potential for a child growing up in a loving environment.

❖

FUTURE DIRECTIONS: IMPROVING PROGRAMS FOR PREVENTING CHILD MALTREATMENT

Because of the nationwide crisis of child abuse and neglect in this country, there is no time to lose in remedying the areas of prevention programming that are underdeveloped. The progress of the field hinges on two important issues that involve policy makers and government support: 1) delineating a consistent definition of child maltreatment utilized in all states and 2) ensuring financial support for ongoing and future prevention programs.

First and foremost, government at the federal and state levels must begin to define more clearly and consistently which behaviors actually constitute child endangerment. Because many programs target for their services families with substantiated reports of maltreatment and also utilize subsequent recidivism rates to evaluate programming effectiveness, it is vital that programs in different geographic locations are held to the same standard, particularly when one program has multiple sites. Without consistency in definitions, clear interpretation of the data becomes questionable and advancements in the field of prevention are hindered.

Government and private agency funders also must rise to the challenge of making adequate investments in prevention programming. Without consistent, long-term financial backing, well-conceived and empirically rigorous programs cannot be carried through to completion nor can their effects be adequately assessed. Funding support is at the crux of ensuring that innovative programs and their subsequent evaluations are implemented in the most needy communities. As the NHVP has shown, program effects are found up to 15 years later; however, without long-term funding commitments, the widespread enduring influence of prevention programs on communities will be limited and may go unnoticed by the public at large. It is not surprising then that consistent funding has been discussed as an essential component for child maltreatment prevention programming (Thompson, 1995).

Increased collaboration between policy makers and child maltreatment researchers will bring prevention programming to a new level and result in programs designed with rigorous methodologies, strong and consistent evaluative standards, and long-term assessment schemes. Stopping violence against children must become a top priority for the nation and for each community within its boundaries.

REFERENCES

Belsky, J. (1993). Etiology of child maltreatment: A developmental-ecological analysis. *Psychological Bulletin, 114,* 413–434.

Bigelow, K.M., & Lutzker, J.R. (1998). Using video to teach planned activities to parents reported for child abuse. *Child and Family Behavior Therapy, 20,* 1–14.

Bolton, F.C. (1990). The risk of child maltreatment in adolescent parenting. *Advances in Adolescent Mental Health, 4,* 223–237.

Bronfenbrenner, U. (1979). *The ecology of human development: Experiments by nature design.* Cambridge, MA: Harvard University Press.

Child Abuse Prevention and Treatment Act of 1974, PL 93-247, 42 U.S.C. 5101 *et seq.*

CNN News. (2005, February 5). *Pair accused of child torture arrested in Utah.* Retrieved March 15, 2005, from http://www.cnn.com/2005/US/02/04/family.torture/index.html

Connell-Carrick, K. (2003). A critical review of the empirical literature: Identifying correlates of child neglect. *Child and Adolescent Social Work Journal, 20,* 389–425.

Daro, D. (1996). Preventing child abuse and neglect. In J. Briere, L. Berliner, J. Bulkley, C. Jenny, & T. Reid (Eds.), *The APSAC handbook on child maltreatment* (pp. 359–382). Thousand Oaks, CA: Sage Publications.

Daro, D.A., & Harding, K.A. (1999). Healthy Families America: Using research to enhance practice. *The Future of Children, 9,* 152–176.

Duggan, A.K., McFarlane, E.C., Windham, A.M., Rohde, C.A., Salkever, D.S., & Fuddy, L., et al. (1999). Evaluation of Hawaii's Healthy Start Program. *The Future of Children: Home Visiting: Recent Program Evaluations, 9,* 66–90.

Eckenrode, J., Laird, M., & Doris, J. (1993). School performance and disciplinary problems among abused and neglected children. *Developmental Psychology, 29,* 53–62.

Eckenrode, J., Zielinski, D., Smith, E., Marcynyszyn, L.A., Henderson, C.R., Kitzman, et al. (2001). Child maltreatment and the early onset of problem behaviors: Can a program of nurse home visitation break the link? *Development and Psychopathology, 13,* 873–890.

Fromm, S. (2001). *Total estimated cost of child abuse and neglect in the United States: Statistical evidence.* Retrieved on May 15, 2005, from http://www.preventchildabuse. org/learn_more/research_docs/cost_analysis.pdf

Galano, J., & Huntington, L. (2004). *Healthy Families Virginia: FY 2000–2004. Executive Summary Statewide Evaluation Report.* Richmond, VA: Prevent Child Abuse Virginia.

Gellis, S., & Feingold, M. (1976). Cao gio: Psuedobattering in Vietnamese children. *American Journal of Diseases of Children, 130,* 857–858.

Gershater-Molko, R.M., Lutzker, J.R., & Wesch, D. (2002). Using recidivism data to evaluate Project Safecare: Teaching bonding, safety, and health care skills to parents. *Child Maltreatment, 7,* 277–285.

Hutchison, E.D. (1990). Child maltreatment: Can it be defined? *Social Service Review,* 60–78.

Jacobs, F., Easterbrooks, M.A., Brady, A., & Mistry, J. (2005). *Healthy Families Massachusetts Final Evaluation Report* (Executive Summary). Medford, MA: Tufts University.

Johnson, C.F. (1996). Physical abuse: Accidental versus intentional trauma in children. In J. Briere, L. Berliner, J.A. Bulkley, C. Jenny, & T. Reid (Eds.), *The APSAC handbook on child maltreatment* (pp. 206–226). Thousand Oaks, CA: Sage Publications.

Kaufman, J., & Cicchetti, D. (1989). Effects of maltreatment on school-age children's socioemotional development: Assessments in a day-camp setting. *Developmental Psychology, 25,* 516–524.

Kempe, C.H., Silverman, F.N., Steele, B.F., Droegemueller, W., & Silver, H.K. (1962). The Battered-Child Syndrome. *Journal of the American Medical Association, 181,* 17–24.

Kendall-Tackett, K., & Edwards, V. (2004, July). *The lifetime health effects of childhood abuse and adversity.* Paper presented at Victimization of Children and Youth: An International Research Conference, Portsmouth, New Jersey.

LeCroy & Milligan Associates, Inc. (2004). *Healthy Families Arizona Evaluation Report.* Tucson, AZ: Author.

Lewis, D.O. (1992). From abuse to violence: Psychophysiological consequences of maltreatment. *Journal of the American Academy of Child and Adolescent Psychiatry, 31,* 383–389.

Lutzker, J.R. (1984). Project 12-Ways: Treating child abuse and neglect from an ecobehavioral perspective. In R.F. Dangel & R.A. Polster (Eds.), *Parent training: Foundations of research and practice* (pp. 260–291). New York: Guilford Press.

Lutzker, J.R., & Bigelow, K.M. (2002). *Reducing child maltreatment: A guidebook for parent services.* New York: Guilford Press.

Lutzker, J.R., Bigelow, K.M., Doctor, R.M., & Kessler, M.L. (1998). Safety, health care, and bonding within an ecobehavioral approach to treating and preventing child abuse and neglect. *Journal of Family Violence, 13,* 163–185.

MacLeod, J., & Nelson, G. (2000). Programs for the promotion of family wellness and the prevention of child maltreatment: A meta-analytic review. *Child Abuse and Neglect, 24,* 1127–1149.

O'Brien, M.P., Lutzker, J.R., & Campbell, R.V. (1993). Consumer evaluation of an ecobehavioral program for families with children with developmental disabilities. *Journal of Mental Health Administration, 20,* 278–284.

Olds, D. (1997). The Prenatal Early Infancy Project: Preventing child abuse and neglect in the context of promoting maternal and child health. In D.A. Wolfe & R.J. McMahon (Eds.), *Child abuse: New directions in prevention and treatment across the lifespan* (pp. 130–154). Thousand Oaks, CA: Sage Publications.

Olds, D.L., Eckenrode, J., Henderson, C.R., Jr., Kitzman, H., Powers, J., Cole, R., et al. (1997). Long-term effects of home visitation on maternal life course and child and neglect: 15-year follow-up of a randomized trial. *Journal of the American Medical Association, 278,* 637–643.

Olds, D.L., Henderson, C.R., Chamberlin, R., & Tatelbaum, R. (1986). Preventing child abuse and neglect: A randomized trial of nurse home visitation. *Pediatrics, 78,* 65–78.

Olds, D.L., Henderson, C.R., Cole, R., Eckenrode, J., Kitzman, H., Luckey, D., et al. (1998). Long-term effects of nurse home visitation on children's criminal and antisocial behavior: 15-year follow-up of a randomized controlled trial. *Journal of the American Medical Association, 280,* 1238–1244.

Olds, D.L., Henderson, C.R., Tatelbaum, R., & Chamberlin, R. (1986). Improving the delivery of prenatal care and outcomes of pregnancy: A randomized trial of nurse home visitation. *Pediatrics, 77,* 16–28.

Olds, D.L., Kitzman, H., Cole, R., Robinson, J., Sidora, K., Lucky, D.W., et al. (2004). Effects of nurse home-visiting on maternal life course and child development: Age 6 follow-up results of a randomized trial. *Pediatrics, 114,* 1550–1559.

Pelton, L.H. (1994). The role of material factors in child abuse and neglect. In G.B. Melton & F.D. Barry (Eds.), *Protecting children from abuse and neglect: Foundations for a new national strategy* (pp. 131–181). New York: Guilford Press.

Prevent Child Abuse America (2001a). *Critical elements: Rationale and supporting research.* Retrieved on August 24, 2005, from http://www.healthyfamiliesamerica.org/down loads/critical_elements_rationale.pdf

Prevent Child Abuse America (2001b). *Network resources: Training.* Retrieved on August 24, 2005, from http://www.healthyfamiliesamerica.org/network_resources/training. shtml

Prevent Child Abuse America (2002a). *Characteristics of effective home visitors.* Retrieved on August 24, 2005, from http://www.healthyfamiliesamerica.org/downloads/home_visi-tors.pdf

Prevent Child Abuse America (2002b). *Healthy families America: A distinctive approach to home visiting.* Retrieved on August 24, 2005, from http://www.healthyfamiliesamerica. org/downloads/hfa_home_visit.pdf

Sedlak, A., & Broadhurst, D. (1996). *Third national incidence study of child abuse and neg-lect (NIS-3)* (Executive Summary). Washington, DC: U.S. Department of Health and Human Services, Administration on Children, Youth and Families.

Teicher, M.H. (2002, March). Scars that won't heal: The neurobiology of child abuse. *Scientific American, 68*–75.

Teicher, M.H., Dumont, N.L., Ito, Y., Vaituzis, C., Giedd, J.N., & Andersen, S.L. (2004). Childhood neglect is associated with reduced corpus callosum area. *Biological Psychiatry, 56,* 80–85.

Thompson, R.A. (1995). *Preventing child maltreatment through social support.* Thousand Oaks, CA: Sage Publications.

Twentyman, C.T., & Plotkin, R.C. (1982). Unrealistic expectations of parents who mal-treat their children: An educational deficit that pertains to child development. *Journal of Clinical Psychology, 38,* 497–503.

U.S. Advisory Board on Child Abuse and Neglect. (1990). *Child abuse and neglect: Critical first steps in response to a national emergency.* Washington, DC: Government Printing Office.

U.S. Advisory Board on Child Abuse and Neglect. (1991). *Creating caring communities: Blueprint for an effective federal policy for child abuse neglect.* Washington, DC: Government Printing Office.

U.S. Department of Health and Human Services, Children's Bureau [USDHHS]. (2004). *Child maltreatment 2002.* Retrieved December 15, 2004, from http://www.acf.hhs.gov/ programs/cb/publications/cmreports.htm

Whitman, T.L., Borkowski, J.G., Keogh, D., & Weed, K. (2001). *Interwoven lives: Adolescent mothers and their children.* Mahwah, NJ: Lawrence Erlbaum Associates.

Wodarski, J.S., Kurtz, P.D., Gaudin, J.M., & Howing, P.T. (1990). Maltreatment and the school-age child: Major academic, socioemotional, and adaptive outcomes. *Social Work, 35,* 506–513.

5

PREVENTING YOUTH VIOLENCE

Shannon S. Carothers and Chelsea M. Weaver

Highly publicized youth-related shootings have sobered communities that may have believed they were immune to youth violence. Once viewed as a problem only in inner-city neighborhoods, youth violence is now perceived as a national crisis, and political, school, and community leaders are eager to find ways to stop it (U.S. Department of Health and Human Services [USDHHS], 2001). The goals of this chapter are to 1) present research found in the extended literature on youth violence, 2) highlight characteristics of specific youth violence prevention programs, and 3) demonstrate ways in which prevention programs geared toward violence can become more effective.

RATIONALE FOR PREVENTING YOUTH VIOLENCE

The Centers for Disease Control and Prevention (CDC; 2000) has defined *youth violence* as "the threatened or actual physical force or power initiated by an individual that results in, or has a high likelihood of resulting in physical or psychological injury or death" (p. 1). It is evident that youth violence threatens the safety and socioemotional well-being of children and adolescents as well as their families (see Osofsky, 2003). Incidences such as child abuse, gang-related deaths, multiple school homicides in Denver, Colorado, and Jonesboro, Arkansas, have detrimental impacts on children's sense of felt security. Donna E. Shalala, former Secretary of Health and Human Services, stated, "In our country today, the greatest threat to the lives of children and adolescents is not disease or starvation or abandonment, but the terrible reality of violence" (USDHHS, 2001).

Incidence of Youth Violence

In 2000, more than 400,000 youth ages 10–19 were injured as a result of violence, and approximately 1 in 28 of these injuries required hospitalization (Centers for Disease Control and Prevention [CDC], 2001). In addition, homicide was reported by the CDC as 1) the second leading cause of death for people ages 10–19 overall, 2) the number one cause of death for African Americans ages 15–24, and 3) the leading cause of death for Hispanic youth. Thornton, Craft, Dahlberg, Lynch, and Baer (2002) reported that the rates of nonfatal victimization for rape, sexual assault, robbery, and aggravated assault were higher among people under age 25 than among other age groups. Although the number of school-associated violent death events has decreased steadily since the 1992–1993 school year, the occurrence of multiple-victim events—those with two or more deaths per event—appear to have increased (CDC).

In an important study of inner-city youth, Cooley-Quille, Boyd, Frantz, and Walsh (2001) found that 46% were exposed to high levels of community violence. Even more striking is the fact that 96% of inner-city males witnessed at least one violent event (e.g., heard guns being shot, seen someone being arrested or killed), and 75% had witnessed four or more violent events (Miller & Wasserman, 1999). Overstreet and Dempsey (1999) reported that 92% of their participants heard gunfire, 83% knew someone who had been killed, and 55% had witnessed a shooting. This frequency of exposure to violence may account, in part, for the high incidence of inner-city children displaying poor socioemotional and behavioral adjustment.

Just as alarming as the number of youth exposed to, and falling victim to, violence is the number of young people who are committing violent acts (Thornton et al., 2002). Since the 1980s, violence in the United States has been at unacceptably high levels (Fields & McNamara, 2003; Kelly, Huizinga, Thornberry, & Loeber, 1997). Reppucci, Woolard, and Fried (1999) reported that juvenile homicide rates (51%) surpassed those of adults (20%), as have rates of juvenile aggravated assault (49% versus 23% for adults) and juvenile robbery (50% versus 13% for adults). In a national survey of tenth- and eleventh-grade boys, Brezina (1999) found that in the past $1\frac{1}{2}$ years, 11% of tenth graders and 7% of eleventh graders committed violence against their parent(s). Furthermore, the Centers for Disease Control and Prevention's (CDC) 2002 study of high school students found that more than 6% of students surveyed had carried a weapon during the preceding 30 days. Similarly, the U.S. Department of Health and Human Services (USDHHS, 1999) reported that by age 17, about 30%–40% of males and 15%–30% of females had committed a serious violent offence.

In summary, unacceptably high rates of children are exposed to shootings, arrests, and deaths on a daily basis within their neighborhoods and communities.

The disturbing trend of increased exposure to violence makes evident the need to ask whether interventions can reduce youth violence in communities most at risk. It is imperative for children's healthy development that violence prevention/intervention programs counteract the increasing exposure, thereby decreasing children's likelihood of emulating the violence they are exposed to on a daily basis. Stopping the *cycle of violence* in which children go from being witnesses to or victims of violence to violence perpetrators is a national priority.

Consequences of Youth Violence

The impact and cost of youth violence can be seen on three levels: victim, perpetrator, and taxpayers. Snyder et al. (2003) observed victimization during early elementary school and found that increased rates of victimization was related to growth in both boys' and girls' antisocial and depressive behavior. In addition to the psychological strains of violence victimization such as trauma, hyperarousal, anxiety, re-experiencing, dissociation, substance abuse, and lack of academic motivation (e.g., Cohen, Berliner, & Mannarino, 2003; Kilpatrick & Arciero, 2003), Fagan (2001) and Osofsky (2003) argued that early repeated exposure to family violence may be a precursor to later violent behaviors in adolescence and adulthood. Moreover, Pearce, Jones, Schwab-Stone, and Ruchkin (2003) found that witnessing of and victimization by community violence were risk factors for conduct problems during the year following the event.

Youth found guilty of violence can be sentenced to a variety of punishments such as community service, boot camp, treatment programs, and/or imprisonment depending on the severity of the crime. With the onset of drug-gang violence and school shootings since the 1990s, lawmakers have sometimes decided that adult prisons should deal with adolescent offenders as well as adult offenders (McQueen, 2000). In fact, as more and more adolescents are prosecuted as adults, those found guilty of committing violent acts are more likely to serve time in prison than in the past. In 1997, 33 youth were sentenced to prison for every 1,000 arrests for violent crimes, up from the 18 per 1,000 in 1985 (McQueen). State prison data reveal that 7 out of 10 youth offenders who received adult punishment have been convicted of violent offenses (Associated Press, 2000).

Taxpayers' money is spent on prevention, criminal justice, and health care systems in an effort to deal with the aftermaths of youth violence. Fields and McNamara (2003) reported that youth violence results in frequent cases of injury, disability, and even death. Relatedly, Anderson, Dyson, and Grandison (1998) pointed out that many victims survive violent criminal episodes and come to depend on health care systems for long-term rehabilitation and therapeutic programs to aid in adjusting to their injuries. In summary, youth violence affects victims' socioemotional adjustment, as well as the perpetrators' personal freedom. Both state and federal funding are required to remedy the consequences of youth violence.

Causes and Correlates of Youth Violence

Since the 1980s, social scientists have made great strides in uncovering the causes and correlates of youth violence (USDHHS, 2001). Most causal factors reside either in the individual youth, the family, or the community at large (Reppucci et al., 1999). Important dispositional factors include sociocognitive components such as attitudes and beliefs favorable toward aggression, poor problem-solving skills, low academic aspirations, alcohol and drug use, and disruptive behavior patterns during the early years (e.g., Chung, Hill, Hawkins, Gilchrist, & Nagin, 2002; Guerra & Slaby, 1990; Hill, Howell, Hawkins, & Battin-Pearson, 1999; Tremblay, Pagani-Kurtz, Masse, Vitaro, & Phil, 1995). Of most importance, aggressive children are at high risk for later serious and chronic violent behavior (Hawkins et al., 1998; Loeber & Stouthamer-Loeber, 1998; Nagin & Tremblay, 1999).

Risk factors at the family level have focused primarily on parental characteristics such as ineffective parenting (Amodei & Scott, 2002; Hill et al., 1999; Tremblay et al., 1995), lack of adequate supervision (Bank & Burraston, 2001), skills deficits (Kalil & DeLeire, 2004), and violent behavior in the household (e.g., Bank & Burraston, 2001; Hill et al., 1999; Osofsky, 2003; Ulman & Straus, 2003; Widom, 1991). There is ample evidence suggesting that violence among family members occurs frequently in homes, suggesting that children have firsthand exposure to violence and its negative effects (Osofsky). Domestic violence in the lives of children frequently leads to an intergenerational cycle of violence: Violent children are often taught models of violent behavior by their parents (Bell, 1995; Ulman & Straus). An important study by Ulman and Straus found that children exposed to corporal punishment were more likely to direct violent behaviors toward their parents, a term referred to as *child-to-parent violence.*

In addition, exposure to violence has been found to relate to bullying among youth (e.g., Cooley-Quille et al., 2001; Miller & Wasserman, 1999; Overstreet & Dempsey, 1999; Shields & Cicchetti, 2001) as well as behavioral problems such as conduct disorders and delinquency (e.g., Flannery, Singer, Williams, & Castro, 1998). In particular, Coie and Dodge (1998) found that children who were abused were less likely to respond to peers with concern and more likely to retaliate or escalate conflict. Other researchers have shown that recurrent exposure to violence was associated with socioemotional outcomes such as lowered self-esteem and higher levels of depression, trauma, aggression, and anxiety (e.g., Singer, Anglin, Song, & Lunghofer, 1995).

In addition to dispositional and family factors, researchers have begun to identify community or contextual factors that place youth at risk for violent behavior (Lowry, Sleet, Duncan, Powell, & Kolbe, 1995). For instance, Guerra, Attar, and Weissberg (1997) identified the stress and violent environment that is characteristic of inner-city communities as critical factors that increase the risk of youth violence as well affect the effectiveness of preventive interventions. Other risk factors for violence include media portrayals and sanctioning of violence, availability of alcohol and drugs, access to weapons, and poor economic conditions such as low socioeconomic status, poverty, and lack of positive opportunities (Hawkins, Catalano, & Arthur, 2002; Reppucci et al., 1999). Other less studied risk factors are peer and school influences such as associating with delinquent friends (Chung et al., 2002; Hill et al., 1999).

PREVENTION PROGRAMS: DESIGN AND IMPLEMENTATION ISSUES

Approaches to reduce the incidence of youth violence sometimes place delinquent youth into boot camps or require mandatory field trips to penitentiaries (Osofsky, 2003). The focus has traditionally been on harsh rehabilitation methods and *scared-straight* tactics. Recently, it has become evident that these strategies do little to actually prevent or deter youth from engaging in delinquency. Although punitive discipline or incarceration is necessary under certain conditions, they produce few positive behavioral changes and should be considered as the treatment of last resort (National Association of School Psychologists, 2003). Dissatisfaction with both the timing and the outcomes associated with the *rehabilitation ideal* has spurred a search for more effective roles for health care in addressing youth violence (USDHHS, 2001).

Design and Implementation

It becomes evident that multiple, rather than single, factors place children at risk for becoming victims or perpetrators of violence (Thornton, Craft, Dahlberg, Lynch, & Baer, 2000). Numerous reviews of prevention research have shown that the targets for prevention and intervention programs should be on both risk and protective factors (e.g., Osofsky, 2003). The complex network of factors that place youth at risk for exposure to, and involvement in, youth violence—at the level of individuals, families, and communities—presents challenges for those who aim to prevent youth violence. As a consequence, effective violence prevention programs usually address multiple risk factors in a variety of ecological settings.

Osofsky (2003) recommended that traditional societal protectors of children, such as schools, community centers, and churches, create violence-free environments for youth. Pathrow-Stith (1987) maintained that to be effective, a national public health strategy to reduce violence would have to employ primary (creating safe environments), secondary (reducing risk), and tertiary (managing crises situations) prevention strategies. Along these lines, the Office of Juvenile Justice and Delinquent Prevention's Study Group on Serious and Violent Juvenile Offenders reported that the most promising prevention and intervention efforts are those modeled on the public health approach of addressing both risk and protective factors (Catalano & Hawkins, 1996; Catalano, Loeber, & McKinney, 1999).

Effective Youth Violence Prevention Programs

It is essential to identify the characteristics of effective prevention programs in an effort to inform future research and practice. Advancements in addressing youth violence require well-designed, executed, and evaluated prevention programs (Fields & McNamara, 2003). Three programs in particular meet the qualifications for an effective prevention program: Oregon Social Learning Multidimensional Treatment Foster Care (MTFC), Multisystemic Therapy (MST), and Families and Schools Together (Fast Track). Each program shares many common features such as targeting both males and females with histories of aggressive and/or violent behaviors, including a focus on families, and demonstrating positive outcomes. Yet, the programs are able to distinguish themselves from other violence prevention programs in critical ways, particularly in the content of their intervention.

The MTFC program places adolescents with histories of violent behavior into the homes of supervised and trained foster parents as a cost-effective alternative to group or residential treatment, incarceration, and/or hospitalization. MST is an intensive family and community treatment program that addresses both behavioral and cognitive determinants of serious antisocial behavior among adolescents. The Fast Track project is comprehensive in that it intervenes with parents, teachers, and children who are at high risk. As opposed to the other two programs, Fast Track places more of an emphasis on prevention as opposed to intervention. The program seeks to increase communication, social, cognitive, and problem-solving skills and improve peer relationships. Table 5.1 more fully presents each program and its defining characteristics.

Table 5.1. Three violence prevention programs and their defining characteristics

	Oregon Multidimensional Treatment Foster Care	Multisystemic Therapy	Fast Track
Targets of intervention	Males and females Teenagers Histories of chronic and severe criminal behavior; at risk of incarceration Offender's family	Male and females Chronic, violent, or substance-abusing offenders Ages 12 to 17 Offender's families	Males and females Rural and urban areas Kindergarten children displaying poor behavior and peer relations Offender's families
Content of intervention	Structured, therapeutic living environment Ongoing supervision of MTFC parents Family therapy Supervised home visits Frequent contact between MTFC case manager, youth's parole officer, teachers, work supervisors, and other involved adults	Strategic family therapy Structural family therapy Behavioral family therapy Cognitive behavior therapy	Parent training Biweekly home visitation Social skills training Academic tutoring Classroom intervention uses the PATHS curriculum
Outcomes of intervention	Youth spend 60% fewer days incarcerated Youth have fewer subsequent arrests Youth are three times less likely to run away from their placements Significantly less hard drug use Quicker community placements for more restrictive settings	25%–70% reduction in re-arrest 47%–64% reduction in out-of-home placements Improved family functioning Decreased mental health problems	Improved teacher and parent rating of children's behavior with peers and adults Improved rating of children's aggressive, disruptive, and oppositional behavior in classrooms Less physical punishment endorsement by parents More appropriate discipline techniques; involvement in school; warmth by mothers
Costs and duration	On average, $18,937 per youth; 7 months	$4,500 per youth; individually tailored	Grades 1–6; 7 years

PREVENTION PROGRAMS AND THEIR EVALUATIONS

The characteristics of three prevention programs and how they influence reductions in youth violence are analyzed in the following sections.

Oregon Social Learning Multidimensional Treatment Foster Care

Multidimensional Treatment Foster Care (MTFC) is a multisystemic, multicontextual clinical intervention that targets teenagers with histories of chronic and severe criminal behavior as an alternative to incarceration, group or residential treatment, and/or hospitalization (Chamberlain & Mihalic, 1998; USDHHS, 2001). The program is an example of a secondary prevention program in that it targets youth who are at high risk for engaging in violence or who have clearly displayed some form of antisocial or delinquent behavior.

Program Description   MTFC grew out of evidence for the effectiveness of behavioral parent training approaches and a clinical need for programs to address the behavior of delinquent adolescents who have been found to be beyond parental control (Moore, Sprengelmeyer Chamberlain, 2001). It starts with a focus on the need to return the adolescent to the family and community; thus, the program stresses the generalization of treatment effects. Youth are placed, usually singly or at most in groups of two, with trained and supervised foster parents for 6 to 9 months; and their own parents also participate in family therapy (Chamberlain & Mihalic, 1998).

The MTFC program uses a comprehensive multimodal (e.g., home, school, peers) treatment model, including

1. Foster parent recruitment and screening
2. Intensive preservice training for both community (foster) families and parents
4. School consultation, individual youth treatment, and family therapy
5. After-care services using *wrap-around* or customized service delivery for the youth and their families (Moore et al., 2001)

Youth who participate in this program also receive behavior management and skill-focused therapy and work with a community liaison who coordinates contacts among case managers and others who have contact with the youth (USDHHS, 2001).

In this family-based treatment model, it is the foster parents, under the close guidance of professional staff, who structure and provide most of the *treatment* for youth in the program. Recruitment for community families is done primarily through word of mouth, particularly from current MTFC foster parents who are paid a finders fee for referring others who become program foster parents (Moore et al., 2001). By using an in-depth 20-hour training model, MTFC parents are taught by staff and an experienced MTFC foster parent to provide structured, individualized home environments designed to build on participant's strengths while maintaining clear rules regarding expectations and limits (Chamberlain & Mihalic, 1998). Foster parents meet daily with the participants to tally points and provide feedback so that they know what was done well and where improvement is needed (USDHHS, 2001).

Foster parents are closely supervised by case managers in teaching and reinforcing skills that facilitate healthy and functional parent–child interactions. More specifically, daily contacts are made by telephone between program parents and staff to collect data on children's behavior, discuss potential problems, and coordinate plans for the following day (Chamberlain & Mihalic, 1998). Supervision and monitoring also are necessary to direct clinical staff and foster parents toward a coherent set of interventions and away from being reactive to isolated situations that may arise (Chamberlain & Mihalic). An adolescent moving back into his or her home does not signify the end of the program; instead, youth and their biological parents continue to attend family therapy sessions.

Treatment activities are organized into a plan that focuses on teaching relevant family living, social, academic, recreational, and vocational skills. Adolescents who are placed in MTFC are given intensive supervision at home, in school, and in the community that enforce clear and consistent limits with follow-through on consequences; positive reinforcement for appropriate behavior; a relationship with a mentoring adult; and separation from delinquent peers. In addition, MTFC foster parents are trained to adapt the general program principles to the specific daily teaching needs of the adolescent. An individualized point-and-level system (or some developmentally appropriate contingency management system such as a start chart for younger children) with daily feedback (point card) is used. The point-and-level system is divided into three levels that gradually give youth more privileges and responsibilities, with the highest level moving youth as far toward independent living as developmentally appropriate (Moore et al., 2001). In addition, youth's biological parents attend weekly treatment sessions that teach them effective methods for supervising, disciplining, and encouraging their children's positive behavior. Parents are able to practice these skills during home visits that allow them the opportunity to run the individualized program currently implemented by the MTFC foster parent. A family therapist works with the family to help advance them toward overnight visits (Chamberlain & Mihalic, 1998).

Program Evaluation Evaluations of program effectiveness use third-party information sources (e.g., official arrest records, school records, a validated measure of postprogram living situation, retention of foster parents, community consumer satisfaction). Chamberlain and Mihalic (1998) compared the effectiveness of two treatment models (therapeutic peer group interactions versus maximizing mentoring adults and prosocial peers while decreasing contact with delinquent peers) on male participants ages 12–17 (M = 14.3) who had an average of 13 prior arrests and 4.6 felonies; half of the participants had committed at least one crime against a person and were identified as chronic offenders.

Evaluations indicated that MTFC can reduce the number of days of incarceration, overall arrests, drug use, and program drop-out rates in treated youth versus group setting controls during the first 12 months after completing treatment; it also can speed the placement of youth in less restrictive community settings (USD-HHS, 2001). More specifically, at 1-year posttreatment, boys in MTFC had less than half the number of arrests as boys in the control (i.e., an average of 2.6 offenses for MTFC boys and 5.4 offenses for control boys); had an 83% higher rate of resistance from arrest than did boys in the control group; were three times less likely to run away or be expelled from their programs than those in group settings (5 out of 36 MTFC boys and 15 out of 38 control boys); spend about twice as many days living with parents or relatives in follow-up than did boys in group settings; and reported committing significantly fewer criminal acts than control boys at 6, 12, and 18 months postenrollment in the study (Chamberlain & Mihalic, 1998). Of most importance, specific treatment components such as supervised discipline, decreased association with delinquent peers, and positive relationships with adults were shown by Eddy and Chamberlain (2000) to mediate the treatment effect of MTFC on outcomes.

In addition, anecdotal reports from a large child care agency in Tennessee using MTFC suggested reduced residential care costs, improved placement stability, and reduced foster parent turnover. Chamberlain and Reid (1998) showed that compared with youth treated in group care settings (residing with other delinquent youth), those treated in the MTFC program were re-arrested significantly less often and were returned home to live with parents or relatives significantly more often. Analyses showed that the treatment condition (i.e., group setting, MTFC) predicted both official and self-reported criminality at follow-up above and beyond other well-known predictors of chronic juvenile offending (i.e., age at first offense, number of previous offenses, age at referral). Chamberlain and Reid's findings implied that treating even older, early onset delinquents with strong, well-trained, and supported MTFC families has the potential to change their delinquent trajectories. The program has also been able to affect similar levels of change in older and younger delinquents (Moore et al., 2001).

The Washington State Institute for Public Policy found an effect size for MTFC to be about −.37 for basic recidivism. Aos, Phipps, Barnoski, and Leib (2001) found that by the time subjects were age 25, MTFC saved taxpayers more than $21,836 compared with usual services (e.g., residential care, institutional settings). Moreover, the analysis revealed that program costs were recaptured within 1 year posttreatment. Initial data from these projects suggest both that the general parameters of MTFC programs are effective with a variety of different, hard-to-treat populations and that important adjustments are necessary to optimize treatment effectiveness.

Critical Analysis of Treatment Characteristics   As a secondary prevention program, the MTFC program is an excellent example of a program that is theory-driven; is comprehensive; utilizes varied teaching methods; and, above all, encourages positive relationships. In particular, the basic premise of the MTFC program was modeled after Social Learning Theory that describes the mechanisms by which individuals learn to behave in social contexts (Chamberlain & Mihalic, 1998). The program acknowledges that negative social interactions with both parents and peers encourage the development and maintenance of antisocial behavior patterns among youth. For instance, parents of aggressive children are thought to inadvertently reinforce antisocial behaviors by *giving in* or *backing off* when their child responds in a coercive manner to parenting requests (Chamberlain & Mihalic).

Taken together with research documenting the relationship between peers who are deviant and elevated rates of aggression and delinquent behavior, the MTFC program seeks to build social skills by providing environments that limit association with peers who are antisocial while simultaneously enhancing opportunities to engage with adults and mentors who are prosocial. By the time youth return home to their parents, parents have improved their ability to provide a successful home environment, and children have been taught behaviors that are conducive to maintaining this environment as well as other social contexts (e.g., peers, schools, community).

Furthermore, the MTFC program is comprehensive and utilizes varied teaching methods. The program is comprehensive in that it includes multiple components within the home and community that are thought to influence the development and maintenance of prosocial behaviors as opposed to aggression and violence. More specifically, the program includes weekly supervision and support meetings for MTFC parents; skill-focused individual treatment for youth; weekly family therapy for biological parents; and frequent contact between youth and their biological/adoptive family members, including home visits; close monitoring of the children's progress in school; coordination with probation/parole officers; and psychiatric consultation/mediation management, when needed (Chamberlain & Mihalic, 1998). In addition, the intervention component of the MTFC is aimed at both the youth and their biological parents. Biological families are taught parenting skills that are practiced during home visits and are provided a help-line for consultation by a family therapist and case manager (Center for Substance Abuse Prevention, 2004).

A critical component of the MTFC program is building positive relationships between youth labeled as *chronic offenders* and foster parents residing within the community. Program initiators point out that the success of the program is greatly dependent on the group of adults (i.e., case manager, family therapist, individual therapist) that work with youth and their parents (both biological and foster) to surround them with positive role models, constructive mentors and provide nondelinquent environments (Chamberlain & Mihalic, 1998). Most important, the MTFC intervention is tailored to each individual participant in that the intervention is contingent on youth's success, or lack thereof, in progressing through the program.

Critical Analysis of Procedural Characteristics   The MTFC program has sufficient dosage, well-trained staff, programmed generalization, and treatment fidelity. Sufficient dosage is evident in that program principles are specifically tailored to youth so enough intervention (not too much or too little) is given to produce desired changes in behavior. As youth progress through the program, treatments are adjusted to their learning needs with the goal of moving them toward independent living and the ability to monitor their own behavior. The feasibility of the MTFC system is dependent on the foster parent's ability to monitor children's progress through the program as well as provide structured home environments with rewards and consequences for behavior. Therefore, families are recruited, trained, and supported by case managers to provide well-supervised placements and treatments (Chamberlain & Mihalic, 1998).

In addition, the MTFC program has taken the necessary steps to ensure treatment fidelity and the generalization of learned social skills. In particular, individual placements are continuously monitored for the precision of their implementation. More specifically, MTFC parents are contacted daily by telephone as a way to gain insights into problematic behavior during the past 24 hours (Chamberlain & Mihalic, 1998). During this call, improvements in behavior and potential problems are discussed as a way for case managers to coordinate treatment plans on the following day (Chamberlain & Mihalic). Programmed generalizations are seen in that multiple teaching settings are used by MTFC parents for the development and maintenance of youth's social competence. Foster care families are recruited, trained, and closely supervised to provide adolescents who are placed in the MTFC program with treatment and intensive supervision at home, at school, and in the community (Chamberlain & Mihalic).

The MTFC program is a secondary prevention program in that it aims to teach adaptive social skills to youth already characterized as chronic offenders in an effort to decrease their incidence of aggressive behavior. The MTFC program does so by reducing the adolescent's interactions with peers who are antisocial and teaching parents ways to interact with and structure home environments for their children. An objective of the MTFC program is to come up with an intervention that provides corrective or therapeutic parenting for adolescents who are antisocial and whose parents, for one reason or another, were unable to do so (Chamberlain & Mihalic, 1998). In contrast, primary prevention strategies are aimed at stopping violent events from taking place before violence actually occurs.

For youth, their family, the community, and taxpayers, it is imperative that prevention programs focusing on violence begin before aggressive behaviors are prominent. The aim should not be on corrective therapy but on preventing aggression among children who are at risk for violence. The MTFC program recognizes that associations with peers who are delinquent as well as lenient parenting contributes to the development and maintenance of aggressive behaviors among children. It would be efficacious to document whether the principles used in the MTFC program could be implemented in home settings prior to the development of inadequate skills, aggressive behaviors, and violence. In particular, principles could be started early that teach the parent how to best manage problems prior to children acting out or displaying aggressive behaviors.

Critical Analysis of Design Characteristics   In terms of methodology, the MTFC program maintains a strong evaluative component that includes clear goals, an active control, and internal validation. Prior to program implementation, program initiators set two main goals and objectives for the MTFC program: 1) to evaluate systematically the immediate and long-term outcomes of the intervention and 2) to assess the contribution of the intervention's key variables to changes in youth's behavioral outcomes (Chamberlain & Mihalic, 1998). The use of such clearly defined goals served as a reference point for the design of the program (i.e., the use of a control group) and the types of analyses used (multiple regression) to address these goals. In short, evaluations have examined the differential impact of the MTFC program versus a matched control group (group care) on youth's behavior such as duration of placement, number of arrests, frequency of program expulsions, school achievement, and engagement in criminal activities after placement. Participants are typically matched on parole/probation supervision, felonies committed, and age.

Moreover, in an effort to fully understand the processes by which the intervention affected youth's behavior, multiple factors (i.e., supervision, discipline, deviant peers) were measured that have been found in the literature to relate to the development of aggression and delinquency among children (Chamberlain & Mihalic, 1998). The ability to prospectively collect various factors allowed the examination of possible mediators of the intervention–behavior relationship. In fact, program evaluations revealed that boys in either the MTFC program or group settings (control group) who received good supervision and consistent, predictable discipline, and who had less association with peers who were delinquent, had fewer arrests in follow-up than those who did not (Eddy & Chamberlain, 2000).

Despite the previous strengths, two precautions must be addressed in reference to design characteristics: effect sizes and cost of implementation. Though a moderate effect size has been documented ($-.37$), the relatively small sample size used in analyses ($N = 32$) makes interpretations of the nature of the intervention as well as component part's effects somewhat problematic; in particular, small sample sizes have been shown to reduce the statistical power necessary to detect true differences (O'Rourke, 2003).

The MTFC program requires large amounts of money and commitment by staff to ensure proper implementation, particularly for the supervision of foster parents. The Center for Substance Abuse Prevention (2004) mentioned that the cost of implementing the MTFC program is dependent on organizational size and how many youth and foster families are participating. Before implementing the MTFC model, consideration must be given as to whether ample personnel are available who are trained to carry out the program. If program staff are not trained, they are required to attend a 1-year training course, during which organizational readiness is addressed; program staff is trained; and foster parents are recruited, certified, and trained. Training costs are approximately $40,000 plus travel and lodging expenses at the OSLC MTFC site. Furthermore, the cost of implementing the program per youth is just as much a financial investment as is the cost of training staff. Individual youth spend an average of 7 months under the care of foster parents at a cost of $2,691 per month (Center for Substance Abuse Prevention). Although MTFC has been shown to save considerable amounts of taxpayer money and is less expensive than placement in group, residential care, or institutional settings (Chamberlain & Mihalic, 1998), the significant financial and staff resources needed should be taken into consideration before implementing the MTFC model in community settings.

Multisystemic Therapy

Multisystemic Therapy (MST) is an indicated program designed to prevent the development of violence perpetration and severe antisocial behavior in youth who are at risk. MST is characterized by a multidimensional therapeutic approach that uses a community perspective in treating youth within their social support systems. Treatment strategies are derived from family, behavioral, and cognitive therapy techniques. Success of MST is measured by decreasing recidivism rates, behavioral problems, and out-of-home placements and by increasing positive family and peer relationships (Henggeler, 1997). MST is relatively short term, with approximately 30 sessions over 4–6 months. Treatment termination is defined by the family's unique gains and indicated needs (Henggeler, Schoenwald, Pickrel, Brandino, & Hall, 1994).

Program Description   MST is based on the premise that to prevent youth violence, one must reduce risk and promote protective factors in multiple settings. Antisocial behavior among youth has been associated with factors within the individual (e.g., poor social skills), the family (e.g., ineffective parenting), the school environment (e.g., academic failure), and the community (e.g., criminality; Henggeler, 1997). Although multiple environmental contexts are targeted during treatment, the initial focus is typically on promoting effective parenting, reducing parental stress, and treating parental substance use when necessary. In addition, protective factors are promoted through building on family competencies to strengthen the family unit and increase the likelihood of long-term success.

MST is a theoretically driven prevention program based on the socioecological model developed by Bronfenbrenner (1979). The individual is viewed as being nested within various social systems, and behavior is considered the antecedent as well as the consequence of complex transactions between multiple levels (proximal and distal) of systems. MST also is rooted in Family Systems Theory of therapy, which views the interaction patterns within the family as the source of dysfunction (Minuchin, 1974). Extending from this paradigm, MST is based on the family preservation model of delivery, which emphasizes the need for intensive, home-based, family-focused, goal-oriented programming (Henggeler, 1997). The advantages of such a design include validity in assessment of maladaptive behavioral contingencies, improved generalization and maintenance of treatment gains, enhanced respect in the family and professional partnership, and the promotion of family cooperation with treatment (Henggeler).

Treatment specificity of MST is achieved through strict adherence to nine principles of intervention:

1. Assessments are conducted to understand how identified problem behaviors fit into the larger ecological context.
2. Therapy is based on emphasizing and utilizing the strengths of the system in order to bring about change.
3. Interventions target increasing responsible behaviors and decreasing irresponsible behaviors of the family members.
4. Interventions are present-focused, action-oriented, and target clear, distinct problems.
5. Interventions target chains of behaviors within or between systems.
6. Interventions are developmentally appropriate and meet the needs of the participants.
7. Interventions must require daily or weekly effort by family members.
8. Efficacy is continuously evaluated from multiple perspectives (e.g., therapist, mother, teacher).

9. Interventions promote generalization and maintenance of therapeutic change (Henggeler et al., 1994).

The nine principles are clearly outlined in the MST treatment manual, which is the foundation on which the clinical intervention trials are built.

Treatment individualization is an important feature of MST that allows the programming to be highly specific and applicable to each family. According to Henggeler (1997), by targeting the unique factors that operate within each individual's social ecology, the probability of successfully decreasing antisocial behaviors is increased. Therapists are trained to assess each family's distinctive strengths to build on and develop them for use in ameliorating their self-defined needs. In addition, families play an integral role in identifying their own strengths and needs, in developing their treatment goals, and in monitoring their progress. Families are empowered with the resources necessary for successful independent functioning in the challenging circumstances of everyday life by facilitating positive relationships within social networks (e.g., church, community center). In addition, MST teaches families and youth the skills needed (e.g., anger management, problem solving) to adaptively function across multiple social contexts.

MST therapists hold master's degrees and typically carry a caseload of four to six families (Henggeler et al., 1994). Therapists are on call 24 hours a day, 7 days a week to assist families in coping with crisis situations. A unique feature of MST is its focus on therapist accountability. When treatment efforts are unsuccessful, participants are not viewed as resistant or labeled the cause of ineffectiveness. According to Henggeler and colleagues, the therapists and supervisors are held responsible for bringing about lasting change within each of the participating families, and they are instructed to do whatever it takes to achieve those changes. Due to such a high standard of accountability, therapists undergo extensive training, have light caseloads, and are highly supervised. Designing the program in such a way promotes positive case outcomes for the therapists and helps prevent negative consequences (e.g., therapist burnout) that frequently accompany working with populations who are at high risk (Henggeler et al.).

Program Evaluation Borduin and colleagues (1995) conducted a study comparing the effectiveness of MST to individual therapy (IT) in a clinical sample of juvenile offenders. Participants were 200 juvenile offenders between the ages of 12 and 17 (M = 14.7, SD = 1.6; 67% male) and their families. The racial composition of the sample was 67% Caucasian and 32.2% African American; 65% were of low socioeconomic status, and 50% lived with two-parent families (e.g., biological, step, foster). The juvenile offenders had an average of four previous arrests, and 61% had been previously incarcerated. Participants were randomly assigned to receive either MST (n = 92) or IT (n = 84); 24 families refused to participate in treatment. IT is characterized by psychodynamic, client-centered, or behavioral orientations toward encouraging change regarding personal, family, and/or school problems. The study yielded five groups: MST completers (n = 77), MST dropouts (n = 15), IT completers (n = 63), IT dropouts (n = 21), and treatment refusers (n = 24). Posttreatment, families receiving MST had significantly increased family cohesion, adaptability, and supportiveness and had decreased hostility as compared with the IT group (Borduin et al., 1995). At a 4-year follow-up, the MST completers had lower rates of recidivism (22.1%) as compared with the MST dropouts (46.6%), the IT completers (71.4%), the IT dropouts (71.4%), and the treatment refusers (87.5%). Furthermore, those arrested in the MST groups were arrested less frequently, for less serious offenses, and for fewer violent crimes than the IT youth (Borduin et al., 1995). In an analysis of violence prevention programs, Aos et al. (2001) reported an adjusted effect size (accounting for small sample size) between the MST and IT groups in recidivism of -0.47 ($p = .000$).

Aos and colleagues (2001) conducted a cost–benefit analysis of MST, adjusting research findings to reflect the 2000 U.S. dollar. The net direct cost of MST was $4,743 per participant; taxpayers save approximately $31,661 in future criminal justice expenses, and crime victims save $131,918 in related costs, yielding a benefit-to-cost ratio of $28.33 for every dollar spent on MST. These findings support the overall treatment and cost effectiveness of MST in treating youth who are at high risk and preventing future violence perpetration. Consequently, MST is currently implemented in more than 25 states and in Canada, England, Ireland, Sweden, Norway, and New Zealand (Substance Abuse and Mental Health Services Administration, n.d.).

Critical Analysis of Treatment Characteristics   MST is a prevention program that is embedded within a strong theoretical framework. The socioecological model of Bronfenbrenner (1979) provided the basis for MST, which views change as resulting from transactions between an individual and his or her social systems. Accordingly, MST incorporates proximal (family and peer) and distal (community and social services agencies) networks in its treatment protocols. MST also features program comprehensiveness, generalization, and sociocultural relevance. In addition to the socioecological model, MST is heavily influenced by family therapy models (Haley, 1976; Minuchin, 1974), which highlight the importance of family processes in initiating individual change (Henggeler, Cunningham, Pickrel, Schoenwald, & Brondino, 1996). Along with behavioral parent training (Munger, 1993) and cognitive–behavioral therapy (Braswell & Kendall, 2001), therapeutic techniques are integrated on an individual basis to form the foundation of the MST program (Henggeler, 1999).

Positive relationships between therapists and clients are critical aspects of prevention programs. A study conducted by Huey, Henggeler, Brondino, and Pickrel (2000) revealed that therapeutic attempts of MST staff to change family interactions before building positive rapport with the family lead to unsuccessful and possibly harmful results. Several MST principles are geared toward promoting positive relationships, thereby decreasing attrition and supporting positive outcomes. Program staff are highly involved with, and available to, families. Respect for families serves as the foundation on which supportive therapeutic relationships are built. In short, MST does an excellent job of employing the treatment characteristics of an ideal violence prevention program.

Critical Analysis of Procedural Characteristics The level of individualization required by MST makes intensive staff training an essential program component. Program therapists, supervisors, and administrators are required to attend a 5-day orientation to the MST model (Henggeler, 1999). Therapists receive on-site supervision a minimum of once per week from an MST supervisor, who adheres to the MST supervisory protocol. In addition, staff receives services from an off-site MST consultant, who promotes treatment fidelity and assists in overcoming barriers with families. The consultant also provides booster sessions and works with administrators to evaluate and address programmatic and organizational issues.

Because MST is based on each family's needs, dosage levels are tailored to meet individual skill deficits. The adequacy of dosage has been supported by evidence on long-term change. For example, in a 4-year follow-up, MST was more effective than individual therapy in preventing criminality, including juvenile offending (Borduin et al., 1995). Long-term maintenance of behavioral gains indicates that 4 months of intensive treatment is sufficient to facilitate lasting change.

A particular strength of the MST program is the emphasis placed on the treatment fidelity of program delivery. Despite intensive staff training and supervision, MST trials have yielded variability in adherence to treatment principles, partly due to the complexity and individualization of the program (Huey et al., 2000). Furthermore, analyses revealed that higher therapist adherence to MST principles decreased delinquency, which was mediated by family and peer factors. Due to the importance of treatment fidelity and its direct impact on dosage level (lack of adherence leads to decreased dosage), an MST consultant provides ongoing services and booster sessions to the treatment team to promote adherence to treatment protocol. In addition, treatment fidelity is measured using a quality assurance procedure, which is a parent-report MST treatment adherence measure (Henggeler, 1999).

A weakness of MST is the timing of program implementation. MST is an indicated program, meaning that the individual must be identified as having serious problems such as violent offending, sexual offending, and substance abuse. Thus, program participants already have salient behavioral problems, a characteristic that typically leads to the classification of MST as a secondary or tertiary program. However, MST includes many characteristics of a primary prevention program—namely, reducing existing risk and promoting protective factors. MST should be implemented with individuals who are at risk for developing serious problems before they become juvenile offenders.

Critical Analysis of Design Characteristics Clinical trials of MST have typically compared treatment participants to individuals who receive another type of therapeutic intervention, such as individual therapy or *typical* services that are in place for offending youth. The presence of active control groups allows for positive outcomes to be attributed to MST rather than to the presence of treatment alone.

Relatedly, treatment outcomes used to evaluate MST efficacy are levels of recidivism and violent offending presented by youth. In treatment, program goals are individualized and developed with each family. Typically, goals address areas such as increasing parental monitoring, dissolving relationships with deviant peers, and increasing educational success (Henggeler et al., 1996). In analyses, these constructs are sometimes used as predictors or mediators of violent outcomes (e.g., Huey et al., 2000), thereby lending support to the process by which individuals achieve and maintain behavioral change as well as the internal validity of MST.

Family and Schools Together (Fast Track)

The Fast Track program represents an excellent example of a theory-based approach to creating preventive interventions that operate in multiple domains of children's lives (Reppucci et al., 1999). It is a community-based, multicomponent intervention designed to prevent the development of conduct disorders among youth who are at risk (Conduct Problems Prevention Research Group [CPPRG], 1992). Based on a prevention-science approach, Fast Track is a developmentally based, long-term program implemented in demographically diverse communities (urban, suburban, and rural) and embedded within family and community contexts.

Program Description Fast Track is based on the idea that multiple causal factors interact within the child, family, peer group, school, and community to influence the development of conduct problems (Conduct Problems Prevention Research Group [CPPRG], 2002a). Research by Patterson (1986) and Moffitt (1993) identified a distinct group of children whose conduct problems began early (as young as age 5) and progressed and/or persisted over time. This conceptual model of early starters assumes that 1) there are a variety of etiological factors at play (e.g., neurological deficits, harsh parenting); 2) the trajectory of the early starter is plastic, leading to differing developmental outcomes; 3) such outcomes depend on experiences in three domains: family, school, and social (Conduct Problems Prevention Research Group [CPPRG], 2002c).

Fast Track targets individual competencies and contextual supports over the span of 10 years (grades 1 through 10); a comparison high-risk control group and a normative comparison group were used at each of the four sites. The program consists of two phases: 1) grades 1 through 5 and 2) grades 6 through 10. Phase 1 is characterized by three levels: universal intervention (school level), standard indicated intervention (for children who are at risk), and individualized indicated intervention (addressed unique needs of those in the at-risk group; CPPRG, 2002a). Phase 2, or the adolescent phase, shifted the emphasis from group-based intervention to individualized programming based on demonstrated need from criterion-based assessments (Conduct Problems Prevention Research Group [CPPRG], 2005). This was done to promote protection and reduce risk while also avoiding the facilitation of engagement with deviant peers.

During Phase 1, universal interventions include the Promoting Alternative Thinking Strategies (PATHS; Kusché & Greenberg, 1994) curriculum, which was taught by trained classroom teachers (CPPRG, 2002a). PATHS facilitates school success through targeting the skills in four domains: 1) prosocial behavior and friendship, 2) emotional understanding and self-control, 3) communication and conflict resolution, and 4) problem solving (see Kusché & Greenberg, 1994). Indicated interventions were provided to students who were identified in kindergarten as high risk according to parent and teacher reports of behavior problems (CPPRG). Children were categorized as high risk if they scored in the top 10% at each site.

Treatment began in first grade with all identified participants receiving intervention to reduce risk and promote protective factors in six domains: 1) parenting, 2) social problem solving and emotional coping, 3) peer relationships, 4) classroom atmosphere and curriculum, 5) academic achievement, and 6) home–school relations. From second through fifth grade, the level of indicated home visits (weekly, biweekly, or monthly), peer pairing, and academic tutoring interventions were individualized to meet the unique needs of the participants. Furthermore, the intensity of interventions targeting parenting, social skills, and parent–child relationships were decreased over time from weekly sessions in first grade and biweekly sessions in second grade to monthly sessions in third through sixth grades.

Program Evaluation   In an evaluation of the PATHS program, investigators found a significant effect on peer ratings of aggression and classroom observations at the end of first grade (CPPRG, 1999a). The quality of program implementation predicted variability in classroom functioning with integration of core concepts into regular teaching practices leading to favorable child outcomes. Furthermore, significant effects on children's peer interactions, social status, behavior problems, and special education use were found at the end of first grade (Conduct Problems Prevention Research Group [CPPRG], 1999b). By the end of third grade, children at high risk who received the intervention were found to have fewer conduct problems and their parents displayed more positive change; however, effect sizes were modest, ranging from 0.14 to 0.27 (CPPRG, 2002b). Fast Track had a significant, yet modest, impact on children's social competence, social cognition, associations with deviant peers, and conduct problems at home and in the community during fourth and fifth grades ($ES = .15$ to $.18$); however, no effect was found for conduct problems demonstrated at school (Conduct Problems Prevention Research Group [CPPRG], 2004). Clinical trials of Fast Track are still underway with some children now attending middle and high schools; however, preliminary evidence supports the overall efficacy of the Fast Track program in changing multiple facets of the participants' lives and decreasing the risk for the development of conduct problems.

Critical Analysis of Treatment Characteristics   The Fast Track program is based on an early starter model, which is in turn based on research that demonstrates early child characteristics (e.g., impulsivity) combined with family stressors (e.g., poverty) as precursors to children's reliance on negative behaviors to meet their wants and needs (CPPRG, 2002a). Furthermore, harmful parent–child interactions compromise children's cognitive and emotional regulation skills, leading to aggressive behavioral strategies, which in turn are exacerbated by negative peer interactions when children enter school. These destructive transactions continue into adolescence, facilitating the development of delinquent behavior (CPPRG, 2002b). Fast Track works to intervene in each of these domains, thereby interrupting the cycle and replacing harmful strategies with constructive, effective regulatory processes. It should be noted that such a complex theoretical model is difficult to test, and significant changes in program participants provide little evidence as to the specific components (or combination of components) of the intervention that are actually promoting behavioral changes.

A significant strength of the Fast Track program is its emphasis on promoting positive relationships among those involved in the program (e.g., participants, school personnel). First, program staff who possess similar sociocultural backgrounds and who are from the same communities as participants are recruited in order to promote relevance for families. Staff are then instructed to allow families to warm up to the program at their own pace and to focus on the goal of establishing and maintaining positive relationships with families rather than highlighting accomplishment of short-term programmatic goals. Within program delivery,

Fast Track emphasizes family and children's strengths, rather than employing a deficit model. In general, the program builds on parents' hopes for their children's success rather than instill fear of the possible consequences of early behavior problems (CPPRG, 2002a).

Critical Analysis of Procedural Characteristics   Fast Track is a violence-prevention program that begins when children are in the first grade. By starting early, skills can be taught and children's strengths can be developed before negative behaviors and patterns of interaction become salient. Program dosage is very good considering the fact that it spans 10 years, covering significant transitions into elementary, middle, and high school (CPPRG, 2002a). In addition, dosage is individualized based on each child's need, thereby making program goals relevant to unique circumstances of each child and their family.

Fast Track staff are highly trained and supervised prior to and during program implementation. Educational Coordinators (EC) were required to have degrees in education (CPPRG, 2002a). Family Coordinators (FC) had backgrounds in social work, counseling, psychology, and/or extensive professional experience working with families at high risk. The codeveloper of PATHS traveled to each site to train teachers in the implementation of the curriculum. In the spring before program initiation, a 4-week pilot program that included all intervention components was implemented with a group of children who were referred by the school at each site. The incorporation of a pilot program is a unique aspect of their training procedure that served to enhance staff readiness and competence in program implementation.

To promote treatment fidelity across sites, ECs, FCs, clinical supervisors, and principal investigators conducted cross-site meetings for 2.5 days each year; cross-site conference calls were conducted weekly for the first 2 years of the program, and then monthly beginning in the 3rd year. Detailed, comprehensive training manuals were developed to guide staff through each of the core intervention components (CPPRG, 2002a). In addition, staff were observed during program delivery by clinical supervisors, who provided feedback regarding adherence to the protocol (CPPRG, 2004). Whereas treatment fidelity was acknowledged by investigators, data on program adherence should be used in analysis of treatment effects. If intervention fidelity is not obtained, then targeted outcomes may be negatively affected and the interpretation of findings may be hindered.

Critical Analysis of Design Characteristics   Fast Track has the clear goal of preventing conduct problems in adolescence by intervening with children early in life. In addition to assessing children's conduct throughout program implementation, potential mechanisms such as parenting techniques and children's social skills also are measured to provide evidence of program success. By testing the process components, investigators shed light on why children are improving based on which mechanisms are associated with positive outcomes. In addition, because preliminary findings regarding process variables are in accordance with expectations based on the theoretical model (CPPRG, 2002b), they also serve to increase the program's internal validity.

Fast Track investigators reported effect sizes for their preliminary outcomes at the end of the first 3 years and found an overall small but significant impact of their treatment (*ES* ranging from .14 to .27; CPPRG, 2002b). It is important to note that the targeted goal of this program is to reduce serious conduct problems in adolescence, and the social significance of a small effect must be weighed. Further, Fast Track is a 10-year prevention program and these 3-year results may be casting a shadow of what is to come; there will likely be a greater benefit as dosage levels accumulate over time.

A drawback of the Fast Track program is the fact that children and families in the control condition received no supports. This leads to the attention provided to intervention families and could be a potential confounding factor. For example, it may be the act of intervening that is prompting behavioral change rather than the actual program content, which is especially concerning due to the complexity of the theoretical model driving the Fast Track project. Future trials should employ active control groups who receive attentional supports, as well as experimental groups that receive only specific components of Fast Track to draw more accurate conclusions regarding the impact of each aspect of the program.

BUILDING A MODEL PROGRAM

The later part of the chapter highlights and discusses characteristics of specific youth violence prevention programs. Through the presentation of a "model" youth violence prevention program, a special emphasis is placed on demonstrating the ways in which prevention programs geared toward violence can become more effective.

A Model Youth Violence Prevention Program

The essential components of a model program designed to prevent youth violence are presented in Table 5.2. Parents and children who are at risk for developing, or who are displaying, violent behaviors (e.g., domestic violence, physical aggression) are candidates for inclusion in the program. Prevention curricula should target social skill-building among children and their families, including domains such as anger management, social competency, problem solving, communication, and decision making. A critical aspect of the model program is the assignment of a case coordinator to integrate multiple environmental and social contexts into prevention programming. For example, case coordinators should teach parenting

Table 5.2. Components of a model youth violence prevention program

Targets of intervention	Males and females
	Families experiencing conflict and/or domestic violence
	Children who display aggression or poor behavior and/ or who are diagnosed with aggressive/hyperactivity disorders
	Offenders' families
	Both general and high-risk populations
Content of intervention	Parent training
	Stress management for parents
	Anger management for parents and children
	Innovative teaching techniques (e.g., role playing)
	Community referrals when necessary (tutoring programs, mentors)
Outcomes of intervention	Reduce incidence of aggressive behavior
	Increase family cohesion
	Increase commitment to school
	Increase appropriate parenting practices
Costs and duration	One year of intense intervention beginning at the onset of aggressive behavior; booster sessions from first through twelfth grades

skills (e.g., discipline practices, appropriate modeling and mentoring techniques, stress management tactics) and social skills to parents and their children, as well as assist teachers in designing and implementing innovative instructional techniques to engage their students. Multiple teaching methods (e.g., role playing, small-group activities) should be employed to respect children's diverse learning styles. In addition, a model program should encourage and assist participants in using resources available in their community such as church organizations, community centers, and after-school programs as a way to increase the amount and types of supports and/or protective factors used by the family.

If implemented correctly, with a high level of treatment fidelity, this model program should prevent the development and/or reduce the incidence of aggressive behaviors both in children in general and children who are at risk. To promote the maintenance of treatment success, booster sessions targeting areas such as anger management tactics training should be taught by both parents and teachers from first through twelfth grades.

Critical Components of a Model Program for Preventing Youth Violence

The planning and implementation of prevention programs for families and children has shifted toward community-based, multicomponent approaches that are rooted in partnerships among diverse stakeholders (Nelson, Amio, Prilleltensky, & Nickels, 2000). Research on youth violence has benefited from integrating the paradigms of several disciplines and subspecialties, including public health as well as developmental, community, and clinical psychology (Reppucci et al., 1999). Most programs for preventing youth violence have been based on the belief that a particular strategy will work to reduce the risk of teenagers engaging in violent behavior and/or to build resilience to protect them from exerting violence (National Youth Violence Prevention Resource Center [NYVPC], 2003).

Experts believe that effective programs build on the understanding that individuals operate within a complex network of individual, family, community, and environmental contexts that affect their capacity to avoid risk (NYVPC, 2003). Solutions, therefore, must be designed to strengthen each of these spheres of influence with the goal of reducing overall risk. Multiple reviews of intervention programs have identified several key characteristics of successful programs: using a broad-based approach; targeting multiple issues in multiple domains; and focusing on behavior in its social context, including coordinating strategies across social domains (Mulvey, Arthur, & Reppucci, 1993; Slaby, 1998; Tolan, Guerra, & Kendall, 1995). Programs modeled on a public health approach to addressing risk factors and introducing new protective factors have been identified by the Office of Juvenile Justice and Delinquency Prevention's Study Group on Serious and Violent Juvenile Offenders as the most promising prevention and early intervention strategy (NYVPC, 2003). Moreover, to be most effective, it is imperative that violence prevention programs incorporate appropriate timing. One such program identified as *promising* by *Youth Violence: A Report of the Surgeon General* (USDHHS, 1999, 2001) places a special emphasis on targeting children prior to the emergence of violent behavior. The next section discusses the Seattle Social Development Project, with a special emphasis on its incorporation of appropriate timing.

The Seattle Social Development Project

The Seattle Social Development Project believes that it is important to build children's decision-making, negotiating, and problem-solving skills prior to, as well as during, children's engagement with antisocial peers. As such, first-grade children are recruited to participate. The program is a prospective, school-based longitudinal study of risk and protective factors, as well as the development of prosocial and antisocial behaviors for urban students who are socioeconomically disadvantaged in first through sixth grades (Chung et al., 2002). The multidimensional intervention has been shown to decrease juveniles' problem behaviors by working with parents, teachers, and children. It incorporates both social control and prosocial bonds, strengthens attachment and commitment to schools, and has been shown to decrease delinquency (Hawkins et al., 1998). Though simple in design, the intervention has shown that school programs focused on improving academic performance and children's bonding to school and family and reducing antisocial behaviors can produce reductions in early aggressiveness and long-term reductions in violent behaviors (Hawkins et al.). In general, the Seattle Social Development Project is an excellent example of a program that has appropriate timing. Though the program has not reached the status of a *model* program, it does highlight possible ways in which future and present youth violence prevention programs can incorporate appropriate timing through a focus on increasing family management practices, communication, and attachment in families prior to the emergence of aggressive behaviors among their children. The remainder of this chapter presents a case study of a child at risk for developing aggressive and/or violent behaviors due to familial circumstances and personal characteristics.

❖

The Jackson Family

The Jackson family has experienced prolonged family conflict stemming from the long hours Mr. Jackson has been devoting to his career. In particular, Steven, age 7, has found himself caught in the middle of his parent's recurring arguments over his mother's inability to parent him appropriately. Steven has begun to resent his diagnosis of attention-deficit/hyperactivity disorder (ADHD) and feels that if he had never been born, his parents wouldn't have reasons to argue and fight with each other. During a recent fight between his parents, Steven was shocked at his own overwhelming urge to scream and lash out at them.

Because of the conflicts with her husband, Mrs. Jackson has found that she doesn't have the energy necessary to take care of a child diagnosed with ADHD. She finds that she has to make repeated requests and demands of Steven. His reaction to this is to whine, yell, or refuse to comply. Mrs. Jackson realizes that she needs to choose her battles and that she all too often decides to *give in* or *back off* in arguments with her son. Just like his father, Steven has recognized that aggressive outbursts are an effective means to get his way with his mother. Mrs. Jackson worries that even though giving in decreases her stress level in the short term, she is reinforcing negative behavior in her child, which may lead Steven to an aggressive disposition, poor social skills, failure in school, peer rejection, and, subsequently, engagement in violent behaviors.

Due to the tensions at home, Steven has found that he doesn't like being around his parents and finds it hard to concentrate on his schoolwork. Though his grades are okay, he is no longer excited about attending school because of how difficult it is for him to mask his feelings about the problems at home. His friends have begun to accuse him of having a short temper and of playing too aggressively; thus, they no longer invite him to play with them during recess or after-school activities. Steven is disappointed because it was only through interacting with friends and playing sports that he felt he was able to relieve the aggression building inside.

Application of the Model Program to the Jackson Family

When Steven began the fourth grade, his teacher announced that they were starting a new program. Each day, the class would spend time talking about different issues that were important to kids. At first, Steven was skeptical. What do adults at school know about his problems? His teacher explained that they would be playing games and role-playing in the classroom. Steven was excited because even if they couldn't help him with his troubles, this would take some time away from *real* school, which seemed to be getting more and more difficult for him.

During the first class activity, the group talked about different emotions that people feel and how they can control themselves in emotional situations. Steven listened to people talk and couldn't believe that other kids had parents who argued a lot too—he thought he was the only one. He began thinking about how he had recently been treating his friends when his feelings overwhelmed him. It made him sad that the other kids didn't ask him to play with them anymore, but now he was starting to understand why.

When Steven got home, his parents asked him about the program at school. He said it was fine and was surprised to hear from them that there were parent meetings at school in the evenings every week. Not only that, but there also was someone called a *case coordinator* from the program who was going to come to his house every month. His parents explained that although every family has its struggles, each one is different, and with the help of the case coordinator, his family was going to start making the most of what their community has to offer.

Before long, Steven started to learn more ways to handle his emotions. He practiced constructive techniques to handle conflict, such as compromising with others and keeping a journal rather than yelling and hitting. He noticed that his mother wasn't giving in to him anymore, even when he made a fuss. Instead, she had been standing her ground and calmly discussing issues with him. He thought this had something to do with the parent meetings they attended. Thanks to his case coordinator, Steven began receiving tutoring and was involved in a mentoring program. He looked up to his mentor and was able to tell him things that he couldn't tell his parents—it was almost like having an older brother. His parents started going to marital counseling so that they could nip their problems in the bud before things got out of control. They also joined a support group for parents of children with ADHD, which helped them connect with others in their community who share the unique challenges of raising a hyperactive child.

The Jackson family continues to participate in the aggression prevention program, and they continue to make progress. They still experience difficult times—Steven sometimes struggles in school and his parents become stressed and argue every once in a while—but they have a greater repertoire of effective tools for coping with these challenging circumstances. For example, Steven can communicate with others regarding his frustrations and address them before they escalate. Rather than fight, Steven's parents calmly discuss their disagreements behind closed doors. Most important, the Jackson family has an extensive support network rooted in their community, which helps them get through times of trouble. The Jackson family is an excellent illustration of success in terms of the goals of effective violence prevention programming.

❖

Improving Violence Prevention Programs

Understandably, the pressure to respond immediately to crisis situations has often resulted in well-intentioned programs that lack a clear theoretical base or evaluative component (Reppucci et al., 1999). Fortunately, each of the three youth violence prevention programs presented in this chapter possesses qualities that set them apart from existing programs. Most important, each prevention program is grounded in existing theories and documents short- as well as long-term program effectiveness such as building positive relationships, training staff, and using varied teaching methods. Nonetheless, each program has an overall shortcoming in one general area: timing of implementation. Research on intervention programs has shown timing to play a major role in the effectiveness of programs (Kirby, 2002). Timing of implementation is particularly important for prevention programs focusing on delinquency and violence prevention in that changes need to be set in place prior to children reaching adolescence (the period children are thought to act on their aggression). In accord with this finding, the Seattle Social Development Project acknowledges the importance of timing; thus serving as a guideline for future youth violence interventions.

REFERENCES

Amodei, N., & Scott, A.A. (2002). Psychologists' contributions to the prevention of youth violence. *The Social Science Journals, 39,* 511-526.

Anderson, J.F., Dyson, L., & Grandison, T. (1998). African-Americans, violence, disabilities, and public policy: A call for a workable approach to alleviating the pains of inner-city life. *The Western Journal of Black Studies, 22,* 94–102.

Aos, S., Phipps, P., Barnoski, R., & Leib, R. (2001). *The comparative costs and benefits of programs to reduce crime: Version 4.0.* Olympia: Washington State Institute for Public Policy.

Associated Press. (2000). *Justice: Youth imprisonment doubles.* Retrieved October, 22, 2004, from http://www.nospank.net

Bandura, A. (1977). *Social learning theory.* Oxford, England: Prentice Hall.

Bank, L., & Burraston, B. (2001). Abusive home environments as predictors of poor adjustment during adolescence and early adulthood. *Journal of Community Psychology, 29,* 195–217.

Bell, C. (1995, January 6). Exposure to violence distresses children and may lead to their becoming violent. *Psychiatric News,* pp. 6–18.

Borduin, C.M., Mann, B.J., Cone, L.T., Henggeler, S.W., Fucci, B.R., Blaske, D.M., et al. (1995). Multisystemic treatment of serious juvenile offenders: Long-term prevention of criminality and violence. *Journal of Consulting and Clinical Psychology, 63,* 569–578.

Braswell, L., & Kendall, P.C. (2001). Cognitive-behavioral therapy with youth. In K.S. Dobson (Ed.), *Handbook of cognitive-behavioral therapies* (2nd ed., pp. 246–294). New York: Guilford Press.

Brezina, T. (1999). Teenage violence toward parents as an adaptation to family strain: Evidence from a national survey of male adolescents. *Youth & Society, 30,* 416–444.

Bronfenbrenner, U. (1979). *The ecology of human development: Experiments by nature and design.* Cambridge, MA: Harvard University Press.

Catalano, R.F., & Hawkins, J.D. (1996). The social development model: A theory of antisocial behavior. In J.D. Hawkins (Ed.), *Delinquency and crime: Current theories* (pp. 149–197). New York: Cambridge University Press.

Catalano, R.F., Loeber, R., & McKinney, K.C. (1999, October). School and community intervention to prevent serious and violent offending. *Juvenile Justice Bulletin,* pp. 1–13.

Centers for Disease Control and Prevention (CDC). (2000). *Youth violence in the United States.* Retrieved December 1, 2003, from http://www.cdc.gov/ncipc/factsheets/yvfacts.htm

Centers for Disease Control and Prevention (CDC). (2001). *Web-based Injury Statistics Query and Reporting System (WISQARS)* [Online]. Retrieved December 1, 2003, from http://www.cdc.gov/ncipc/wisquars

Centers for Disease Control and Prevention (CDC). (2002). *Web-based Injury Statistics Query and Reporting System (WISQARS)* [Online]. Retrieved December 1, 2003, from http://www.cdc.gov/ncipc/factsheets/yvfacts.htm

Center for Substance Abuse Prevention (2004). *Multidimensional treatment foster care program.* Retrieved February 3, 2004, from http://casat.unr.edu/westcapt/bestpractices/view.php?program=60

Chamberlain, P., & Mihalic, S.F. (1998). *Blueprints for violence prevention: Book eight: Multidimensional treatment foster care.* Boulder, CO: Center for the Study and Prevention of Violence.

Chamberlain, P., & Reid, J.B. (1998). Comparison of two community alternatives to incarceration for chronic juvenile offenders. *Journal of Consulting and Clinical Psychology, 66,* 624–633.

Chung, I., Hill, K.G., Hawkins, J.D., Gilchrist, L.D., & Nagin, D.S. (2002). Childhood predictors of offense trajectories. *Journal of Research in Crime and Delinquency, 39,* 60–90.

Cohen, J.A., Berliner, L., & Mannarino, A.P. (2003). Psychosocial and pharmacological interventions for child crime victims. *Journal of Traumatic Stress, 16,* 175–186.

Coie, J.K., & Dodge, K.A. (1998). Aggression and antisocial behavior. In W. Damon & N. Eisenberg (Eds.), *Handbook of child psychology: Social, emotional, and personality development* (5th ed., Vol. 3, pp. 779–862). New York: John Wiley & Sons.

Conduct Problems Prevention Research Group (CPPRG). (1992). A developmental and clinical model for the prevention of conduct disorders: The Fast Track program. *Developmental and Psychopathology, 4,* 509–527.

Conduct Problems Prevention Research Group (CPPRG). (1999a). Initial impact of the Fast Track prevention trial for conduct problems: I. The high-risk sample. *Journal of Consulting and Clinical Psychology, 67,* 631–647.

Conduct Problems Prevention Research Group (CPPRG). (1999b). Initial impact of the Fast Track prevention trial for conduct problems: II. Classroom effects. *Journal of Consulting and Clinical Psychology, 67,* 648–657.

Conduct Problems Prevention Research Group (CPPRG). (2002a). The implementation of the Fast Track program: An example of a large-scale prevention science efficacy trial. *Journal of Abnormal Child Psychology, 30*(1), 1–17.

Conduct Problems Prevention Research Group (CPPRG). (2002b). Evaluation of the first 3 years of the Fast Track prevention trial with children at high risk for adolescent conduct problems. *Journal of Abnormal Child Psychology, 30*(1), 19–35.

Conduct Problems Prevention Research Group (CPPRG). (2002c). Using the Fast Track randomized prevention to test the early starter model of the development of serious conduct problems. *Development and Psychopathology, 14,* 925–943.

Conduct Problems Prevention Research Group (CPPRG). (2004). The effects of the Fast Track program on serious problem outcomes at the end of elementary school. *Journal of Clinical Child and Adolescent Psychology, 33,* 650–661.

Conduct Problems Prevention Research Group (CPPRG). (2005, May). *Fast Track program overview.* Retrieved September 5, 2005, from http://www.fasttrackproject.org/fasttrackoverview.htm

Cooley-Quille, M., Boyd, R.C., Frantz, E., & Walsh, J. (2001). Emotional and behavioral impact of exposure to community violence in inner-city adolescents. *Journal of Clinical Child Psychology, 30,* 199–206.

Eddy, J.M., & Chamberlain, P. (2000). Family management and deviant peer association as mediators of the impact of treatment condition on youth antisocial behavior. *Journal of Consulting and Clinical Psychology, 68,* 857–863.

Fagan, A.A. (2001). The gender cycle of violence: Comparing the effects of child abuse and neglect on criminal offending for males and females. *Violence and Victims, 16,* 457–474.

Fields, S.A., & McNamara, J.R. (2003). The prevention of child and adolescent violence: A review. *Aggression and Violent Behavior, 8,* 61–91.

Flannery, D.J., Singer, M., Williams, L., & Castro, P. (1998). Adolescent violence exposure and victimization at home: Coping and psychological trauma symptoms. *International Review of Victimology, 6,* 63–82.

Guerra, N.G., Attar, B., & Weissberg, R.P. (1997). Prevention of aggression and violence among inner-city youths. In D.M. Stoff, J. Breiling, & J.D. Maser (Eds.), *Handbook of Antisocial Behaviors* (pp. 375–383). New York: John Wiley & Sons.

Guerra, N.G., & Slaby, R.G. (1990). Cognitive mediators of aggression in adolescent offenders: II. Intervention. *Developmental Psychology, 26,* 269–277.

Haley, J. (1976). *Problem solving therapy.* San Francisco: Jossey-Bass.

Hawkins, J.D., Catalano, R.F., & Arthur, M.W. (2002). Promoting science-based prevention in communities. *Addictive Behaviors, 27,* 951–976.

Hawkins, J.D., Herrenkohl, T., Farrington, D.P., Brewer, D., Catalano, R.F., & Harachi, T.W. (1998). A review of predictors of youth violence. In D.P. Farrington & R. Loeber (Eds.), *Serious and violent juvenile offenders: Risk factors and successful interventions* (pp. 106–146). Thousand Oaks, CA: Sage Publications.

Henggeler, S.W. (1997). *Treating serious antisocial behavior in youth: The MST approach.* Washington, DC: U.S. Department of Justice, Office of Juvenile Justice and Delinquency Prevention.

Henggeler, S.W. (1999). Multisystemic therapy: An overview of clinical procedures, outcomes, and policy implications. *Child Psychology and Psychiatry Review, 4,* 2–10.

Henggeler, S.W., Cunningham, P.B., Pickrel, S.G., Schoenwald, S.K., & Brondino, M.J. (1996). Multisystemic therapy: An effective violence prevention approach for serious juvenile offenders. *Journal of Adolescence, 19,* 47–61.

Henggeler, S.W., Schoenwald, S.K., Pickrel, S.G., Brandino, S.J., & Hall, J.A. (1994). *Treatment manual for family preservation using multisystemic therapy.* Charleston: South Carolina Health and Human Services Finance Commission.

Hill, K.G., Howell, J.C., Hawkins, J.D., & Battin-Pearson, S.R. (1999). Childhood risk factors for adolescent gang membership: Results for the Seattle Social Development Project. *Journal of Research in Crime and Delinquency, 36,* 300–322.

Huey, S.J., Henggeler, S.W., Brondino, M.J., & Pickrel, S.G. (2000). Mechanisms of change in Multisystemic therapy: Reducing delinquent behavior through therapist adherence and improved family and peer functioning. *Journal of Consulting and Clinical Psychology, 68,* 451–467.

Kalil, A., & DeLeire, T. (2004). *Family investments in children's potential: Resources and parenting behaviors that promote success.* Mahwah, NJ: Lawrence Erlbaum Associates.

Kelly, B.T., Huizinga, D., Thornberry, T., & Loeber, R. (1997). *Epidemiology of serious violence.* Washington, DC: Office of Juvenile Justice and Delinquency Prevention.

Kirby, D. (2002). Effective approaches to reducing adolescent unprotected sex, pregnancy, and childbearing. *The Journal of Sex Research, 39,* 51–57.

Kirkpatrick, D.G., & Acierno, R. (2003). Mental health needs of crime victims: Epidemiology and outcomes. *Journal of Traumatic Stress, 16,* 119–132.

Kusché, C.A., & Greenberg, M.T. (1994). *The PATHS curriculum.* Seattle, WA: Developmental Research and Programs.

Loeber R., & Stouthamer-Loeber, M. (1998). Development of juvenile aggression and violence: Some common misconceptions and controversies. *American Psychologist, 53,* 242–259.

Lowry, R., Sleet, D., Duncan, C., Powell, K., & Kolbe, L. (1995). Adolescents at risk for violence. *Educational Psychological Review, 7,* 7–39.

McQueen, A. (2000). *Report: Youth imprisonment doubles.* Retrieved October 22, 2004, from http://www.commondreams.org/headlines

Miller, L.S., & Wasserman, G.A. (1999). Witnessed community violence and antisocial behavior in high-risk, urban boys. *Journal of Clinical Child Psychology, 28,* 2–11.

Minuchin, S. (1974). *Families and family therapy.* Cambridge, MA: Harvard University Press.

Moffitt, T.E. (1993). Adolescence-limited and life-course-persistent antisocial behavior: A development taxonomy. *Psychological Review, 100,* 674–701.

Moore, K.J., Sprengelmeyer, P.G., & Chamberlain, P. (2001). Community-based treatment for adjudicated delinquents: The Oregon Social Learning Center's "Monitor" Multidimensional Treatment Foster Care Program. *Residential Treatment for Children and Youths, 18,* 87–97.

Mulvey, P.D., Arthur, M.W., & Reppucci, N.D. (1993). The prevention and treatment of juvenile delinquency: A review of the research. *Clinical Psychological Review, 13,* 133–167.

Munger, R.L. (1993). *Changing children's behavior quickly.* Lanham, MD: Madison Books.

Nagin, D., & Tremblay, R.E. (1999). Trajectories of boys' physical aggression, opposition and hyperactivity on the path to physically violent and nonviolent juvenile delinquency. *Child Development, 70,* 1181–1196.

National Association of School Psychologists. (2003). *Preventing youth violence.* http://www.naspoline.org/advocacy/youth_violence

National Youth Violence Prevention Resource Center. (2003). *Youth violence prevention and intervention.* Retrieved December 1, 2003, from http://www.safeyouth.org/topics/intervention

Nelson. G., Amio, J.L., Prilleltensky, I., & Nickels, P. (2000). Partnerships for implementing school and community prevention programs. *Journal of Educational and Psychological Consultation, 11,* 121–146.

O'Rourke, T.W. (2003). Methodological techniques for dealing with missing data. *American Journal of Health Studies, 18,* 165–168.

Osofsky, J.D. (2003). Prevalence of children's exposure to domestic violence and child maltreatment: Implications for prevention and intervention. *Clinical Child and Family Psychology Review, 6,* 161–170.

Overstreet, S., & Dempsey, M. (1999). Availability of family support as a moderator of exposure to community violence. *Journal of Clinical Child Psychology, 28,* 151–159.

Pathrow-Stith, D. (1987). *Violence prevention curriculum for adolescents.* Newton, MA: Education Development Center.

Patterson, G.R. (1986). Performance models for antisocial boys. *American Psychologist, 41,* 432–444.

Pearce, M.J., Jones, S.M., Schwab-Stone, M.E., & Ruchkin, V. (2003). The protective effects of religiousness and parent involvement on the development of conduct problems among youth exposed to violence. *Child Development, 74,* 1682–1696.

Reppucci, N.D., Woolard, J.L., & Fried, C.S. (1999). Social, community, and preventive interventions. *Annual Reviews Psychology, 50,* 387–418.

Shields, A., & Cicchetti, D. (2001). Parental maltreatment and emotion dysregulation as risk factors for bullying and victimization in middle childhood. *Journal of Clinical Child Psychology, 30,* 349–363.

Singer, M.I., Anglin, T.M., Song, L.Y., & Lunghofer, L. (1995). Adolescents' exposure to violence and associated symptoms of psychological trauma. *Journal of the American Medical Association, 273,* 477–482.

Slaby, R.G. (1998). Preventing youth violence through research-guided intervention. In P. Trickett & C. Schellenbach (Eds.), *Violence against children in the family and the community* (pp. 371–399). Washington, DC: American Psychological Association.

Snyder, H., & Sickmund, M. (1995). *Juvenile offenders and victims: 1995 national report.* Washington, DC: Office of Juvenile Justice and Delinquency Prevention.

Snyder, J., Brooder, M., Patrick, M.R., Snyder, A., Schrepferman, L., & Stoolmiller, M. (2003). Observed peer victimization during early elementary school: Continuity, growth, and relation to risk for child antisocial and depressive behavior. *Child Development, 74,* 1881–1898.

Substance Abuse and Mental Health Services Administration. (n.d.). *Multisystemic therapy: Model programs.* Retrieved December 15, 2003, from http://model programs.samhsa. gov/template_cf.cfm?page=model&pkProgramID=21

Thornton, T.N., Craft, C.A., Dahlberg, L.L., Lynch, B.S., & Baer. K. (2000). *Best practices of youth violence prevention: A sourcebook for community action.* Atlanta, GA: Centers for Disease Control and Prevention, National Center for Injury Prevention and Control.

Thornton, T.N., Craft, C.A., Dahlberg, L.L. Lynch, B.S., & Baer. K. (2002). *Best practices of youth violence prevention: A sourcebook for community action* (Rev. ed.). Atlanta, GA: Centers for Disease Control and Prevention, National Center for Injury Prevention and Control.

Tolan, P.H., Guerra, N.G., & Kendall, P.C. (1995). A developmental-ecological perspective on antisocial behavior in children and adolescents: Towards a unified risk and intervention framework. *Journal of Consulting and Clinical Psychology, 63,* 560–568.

Tremblay, R.E., Pagani-Kurtz, L., Masse, L.C., Vitaro, F., & Phil, R.O. (1995). A bimodal-preventive intervention for disruptive kindergarten boys: Its impact through mid-adolescence. *Journal of Consulting Clinical Psychology, 65,* 579–584.

Ulman, A., & Straus, M.A. (2003). Violence by children against mothers in relation to violence between parents and corporal punishment by parents. *Journal of Comparative Family Studies, 34,* 41–60.

U.S. Department of Health and Human Services (USDHHS). (1999). *Youth violence: A report of the Surgeon General: Executive summary.* Rockville, MD: U.S. Department of Health and Human Services, Centers for Disease Control and Prevention, National Center for Injury Prevention and Control; Substance Abuse and Mental Health Services, Center for Mental Health Service; and National Institutes of Health, National Institute of Mental Health.

U.S. Department of Health and Human Services (USDHHS). (2001). *Youth violence: A report of the Surgeon General: Executive summary.* Rockville, MD: U.S. Department of Health and Human Services, Centers for Disease Control and Prevention, National Center for Injury Prevention and Control; Substance Abuse and Mental Health Services, Center for Mental Health Service; and National Institutes of Health, National Institute of Mental Health.

Widom, C.S. (1991). Childhood victimization: Risk factor for delinquency. In M.E. Colton, & S. Gore (Eds.), *Adolescent stress: Causes and consequences* (pp. 201–221). New York: Aldine de Gruyter.

6

PREVENTING ADOLESCENT SUBSTANCE ABUSE

Amber M. Grundy and Stacey B. Scott

Avoiding substance abuse is "one of the fundamental challenges faced by adolescents in modern society" (Simons-Morton & Haynie, 2003, p. 109). Monitoring the Future, a federally sponsored annual national survey of adolescents, found that nearly 50% of eighth-grade students reported having used alcohol at least once in their lifetime (Johnston, O'Malley, & Bachman, 2003). Furthermore, more than one fifth reported having been drunk by the eighth grade (Johnston et al., 2003). The Office of National Drug Control Policy (ONDCP, 2000) estimated that the cost of drug abuse to society was $143.4 billion in 1998, with an expected increase of 5.9% each year. The majority of these costs were the result of loss of productivity due to incarceration, crime careers, drug abuse related illness, and premature death (ONDCP, 2000). Most programs to prevent substance abuse are targeted at youth because early use of drugs has been identified as a risk factor for later use and associated criminal activity (Center for Substance Abuse Prevention [CSAP], 1999).

PREVENTION PROGRAMS: DESIGN AND IMPLEMENTATION ISSUES

Both federal and private funding agencies have placed an emphasis on science-based prevention programs. Despite this focus and the funding attached to it, many communities, and even the federal government, continue to invest in programs with limited demonstrated effectiveness (Hawkins, Catalano, & Arthur,

2002). In 2003, the National Institute of Drug Abuse (NIDA) reported that only one in seven schools utilize prevention programs that include components and present content that have been found to be effective (Zickler, 2003). Blanket funding has been granted to school-based programs such as Drug Abuse Resistance Education (DARE) that have proven to be ineffective (Ennet, Tobler, Ringwalt, & Flewelling, 1994).

Making Prevention Programs Work in Schools

Effective prevention programs share some common characteristics such as the use of control groups and pretesting. Using comparison samples and pretest information is critical because they allow substance abuse prevention programs to examine the effects of the program while controlling for other factors such as simply being involved in a program or age differences. Specifically, the control groups should be *active controls* so that the program effects can be distinguished from the effects of just receiving increased attention. Mass media campaigns targeting substance abuse such as the ongoing "Partnership for a Drug Free America" are problematic because they have no control group and typically have no pretest data against which they can compare results (Crano & Burgoon, 2002).

School is the most common environment in which youth encounter drug prevention. The most successful programs do not target specific drugs or populations at risk; instead, effective school-based prevention programs are aimed at increasing general life skills; promoting protective factors; and diminishing risk factors such as a family history of drug and alcohol abuse, conduct problems at home and at school, ineffective family communication, or negative peer influence (RAND, 2002). The leading paradigm for school-based programs in the United States is a life skills training approach, which focuses on the promotion of refusal skills to deal with pressure to use drugs as well as personal development to offset risk factors motivating drug use (Roe & Becker, 2005).

Although schools are common sites for prevention programs, youth live, learn, and make choices in environments outside of school. Peer influence is a major factor in problem behavior onset in youth (Johnston et al., 2003). Parents also play a role in the initiation of problem behaviors. Avoiding alcohol and drug use has been linked to concern over parental disapproval of substance use (Kumpfer & Alvarado, 2003). Furthermore, researchers have found that a family environment made up of positive parent–child relationships, parental supervision, and consistent discipline, combined with communication of family values, is the major reason youth do not engage in delinquent or unhealthy behaviors (see Kumpfer & Alvarado). Thus, it is important for prevention programs to impact all aspects of the lives of youth, including school, home, and community environments.

Both the Substance Abuse and Mental Health Services Administration (SAMHSA) and NIDA regularly publish lists describing promising, exemplary, and model programs to promote the use of research-based findings in communities; however, the effectiveness of the *model* programs are not undisputed (e.g., Gorman, 2002). Disagreements over what qualifies as a model program have led agencies to use disparate criteria for evaluation and thus frequent promotion of different prevention curricula.

Although research-based prevention and intervention programs represent an important move forward in promoting positive youth development, simply choosing an empirically based curriculum does not guarantee successful outcomes. The match between the prevention method chosen and the community is also an important consideration. Regardless of whether the program selected is implemented at the school, family, or community level, the research-based intervention must fit the needs of the community. Although it is unlikely that a panacea will ever be developed, it is clear that the most effective method for preventing maladaptive outcomes involves choosing an individual curriculum for a particular target group that is best suited to that group's unique risk and protective factors (Kumpfer, n.d.).

Making Prevention Programs Work in Communities

Community groups may be a key to making science-based prevention work. Grass roots organizations are made up of stakeholders in the community who are familiar with the unique characteristics of the target group (Kumpfer, Turner, Hopkins, & Librett, 1993). Since its founding in 1992, the Community Anti-Drug Coalitions of America (CADCA) has grown to more than 5,000 coalitions (CADCA, n.d.; Ellis & Lenczner, 2000), providing a formalized forum for grass roots action. CADCA offers support for its members on topics ranging from starting a coalition to suggestions for proposal writing and funding sources. It also collects outcome data from coalitions. National sharing conferences and institutes allow coalition members to meet with other members, receive training, and learn about research-based programs synthesized by a scientific advisory panel (CADCA, 2003).

A second issue in the gap between science and practice is that of scaling up prevention programs. Schinke, Cole, Diaz, and Botvin (1997) highlighted the importance of developing techniques for translating effective programs and components into consistent successes outside of empirical trials. CADCA materials and guides such as Borkowski and Weaver's (2006) bring science-based programs to community groups in an accessible format. Beyond choosing an empirically based program, community-based prevention efforts often struggle due to a lack of tools and training that would allow them to increase involvement, effectively define their goals, and track their progress (Hawkins et al., 2002). Communities need resources and support to make what has been demonstrated in scientific trials work in their own communities. Biglan, Flay, and Foster (2003) concurred, suggesting that if communities hope to replicate the effects found in prevention research, they need similar services, supports, and monitoring so that the programs are implemented as designed.

Prevention operating systems such as Communities That Care (CTC; Hawkins et al., 2002) have emerged as intensive support and guidance systems for communities planning, implementing, and evaluating prevention programs. CTC is commercially available and uses a system of strategies for motivating communities to use prevention science in their planning and implementation of community prevention programming (CTC, 2003). In the early phases, community leaders and stakeholders assess the community's readiness for change and receive training in tenets of community- and research-based prevention, including community mobilization skills and interpreting profiles of their community's risk and protective factors. Community board members work to take advantage of existing policies, programs, and services and identify gaps to address the risk and protective factors identified by the epidemiological data. The board then develops an action plan using the baseline assessment data to define clear and measurable goals. The board learns about tested policies, programs, and actions that have been effective for creating change in the areas they have selected. Programs are chosen from the CTC guide to research-based programs and coordinated with existing programs and resources. Special attention is paid to planning for monitoring implementation and assessing progress.

The services provided by CTC and similar consulting systems offer essential supports for community-based prevention efforts. However, the monetary costs of such consultations may not be feasible for grass roots, volunteer-based groups such as coalitions. Although CADCA provides information on a variety of relevant topics, including grant writing, hands-on consultation such as that exemplified by CTC is not readily available. For science-based prevention to work, programs need to both fit their target and be implemented effectively. Responding to both of these needs requires the involvement of committed parties with detailed knowledge of the community and a systematic method of developing and completing a project.

PREVENTION PROGRAMS AND THEIR EVALUATIONS

To facilitate this next step, four prevention programs are identified in this chapter and are evaluated in terms of their treatment, procedural, and design characteristics. The programs included in this review were chosen based on their exemplary characteristics, comprehensiveness, and documented outcomes. Two school-based programs, Life Skills Training (LST) and Promoting Alternative Thinking Strategies (PATHS); one family-based program, Strengthening Families Program (SFP); and one combined school- and family-based program, the Incredible Years Series (IYS), are detailed and evaluated in this chapter to scaffold careful choice, implementation, and evaluation of research-based programs. The essential characteristics of these programs are summarized in Table 6.1.

Life Skills Training

Life Skills Training (LST) is a universal, school-based program that aims to influence the chief social and psychological factors that promote the initiation and early use of substances (Botvin & Griffin, 2004; Schinke, Brounstein, & Gardner, 2002). The primary goals of the program are to promote skill development (e.g., drug resistance, self-management) and to provide a broader knowledge base concerning substance abuse (Trudeau, Spoth, Lillehoj, Redmond, & Wickrama, 2003).

Program Description　LST is based on the principles of social learning theory (Bandura, 1977) and problem behavior theory (Jessor & Jessor, 1977). These theoretical underpinnings direct LST's aims: 1) to provide adolescents with the necessary knowledge and skills to resist social influences to use tobacco, alcohol, and other drugs and 2) to reduce potential motivation to use substances by increasing personal and social competencies (Botvin, 1986). LST curriculum teaches students cognitive–behavioral skills to build self-esteem, resist advertising pressure, manage anxiety, communicate effectively, develop personal relationships, and assert their rights—skills related empirically and conceptually to lower use of tobacco, alcohol, and other drugs (Botvin, Griffin, Diaz, & Ifill-Williams, 2001).

Typically, trained classroom teachers deliver the LST curriculum over 3 years. The role of the teacher is that of a skills trainer or coach, using instruction, demonstration, rehearsal, feedback, praise, and behavioral homework practice to teach cognitive-behavioral skills. The program also has been successfully implemented by trained outside professionals and older peer leaders. Teachers or leaders attend a 2-day workshop by a certified Life Skills trainer to promote program fidelity and effectiveness (Botvin, Mihalic, & Grotpeter, 1998).

LST provides skills training in three domains: drug resistance, personal self-management, and general social. Drug resistance training targets misconceptions about tobacco, alcohol, and other drugs. In this component, teachers use coaching to help youth learn accurate information about drugs as well as develop and practice skills for overcoming the pressure to use substances from sources such as their peers and the media (Botvin et al., 1998). Personal self-management training focuses on examining self-image, decision making, and stress and setting goals

Table 6.1. Four substance abuse prevention programs and their defining characteristics

	Life Skills Training (LST)	Promoting Alternative Thinking Strategies (PATHS)	Strengthening Families Program (SFP)	Incredible Years Series (IYS)
Targets of intervention	Males and females	Males and females	Males and females	Males and females
	Grade 3 or 4	Kindergarten through sixth grade	Children ages 6–12 years and their parents	Children at risk ages 2–8 years
	Grade 6 or 7	School based	Family based	Parents
	Booster sessions after middle school			Teachers
	School based			School and family
Content of intervention	Provide adolescents with the knowledge and skills to resist social influence to use alcohol and drugs	Training in:	Goals:	Videotaped vignettes
		Emotional understanding	Communication skills	Home workbooks
		Self-control	Effective discipline strategies	Group sessions
	Reduce motivation to use alcohol and drugs by increasing personal and social competencies	Peer relationships	Problem-solving skills	Classroom management training
		Family communication skills	Understanding and controlling emotions	Child training in:
		Classroom behavior	Peer pressure resistance	Emotional literacy
	Optional violence prevention component		Methods:	Conflict management
			Family activities	Problem-solving skills
			Observation and role play	Positive peer interactions
			Videotapes	

Outcomes of intervention	Reduced drug use and polydrug use 6 years after completion of the program Lower rates of drinking frequency, drunkenness frequency, and drinking quantity Lower rates of smoking, marijuana use, and inhalant use	Improved scores on self-control, understanding and recognition of emotions, and ability to tolerate frustration More effective conflict resolution strategies Increased planning skills Decreased rates of aggression and conduct problems Cognitive gains Decreased depression	Reduced rates of conduct disorder Increased social competency Improved family relationships Improved communication Delayed initiation of substance use	Reduced child aggression Increased prosocial behavior Decreased criticism and increased praise of children by parents Increased use of constructive behaviors Decreased total problem behavior Improved classroom management behaviors
Cost and/or Duration	3 years during elementary and middle school	7 years, beginning in kindergarten	Fourteen-session program Up to $9.60 benefit-to-cost ratio per $1	Parent program: up to 30 weeks Teacher program: 42-hour workshop Child program: 22–24 2-hour sessions

and keeping track of progress. General social training concentrates on effective communication to help students overcome shyness, avoid misunderstandings, utilize verbal and nonverbal assertiveness skills, and develop positive responses rather than aggression and passivity in difficult situations.

LST has distinct elementary and middle school curricula. The elementary school LST curriculum is designed for implementation in either third or fourth grade. It consists of 24 30- to 45-minute class sessions delivered over 3 years. All of the LST skill areas are covered in the 1st year during eight class sessions. Eight booster sessions during the 2nd and 3rd years are designed to present opportunities for additional skill development and practice in key areas. The middle school LST curriculum is designed to be implemented initially with sixth- or seventh-grade students and consists of 15 45-minute sessions during the 1st year. The participants then receive 10 LST booster sessions during the next 2 years. In the 3rd year, there are five additional booster sessions. An optional violence prevention component can be added to the middle school curriculum through three additional sessions during the lst year and two additional sessions each during the 2nd and 3rd years. Both the elementary and middle school curricula can be taught over an intensive (daily or two to three times a week) or extended (once a week) schedule; there is evidence of equal effectiveness for both programs (Schinke et al., 2002).

Program Evaluation   More than a dozen evaluations of LST have been conducted since the mid-1980s, making it one of the most extensively evaluated school-based drug and alcohol use prevention programs. Studies have examined the effects of LST in schools consisting of students who were Caucasian and from middle-class families, ethnic minorities (primarily African American and Hispanic), youth from the inner city, and students who lived in the suburbs and in rural areas (Schinke et al., 2002; Vicary et al., 2004).

Botvin, Baker, Dusenbury, Botvin, and Diaz (1995) examined the long-term efficacy of LST through a randomized trial involving 3,597 twelfth-grade students who were predominately Caucasian at 56 suburban and rural public schools in New York State. Follow-up data were collected 6 years after baseline using school, telephone, and mailed surveys concerning frequency and amount of tobacco, alcohol, and marijuana use. Implementation fidelity in the treatment groups was monitored in randomly selected classes. Botvin et al. (1995) found prevention effects for variables assessing drug use and polydrug use. They also found even stronger prevention effects for drug use and polydrug use in analyses of the subsample that received a relatively complete version of the prevention program, the high fidelity sample (Botvin et al.).

Six and a half years after baseline, Botvin et al. (2000) examined the effects of LST on illicit drug use with a subsample of the original New York State sample. Follow-up questionnaires asked participants how often they used any illicit drugs belonging to 13 different categories (marijuana, cocaine, amphetamines, Quaaludes, barbiturates, tranquilizers, heroin, narcotics other than heroin, inhalants, amyl or butyl nitrates, LSD, PCP, and MDMA). Only 5% of the entire sample had ever used marijuana at baseline; however, at follow-up, the LST group reported significantly lower than the *treatment as usual* control group on heroin and other narcotic use, hallucinogenic use, total illicit substance abuse, and total illicit substance abuse other than marijuana (Botvin et al.).

To examine the effectiveness of LST with other populations, Botvin et al. (2001) conducted a randomized trial of LST with 3,621 minority students from low-income families in 29 New York City middle schools. No significant differences were found for any of the substance use variables at baseline; however, at 3 months posttreatment, the LST group had significantly lower scores than the control group on each of the alcohol measures including drinking frequency, drunkenness frequency, and drinking quantity. Significant effects also were found for lifetime polydrug use, with lower use reported by the LST intervention group than the control group.

At 1-year follow-up, students who participated in LST as well as booster sessions had significantly lower smoking frequency, smoking quantity, drinking frequency, frequency of getting drunk, and number of drinks per episode compared with the control groups. Significant prevention effects for the LST group also were found for frequency of marijuana use, getting high, and inhalant use. Students who received LST reported less lifetime polydrug use and current polydrug use than students in the control condition. In addition, intervention students reported lower normative expectations for smoking and drinking by peers and adults and scored higher than the control group on drug refusal skill efficacy than the control group. They also scored lower on risk taking and delinquency variables than students in the control condition (Botvin et al., 2001).

Spoth, Redmond, Trudeau, and Shin (2002) examined the effect of providing both family and child skill training in 10- to 14-year-old rural children by implementing both LST and SFP (detailed in this chapter). Compared with LST alone and a control group, students who participated in LST and SFP showed the lowest new-user rate. In addition, for students in the combined LST and SFP condition, there was a 30% relative reduction rate for alcohol initiation as compared with a 4.1% reduction in the LST-only condition. Both the LST-only and combined conditions had significantly lower new-user rates for marijuana than the control group. The desired effects may be magnified by providing substance use prevention both in school and within the family. With the current emphasis on achievement and accountability in schools, dedicating time solely to prevention may prove difficult. A recent evaluation of LST responded to this need with an infused teaching option, wherein teachers receive training to integrate LST principles into curricular content areas (Smith et al., 2004). In a 2-year comparison of the infused and traditional LST programs in nine rural school districts, the programs were nearly equally effective at 1 year, but LST was more cost-effective (Swisher, Smith, Vicary, Bechtel, & Hopkins, 2004). At 2 years, the infused program was more costly but also more cost-effective because it was the only approach with any effects. This teaching method has not yet been replicated but provides potential choices for districts without the flexibility to have stand-alone prevention programming.

Critical Analysis of Treatment Characteristics　The LST curriculum is directed by its roots in social learning theory and problem behavior theory. LST, therefore, focuses on building the individual student's cognitive and behavioral skills to resist substances and increase personal and social competencies. In addition to being theory driven, LST employs a variety of teaching techniques to help students learn, practice, and use these skills. Group discussions, demonstrations, modeling, behavioral rehearsal, feedback and reinforcement, and out-of-class behavioral assignments provide students with multiple opportunities to work on their skills for resisting substances.

This prevention program lacks strong efforts to promote positive relationships, particularly with adults, and attempts to address community and family factors. Life skills should be taught in and applied to all areas of the students' lives, rather than solely in the classroom sessions. An at-home video-based parent component is available through the LST publisher; however, it has not been examined empirically nor does it display the interactive teaching methods or program monitoring that are characteristic of effective interventions. Integrating families and the community into the individual, focused prevention is an important area for future development of this program. Intervening at both the individual and family levels, as Spoth, Redmond et al. (2002) examined with LST and SFP, would increase comprehensiveness and may magnify the effects of LST.

Critical Analysis of Procedural Characteristics　Both the elementary and middle school versions of LST provide sufficient dosage through curriculum spread over multiple years and the use of booster sessions. Booster sessions reinforce the goals of the previous years' sessions, focusing on skill development in social resistance, self-management, and global social skills (Spoth, Redmond et al., 2002). These booster sessions also provide an opportunity for staff to monitor students' understanding and for students to practice their skills.

Although the elementary school version has not been tested as extensively as the middle school version, the development of a substance abuse prevention curriculum for younger students based on a well-researched existing program is encouraging and potentially important for addressing concerns of effective timing of prevention programs. LST puts a strong emphasis on staff training in order to promote successful implementation and treatment fidelity. Technical support, including site visits and telephone and e-mail support, is available to staff who have attended the LST training.

Critical Analysis of Design Characteristics   Employing active control groups lends strength to LST's interpretative standards. For example, in addition to a *treatment-as-usual* control group, Botvin and colleagues (1995) included two treatment groups: a formal workshop training with project staff feedback group and a videotape training with no feedback group. By including these differentially trained treatments and an active control, the researchers were able to examine both the effect of treatment on behavior and the effect of training on treatment. Unfortunately, effect sizes were not provided in the LST research reviewed. However, when comparing treatment and control groups on an outcome, it is important to keep in mind that although the absolute difference between the groups may seem small, the social significance may be of great magnitude. For example, Botvin and colleagues (1995) found that rates of heavy cigarette smoking was 25% lower, and monthly and weekly cigarette smoking were 15%–27% lower among the intervention group as compared with the control group, suggesting the long-term prevention of 60,000 to 100,000 deaths per year (Botvin et al.).

Promoting Alternative Thinking Strategies

The Promoting Alternative Thinking Strategies (PATHS) curriculum was developed by Kusché and Greenberg (1994) and is intended for children in kindergarten through sixth grade. PATHS is based on five conceptual models: Affective-Behavioral-Cognitive-Dynamic model (ABCD), ecobehavioral systems model, neurobiology and brain structuralization/organization model, psychodynamic education model, and a model involving psychological issues related to emotional awareness and intelligence (Kusché & Greenberg). The ABCD model centers on the development of emotion-related language and cognitive understanding of emotions to promote social and emotional competence. The PATHS curriculum helps children develop greater emotional competence in these areas by increasing self-control, emotional awareness, and social problem solving.

Program Description   The PATHS curriculum has adopted an eco-behavioral systems orientation, with the goal of promoting the developmental skills of the child while developing a healthy and supportive classroom and school environment (Kusché & Greenberg, 1994). Teaching children to generalize these newly learned skills to other situations and settings is a particular focus in the curriculum. The PATHS curriculum focuses on improving or facilitating the growth of developmentally appropriate skills and abilities. Greenberg, Kusché, and Mihalic (1998) asserted that around age 5, children are ready for training in strategies to help them develop better impulse control. In addition, their brain development is at a point where they can benefit from training in the identification and labeling of emotions. The PATHS curriculum also uses psychodynamic educational strategies to enhance emotional growth, improve school functioning, and optimize mental health (Kusché & Greenberg, 1994). One of the major components is teaching educators to express interest in children's feelings, emotions, and opinions to build positive relationships between students and teachers. The key focus for children is on development of self-control, self-motivation, and self-responsibility for actions.

An important aspect of emotional intelligence is the ability to recognize emotional responses in oneself, in others, and in situations and to use this knowledge in effective ways such as managing emotional responses and handling relationships (Goleman, 1995; Mayer & Salovey, 1997). By preschool, most children can both exhibit and interpret emotional displays. In particular, children at this age are learning new ways to cope with their unpleasant emotions as well as ways to express their emotions verbally. The PATHS curriculum encourages children to discuss their feelings, opinions, and experiences as one way of increasing the support they receive from teachers and peers. In addition, children are taught to listen to and respect the feelings, experiences, and opinions of others.

The PATHS curriculum targets a wide variety of protective factors while reducing risk factors to promote optimal development. The targeted protective factors fall under the domains of 1) individual (e.g., emotional understanding, self-control, empathy development, emotional regulation, problem solving, communication, cognitive and academic skills), 2) peers (e.g., positive peer relationships), 3) family (e.g., family communication skills), and 4) school (e.g., positive classroom environment, teacher management, teacher–student relationships). Categories of targeted risk factors are individual (e.g., impulsivity, aggression, internalizing problems), peer (e.g., poor peer relationships), and school (e.g., disruptive classroom behaviors, chaotic classroom atmospheres; Kusché & Greenberg, 1994).

The PATHS curriculum is divided into two units: the Turtle Unit designed for kindergarten students and the Basic Unit for grades 1 through 6. The major focus of the Turtle Unit is the development of self-control, which is taught through the use of a story about a young turtle whose academic and social difficulties stem from his aggressive behavior and lack of self-control. The Turtle Unit kit includes an instructor's manual, the curriculum manual containing 12 turtle lessons and scripts, a turtle puppet, a turtle stamp, and a poster with the turtle story. Alternately, the Basic Unit consists of five volumes: three feelings and relationships units (56 total lessons), a problem-solving unit (33 lessons), and a supplementary unit to reinforce the previously taught skills (30 lessons). Methods include storytelling, games and activities, parent letters, handouts, and home activities. The Basic Unit includes an instructor's manual, five curriculum manuals, a set of *feelings* photographs, a set of *feelings* face cards, two wall charts, and four full-color posters.

The preschool PATHS Curriculum (Domitrovich, Greenberg, Kusché, & Cortes, 2004) was adapted from the original K–6 PATHS curriculum. The original concepts were preserved, but the material was modified to be developmentally appropriate for younger children. Preschool PATHS is divided into thematic units that include lessons on such topics as complimenting, basic and advanced feelings, a self-control strategy called "The Turtle Technique" (Robin, Schneider, & Dolnick, 1976), manners, and problem solving. Various puppets, as well as pictures, photographs, and feeling faces, are used in the lessons to introduce and illustrate the concepts. In addition, Preschool PATHS is designed to integrate effectively with early childhood programs. Preschool PATHS contains 30 lessons that are delivered weekly by early childhood educators during *circle time* sessions. In each lesson, the teacher introduces new ideas and materials. Over the next few days, the content of that lesson is practiced through the use of extension activities (e.g., group games, art projects, music, storytime). Some of these generalization strategies are undertaken in a group format, but many are integrated into the existing *center* structure of typical preschool programs. In this way, Preschool PATHS combines the direct teaching skills with meaningful opportunities to apply and practice them. This paradigm further promotes the establishment of optional structures in which teachers can provide positive reinforcement for effective skill application.

Program Evaluation   Evaluations of the PATHS curriculum have been conducted in studies of first-grade children in general education classrooms (Greenberg & Kusché, 2003), youth with special needs (Kam, Greenberg, & Kusché, 2004), and youth with hearing impairments (Greenberg & Kusché, 1998). Compared with control groups who received no intervention, use of the PATHS curriculum has resulted in improved self-control, improved understanding and recognition of emotions, increased ability to tolerate frustration, more effective conflict resolution strategies, improved thinking and planning skills, and decreased conduct problems including aggression (Greenberg et al., 1998). At 1-year posttreatment, teachers reported decreased anxiety and depression in the intervention children, and children reported lower rates of sadness and depression.

For the students in regular education programs, postintervention results showed significantly improved social problem-solving skills, increased emotional understanding, and significant improvement on cognitive ability tests, the vocabulary, coding, and block design subscales of the Wechsler Intelligence Scale for

Children–Revised (WISC-R; Wechsler, 1974). In addition, the intervention group was less likely to provide aggressive solutions and more likely to provide prosocial solutions to interpersonal conflict, as compared with the control group. One-year follow-up results indicated significant effects on the emotional understanding and interpersonal problem-solving skills tests. In addition, significant results were obtained for a task involving social planning, compared with the control children. Two-year follow-up results showed significant differences on teacher reports of the Child Behavior Checklist (CBCL; Achenbach, 1991), with the treatment group showing lower scores for externalizing behavior and higher scores on the total adaptive functioning subscales, and child reports indicated lower rates of conduct problems (Greenberg & Kusché, 2003).

Among children with special needs, there were postintervention results indicating significant differences in both internalizing and externalizing behavior problems between the intervention group and a control group consisting of other children with special needs. At the 2-year follow-up, teachers reported significant differences on both the internalizing and externalizing subscales of the CBCL. The intervention students showed less increase in both internalizing behaviors than the control group and decreases in externalizing behaviors, whereas the control group showed increases in reports of externalizing (Kam et al., 2004). Student self-reports of depression also showed a decline in depression for children in the intervention group, whereas the control group children showed a slight increase in depression (Kam et al.). However, teachers reported no differences between the groups in social competence, although intervention children were slightly more likely to provide prosocial, rather than aggressive, solutions to interpersonal situations (Kam et al.). Effect sizes for this study ranged from a Cohen's d value of .18 to .54, indicating a small to medium effect of the intervention.

For the children with hearing impairments, the posttest revealed improvements in problem-solving skills, emotional recognition and understanding, and higher teacher and parent reports of social competence (Greenberg & Kusché, 1998). Specifically, intervention children generated a greater number of alternatives for dealing with angry situations, and of these alternatives, a greater percentage was judged to be prosocial, compared with the control children (Greenberg & Kusché). In addition, the intervention children showed improved emotion recognition skills and were better able to appropriately label emotions in others (Greenberg & Kusché). Both the 1- and 2-year follow-ups indicated maintenance of all effects, with the exception of teacher-reported emotional adjustment, which showed a decline at the 1-year follow-up and then increased again at the 2-year follow-up (Greenberg & Kusché). In addition to these three trials, a first-grade version of PATHS curriculum has been implemented as a part of the multisite Fast Track Program that is designed to prevent the development of conduct problems (Conduct Problems Prevention Research Group, 1999a, 1999b). Findings included lower peer reports of aggression and hyperactive-disruptive behavior as well as higher quality of classroom atmosphere based on observer reports (also see Chapter 7).

The effects of Preschool PATHS were evaluated using a randomized trial design that included 20 Head Start classrooms located in urban and rural Pennsylvania (Domitrovich, Cortes, & Greenberg, 2004). Following random assignment, half of the teachers implemented the Preschool PATHS curriculum, whereas the other half continued to conduct their classes as usual with the standard Head Start protocol. A total of 248 children were evaluated in a sample that consisted of 47% African American, 38% European American, and 10% Hispanic children. There were four sets of findings (Domitrovich, Cortes, & Greenberg). First, it was shown that Head Start teachers, with appropriate support, can effectively implement Preschool PATHS. Second, outcome data at the end of 1 year indicated that children who received Preschool PATHS had improved outcomes as reported by both teachers and parents. More specifically, children who received Preschool PATHS were described by their teachers and their parents as more socially skilled than children in the regular Head Start comparison classrooms. Third, measures collected directly with the children indicated significant improvements in their emotional understanding with regard to both expressive and receptive abilities to identify emotions. Furthermore, the intervention children were less likely than the regular Head Start control children to misidentify facial expressions as being angry. Finally, no child characteristics moderated the effects of the intervention, suggesting that Preschool PATHS was equally effective for both genders and at all levels of risk.

Critical Analysis of Treatment Characteristics   The PATHS program is theory based, with components of five different models contributing to the overall theory of the program. These multiple theories guide the program in the use of multiple strategies for the delivery of treatment components. In particular, the ABCD model drives the emotional development focus of the PATHS model (Greenberg et al., 1998). The ecobehavioral aspect of the program emphasizes the development of a healthy and supportive environment in addition to teaching the program skills to participants. The PATHS program employs many mediums by which the skills are taught and integrates these methods into the daily educational schedule of the participants. For instance, puppets, storytelling, posters, games, and parent–child activities to be completed at home are all utilized as part of the program. The program is designed to target multiple risk factors in individual, peer, and school domains; in addition, it seeks to enhance protective factors in the individual, peers, family, and school (Kusché & Greenberg, 1994). Thus, the PATHS program is comprehensive in its focus on multiple important domains that affect children. Furthermore, by teaching children ways to appropriately express their emotions and interact with others, the program helps to build positive relationships between the children and their peers, teachers, and family.

Critical Analysis of Procedural Characteristics The program is implemented over the course of the first 7 years of formal education, starting in kindergarten and continuing through the sixth grade. According to Greenberg et al. (1998), the program is designed to begin at an age when children are developmentally ready for the emotional training given by the PATHS program. It also is important that a program to prevent adolescent substance abuse begin before the individual is actually exposed to the types of situations that may lead to substance use. Because this program begins in kindergarten and continues until the beginning of the transition to adolescence, it is well timed for the prevention of substance abuse. In addition, the long-term nature of PATHS and its age-appropriate curriculums make it a particularly useful as a prevention program.

Under optimal conditions, teachers receive training for the PATHS curriculum during a 2- to 3-day workshop and in weekly meetings with a curriculum consultant. These meetings are used to promote treatment fidelity by providing teachers with feedback throughout the program and also through modeling and coaching the teachers on the program components. In addition, there was a trained PATHS observer who visited the classrooms of the teachers administering the program once a month to rate them on how well they were teaching the skills of the curriculum and also on how well the teacher helped the children generalize the skills throughout the day (Kam, Greenberg, & Walls, 2003). Follow-up studies have shown that treatment effects continue to be significant at 1- and 2-years posttreatment (Greenberg & Kusché, 1998, 2003; Greenberg et al., 1998; Kam et al., 2004). However, longer-term follow-ups, booster sessions to address issues of dosage, and additional teacher training workshops to facilitate treatment fidelity would be useful for monitoring the impact of the program.

Critical Analysis of Design Characteristics Randomized control groups have been used in each of the program evaluations, and the results indicate that the program is effective in increasing social competence, as well as in decreasing aggression, anxiety, depression, and other problem behaviors (Greenberg & Kusché, 2003). However, these control groups received no intervention or any sort of treatment at all. Active control groups receiving some form of intervention would be recommended for future replications of the program. Active control groups make it possible to determine whether the effects shown by the intervention group are due to the actual treatment they are receiving or simply due to the increased attention they get from the treatment providers. If the control group receives attention in some form, but does not participate in the intervention curriculum, then any differences between the groups can be attributed to the actual treatment received by the intervention group.

The PATHS program also has been implemented in multiple sites and with multiple populations, including students in general education, students with special needs, and students with hearing impairments. The program has been successful in improving self-control, increasing understanding and recognition of emotion in self and others, and helping children develop effective conflict strategies (Greenberg et al., 1998). Intervention children also have shown increases in ability to tolerate frustration and to hone planning skills and have shown decreases in conduct problems (Greenberg et al.). Although these skills are likely important for the prevention of substance abuse, there has been no explicit test of the program's efficacy in the domain of substance use and abuse. Follow-up studies of the youth who received the PATHS curriculum would be useful for determining the effect of the program on substance use. Future studies of the PATHS curriculum should also focus on internal validation; specifically, replications need to test the relations between the improvements in skills targeted by the program and actual adolescent substance abuse. One other notable limitation is that only one published analysis of the PATHS program has explicitly indicated effects sizes (Kam et al., 2004), which are important for understanding the practical difference between the control groups and the intervention groups. Reporting of effect sizes would allow examination of exactly how great an impact the intervention has on the children who receive the program.

Strengthening Families Program

The primary goal of Strengthening Families Program (SFP) is building positive relationships within families to prevent drug use and delinquency among children. SFP was originally developed as a selective prevention program for 6- to 12-year-old children of parents in substance abuse treatment; however, it is widely used with children from non–substance-abusing families through universal prevention programs in schools or selective prevention programs conducted through family and youth service agencies in neighborhoods, faith-based communities, juvenile justice centers, prisons, and treatment centers.

Program Description   The Biopsychosocial Vulnerability Model is the theoretical basis of SFP (DeMarsh & Kumpfer, 1985) and targets both reducing family risks and promoting family protective and resiliency processes (Molgaard & Spoth, 2001). In addition to selective programs for 6- to 12-year-old children at risk for substance abuse, and more broad school interventions, other versions of SFP include a seven-session video-based version for youth ages 10–14 years and their parents, (Kumpfer, Molgaard, & Spoth, 1996; Molgaard & Spoth, 2001), SFP 3–5 years for preschoolers, and SFP 13–17 years for older youth who are at risk and in foster care or treatment centers. Language translations are available in

Spanish, Swedish, Dutch, and Russian (K.L. Kumpfer, personal communication, November 5, 2004). Because SFP is an evidence-based model program, it is currently implemented by more than 3,000 agencies nationwide and a number of foreign countries (Canada, Australia, Spain, Netherlands, Britain, Sweden, and Costa Rica).

SFP targets both the individual and the family through a 14-session behavioral skills training program. Each session is 2 hours in duration and begins with the families eating an evening meal together at the program site. Separate parent and child meetings are held during the first hour after the dinner. The parent meeting, led by two group leaders, focuses on instructing parents on how to promote desired behaviors in their children by increasing attention and rewards for positive behaviors (Schinke et al., 2002). Clear communication, effective discipline, substance use, problem solving, and limit setting are among the other topics covered during the parent training component of each session. Parents learn through observation, practice with feedback from trainers and videotapes, and work with the child and trainer on following the child's lead to improve positive play (Kumpfer & Alvarado, 2003). While the parents meet with their leaders, the children meet separately with two children's trainers. The trainers work with the children on understanding feelings, controlling anger, resisting peer pressure, complying with parental rules, solving problems, and communicating effectively. The development of social skills and teaching about the consequences of substance abuse also are foci of the children's skills component of each session.

During the second hour, parents and children meet jointly to participate in structured family activities, conduct family meetings, and plan family activities. The Family Life Skills Training component of each session allows the families to work together on the skills developed separately during the first hour by collaboratively learning communication skills, practicing effective discipline, and reinforcing positive behaviors in each other. Four trained group leaders and a site coordinator are necessary for program implementation. SFP matches recruitment and retention strategies to meet the needs of the participating families (Department of Health Promotion and Education: University of Utah, n.d.). Aiding recruitment and retention, the program goals promote outcomes that families are likely to value: improvements in family relations, parenting skills, youth behaviors, and grades. Incentives and rewards encourage families to stay in the program, whereas the provision of meals, child care, and transportation additionally reduce barriers to attendance (Schinke et al., 2002). Three-hour booster session reunions following graduation from SFP are held every 3 months, followed by family outings.

Program Evaluation A needs assessment is conducted for each family prior to the initiation of an SFP program. Following the program, an evaluation is conducted using standardized family, parent, and child outcome measures (Department of Health Promotion and Education: University of Utah, n.d.). Outcome studies of SFP conducted in the early 1980s used a randomized control trial with a four-group dismantling design to examine the outcomes of SFP components (DeMarsh & Kumpfer, 1985; Kumpfer & Alder, 2003). The findings of these studies suggested that the parent training component resulted in a reduction of conduct disorders among their children. It also was found that children's skills training directed improvement in children's social competency, and the joint family practice sessions brought about increases in positive family communications and relationships. These outcomes fit well with the program goal of building positive relationships within families. The extent to which these positive relationships offset risk factors present in a family may be particularly important for preventing early starters and redirecting their developmental trajectories (Kumpfer, Alvarado, Tait, & Turner, 2002).

Spoth, Redmond, and Shin (1998) initiated a large-scale prevention trial comparing SFP with an active control (Preparing for the Drug Free Years [PDFY]; see Kosterman, Hawkins, Spoth, Haggerty, & Zhu, 1997) and a minimal contact condition in 19 counties in the rural Midwest. Longitudinal follow-ups of SFP at 18, 48, and 72 months measured substance use related outcomes directly, including lifetime use (alcohol, alcohol without parental permission, drunkenness, cigarette, and marijuana) and frequency of current use (Spoth, Redmond, & Lepper, 1999; Spoth, Redmond, & Shin, 2001; Spoth, Redmond, Shin, & Azevedo, 2004). Following developmental expectations for age of initial use, significant intervention control differences were detectable at 18-month follow-up. Children in the SFP group who had not initiated substance use at 18 months postintervention were significantly less likely to begin using substances 2½ years after the program as compared with the control group (Spoth, Reyes, Redmond, & Shin, 1999).

Both SFP and PDFY showed significant effects at 4 years postintervention; a larger number of significant effects were found for SFP—likely due to its more intensive curriculum (Spoth et al., 2001). In comparison with the minimal contact control, SFP participants showed significantly delayed initiation of alcohol, tobacco, and marijuana use and lower frequency of alcohol and cigarette use at the 4-year follow-up. Spoth et al. (2001) reported effect sizes for both SFP and PDFY on frequency of drinking in past month (.26 and .28, respectively) and frequency of cigarette use in past month (.31 and .12, respectively) at the 4-year follow-up.

At the 6-year follow-up, results suggest a significant effect for delaying initiation of substance use for both intervention groups (Spoth et al., 2004). However, PDFY showed delayed growth effects only for tobacco use, whereas SFP showed delayed growth effects for alcohol use without parental permission, drunkenness, and cigarette use. Comparing SFP with the control group, Spoth et al. found that 40% of the control group participants had started drinking without parental permission at 14.7 years of age, whereas only 18% of the SFP participants had done so at this age. This difference represents a 55% relative reduction rate in initiation (Spoth et al.).

At the 2-year follow-up, a rural school model of SFP was found to be highly effective with effect sizes of .85 to 1.11 in decreasing antisocial behaviors, conduct disorders, and aggression (Office of Juvenile Justice and Delinquency Prevention, 1999). In a 4-year longitudinal follow-up of a program combining SFP with a compatible school-based social skills training program, I Can Problem Solve (ICPS), Kumpfer, Alvarado, Tait, and Turner (2002) found larger effect sizes over the no-treatment control group and larger additive effect sizes in school bonding (1.26), parenting skills (1.21), social competence (.35), family relationships (.37), and self-regulation (.69) for the combined programs. SFP's effects improved with time, whereas ICPS's results decreased with time. This trend suggests the importance of changing the parent–child relationship and parenting skills on long-term positive impacts.

In its systematic review of 56 alcohol prevention studies, International Cochrane Collaboration recommended SFP over all other programs examined (including LST) for its rigorous evaluation and prevention effects (Foxcroft, Ireland, Lister-Sharp, Lowe, & Breen, 2003). In their review, Foxcroft and colleagues re-analyzed programs in terms of their intention-to-treat. Examining the results from several SFP evaluations (Spoth et al., 2001; Spoth, Kavanagh, & Dishion, 2002), they found that for every nine individuals who participated in SFP, there will be one fewer person reporting to have ever used alcohol, used alcohol without permission, or ever been drunk 4 years later.

Although cost–benefit studies for prevention programs are not yet commonly published, these evaluations can be invaluable for making policy decisions and choosing interventions. Spoth, Guyll, and Day (2002) conducted a cost–benefit analysis on ISFP (adapted version for rural Iowa) and PDFY. A $9.60 benefit–cost ratio per $1 invested was found for ISFP, in comparison to a $5.85 benefit–cost ratio for PDFY. These analyses may provide helpful perspective in funding prevention programs by demonstrating that in proportion to the costs of alcohol-related problems to society, the cost of prevention programs are relatively small.

Critical Analysis of Treatment Characteristics   One of the unique features of SFP is its ability to be modified to fit local populations. SFP has been culturally adapted and evaluated in urban and rural communities with Hispanic, Asian and Pacific Islander, Native American, and African American families (see Spoth, Guyll, Chao, & Molgaard, 2003). Implementation and evaluation support is available from the SFP staff. Although SFP is culturally adapted and Spanish language versions of the program are available, SFP staff also provide support in tailoring manuals and videos to make the program even more locally relevant to the particular target population. Modifications in language and audiovisual materials to the targeted population can increase acceptability, recruitment, and retention (Department of Health Promotion and Education: University of Utah, n.d.). Spoth, Kavanagh, and Dishion (2002) encouraged attention to cultural sensitivity in the adaptation of existing programs or the design of new programs for diverse communities. Adapting programs, however, must be done with careful attention to maintaining core elements. Culturally adapted versions of SFP that eliminate core content or reduce dosage can increase family retention rates up to 40%, but also decrease positive outcomes (Kumpfer, Alvarado, Smith, & Bellamy, 2002). This finding suggests that a key component of making research-based programs successful in community settings may be balancing cultural or community adaptations with curriculum fidelity.

SFP curriculum is theory driven (Molgaard & Spoth, 2001), emerging from the Biopsychosocial Vulnerability Model (Kumpfer, Trunnel, & Whiteside, 1990) and other research on family risk and protective factors (Kumpfer et al., 1996). This theoretical framework views a child's vulnerability to substance use or addiction as influenced not only by risks from heredity (e.g., genetic risk for addiction), family environment (e.g., alcoholic parent), and sociocultural mores (e.g., excessive drinking common at community events) but also by a lack of protective factors in these domains (e.g., giftedness in sports, strong grandparent involvement, church committed to youth development). A central goal of the program is building positive relationships within families in order to prevent drug use and delinquency. A focus on risk and protective factors within the family is likely to be especially important for targeting both early starters and the general population.

Critical Analysis of Procedural Characteristics   SFP staff participate in a 2-day on-site training prior to program implementation (Molgaard & Spoth, 2001). Training consists of both general (background, content, goals, and evaluation) and applied (program activities, implementation, and recruitment) information. Trained staff can contact facilitators via telephone and e-mail for consultation and technical assistance throughout the program free of charge. Training and support aid treatment fidelity by providing program staff with a thorough knowledge base and consultations to keep them on track with SFP goals. Treatment fidelity could be further enhanced through consistent monitoring by SFP facilitators. Programmed generalizations also are part of SFP. Booster sessions following graduation help families stay in touch with each other and the staff and provide opportunities for skill maintenance. Although attention to recruiting and retaining participants is not part of the evaluation criteria, SFP's emphasis and strategies for enrolling and keeping families in the program is a notable strength of the program.

SFP engages families together, rather than solely targeting the student in the classroom. The purpose of providing training to parents and children separately and the family as a whole is to promote positive family relationships and build the protective factors the family members can offer one another. This comprehensiveness may be especially useful given the finding that avoiding alcohol and drug use is primarily linked to concern over parental disapproval of substance use (Kumpfer & Alvarado, 2003).

Critical Analysis of Design Characteristics   Evaluations of SFP have included both active control groups and longitudinal follow-ups to study the effects of the program. In addition, SFP is one of the few prevention programs that has undergone a componential analysis, which lends support to the internal validity of the program. This feature allows for a better understanding of which components of SFP make a difference on specific outcomes. With this knowledge, it is possible to target outcomes, such as decreasing conduct problems, with appropriate interventions, such as the SFP parent component. SFP is also one of the few programs to report effect sizes (see Spoth et al., 2001) and to compare them with an active control group. The cost–benefit analysis conducted by Spoth, Guyll, and Day (2002) and the number needed to treat analysis by Foxcroft, Ireland, Lister-Sharp, Lowe, & Breen (2003) represented sophisticated examinations and may encourage improved evaluations throughout the prevention field. The rigorous design features (i.e., sample sizes, randomized controls, evaluation techniques) of SFP are noteworthy and provide an example of the advanced and analytical evaluations needed in prevention research.

Incredible Years Series: Comprehensive School and Family Focus

The Incredible Years Series (IYS) is a three-part comprehensive program for parents, teachers, and children designed to prevent and reduce behavioral and emotional problems in young children, as well as to promote emotional and social competencies. The IYS is a selective program that focuses on children from 2 to 8 years of age who have been identified by parents and teachers as at risk for or already exhibiting conduct problems (Webster-Stratton et al., 2001). Webster-Stratton and Taylor (2001) suggested that there are four major risk factors that must be addressed by a successful intervention in order for it to impact later substance abuse or delinquency: relationships with peers who are deviant, harsh and inconsistent parenting, lack of monitoring, and academic difficulties. The IYS curriculum aims to prevent or reduce each of these risk factors.

Program Description   The IYS is based on Patterson, Reid, and Dishion's (1992) model of coercive family process and the belief that early conduct problems and poor parenting are significant predictors of later substance abuse, violence, and delinquency (Dishion & Loeber, 1985). In addition, other family factors such as marital conflict (e.g., Emery, 1982) and parental depression (e.g., Gondoli & Silverberg, 1997) have been shown to disrupt parenting and contribute to negative affect, inconsistent parenting, emotional unavailability, and lack of monitoring. This research suggests that along with parent training targeting effective child management skills, preventive interventions should help parents cope with other life stressors that may affect their parenting abilities. Children with behavior problems often have negative academic and social experiences (e.g., school failure, peer rejection), which often lead to further behavior problems (Patterson et al., 1992) as well as associations with other children who are disruptive or deviant. Once these relationships have been formed, the risk for becoming involved in alcohol, drugs, and other delinquent behaviors becomes elevated (Patterson et al.). These findings clearly indicate a need for training that focuses on reducing aggression and building social and academic competencies among children displaying early risk factors.

In the school domain, Rutter, Tizard, Yule, Graham, and Whitmore (1976) found that aggressive and delinquent behaviors by children were related to teachers' lack of warmth and supportiveness in the classroom. Walker (1995) reported that children who were antisocial were less likely to receive praise for appropriate behavior and were more likely to be punished for problem behavior than other children in the classroom. Teachers need to be properly trained in classroom management skills that promote appropriate social behavior, problem-solving, and self-management skills among children through the use of consistent response patterns, praise and encouragement, and rewards for appropriate behaviors, as well as loss of privileges for inappropriate behaviors.

The parent program consists of three parts: BASIC, SCHOOL, and ADVANCE. The BASIC program is implemented first in the series. It consists of a 12- to 14-week group program led by trained facilitators and a series of 250 video vignettes. The major focus of the training is to teach parents to engage in child-directed play, empathy, and reinforcement skills, with the goal of developing a realistic and developmentally appropriate understanding of children. The program also teaches parents to use nonviolent discipline, problem solving, appropriate monitoring, and strategies for responding to children in clear and predictable ways. There are two versions of the BASIC programs: one for parents of children ages 2–6 years and one for parents of school-age children ages 6–10. The SCHOOL program is designed to promote and develop connections between the home and school environments and to help parents promote academic success and reading skills. The program helps parents form relationships with their children's teachers in an attempt to get parents more involved in the educational environment. Finally, the ADVANCE program consists of a 10- to

12-week series of group discussions, videotapes, audiotapes, and home workbook activities focused on dealing with family risk factors such as depression, marital discord, poor coping skills, and lack of parenting support. Parents also are taught cognitive self-control strategies and problem-solving and communication skills as well as ways to give and receive support. Other program materials include facilitator manuals, parent books, videotapes, audiotapes, and refrigerator magnets. In addition, group leaders telephone participants at least once every 2 weeks to assess their satisfaction with the program and to work out individual issues with the participants. Participants also fill out brief evaluations of the program components at the beginning of the session following their introduction to the skills. To further engage the parents in the training program, participants are assigned a *buddy* whom they are instructed to call after each session to discuss the skills learned and to talk about their use of the skills at home. If a parent misses a session, then both the group leader and the buddy call him or her to set up a time to make up the session (leader) and to discuss what was missed in the session (leader and buddy; Webster-Stratton, Mihalic, et al., 2001).

In addition to the three-part parent training program, the IYS curriculum has a teacher training component. The teacher training program is a 6-day, 42-hour workshop targeting teachers and other school personnel. The program involves group-based training sessions dealing with effective classroom management, promoting positive relationships with students, strengthening social skills in the classroom and other school settings, and promoting collaboration and positive communication between teachers and parents. For children identified as at risk for or exhibiting conduct disorders, teachers learn to develop behavior plans and to collaborate with parents to develop strategies and goals that will be coordinated from school to home. Teachers learn skills for being sensitive and responsive to developmental differences in positive and consistent ways. Teachers also learn to prevent peer rejection by teaching children appropriate social skills and helping children learn to respond appropriately to peer aggression.

Finally, there is a child training series called the Dina Dinosaur's Emotion, Social Skills and Problem-Solving Curriculum. Its goal is to promote appropriate classroom behaviors, social skills, emotional literacy, positive peer interactions, conflict management strategies, and problem-solving skills. The treatment version of the program is designed as a *pull-out* program for small groups consisting of five to six children of the same age who have been identified as being at risk for or as having conduct problems. The program has been offered in 22–24 2-hour weekly sessions when offered in mental health centers. If offered in schools, it can be delivered twice a week for 1-hour sessions. There also is a classroom prevention version of the program that is delivered to all students in the classroom 2–3 times a week. There are 60 lessons for each year of the curriculum including preschool, kindergarten, and grades 1 and 2.

Program Evaluation   The parenting series of the IYS has been replicated in several different studies by the developer (Webster-Stratton, 1981, 1982a, 1982b, 1984, 1994; Webster-Stratton & Hammond, 1997; Webster-Stratton, Kolpacoff, & Hollinsworth, 1988; Webster-Stratton, Reid, & Hammond, 2004), all of which focused on parents of children who had previously been identified as at risk for or having conduct problems. In addition, three independent replications have been conducted in mental health clinics for parents of children with conduct problems (Scott, Spender, Doolan, Jacobs, & Aspland, 2001; Spaccarelli, Cotler, & Penman, 1992; Taylor, Schmidt, Pepler, & Hodgins, 1998).

The BASIC parenting program was independently evaluated in a selective prevention program with Head Start families (Webster-Stratton, 1998; Webster-Stratton & Hammond, 1997), in a study with inner-city Hispanic families in New York (Miller & Rojas-Flores, 1999), and in a trial with African American mothers of low socioeconomic status in Chicago (Gross, Fogg, & Tucker, 1995; Gross et al., 2003). A videotape series, designed originally for use as a control condition, also has been developed to allow parents to self-administer the program (Webster-Stratton et al., 1988).

For all replications conducted by the developers, data for the parent series were based on parent and teacher reports, home observation, laboratory observation, and child reports. Webster-Stratton and Hammond (1997) also collected observational data on child–peer interactions, and Webster-Stratton and Reid (1999b) conducted classroom observations. In addition, marital problem-solving strategies and collaboration were observed by Webster-Stratton (1994) and Webster-Stratton and Hammond. Child outcomes included reduced aggression and destructive behavior by children, increases in prosocial behaviors, increased social competence, and decreases in oppositional and defiant behavior. Follow-ups 1 year and 3 years later showed continued effects. There were no specific evaluations of substance use or abuse, most likely because of the age of the children at the completion of the programs. Parent outcomes for the BASIC program included reductions in spanking and corporal punishment, fewer critical statements directed at the children, increases in effective discipline strategies, and increased use of praise. Parent outcomes from the ADVANCE program included increased marital problem-solving behaviors, and their children showed increased use of social problem solving.

Two trials of the child training series have been completed (Webster-Stratton & Hammond, 1997; Webster-Stratton et al., 2004). Measures included parent and teacher reports; home observations; laboratory observations; and child social skills, attribution, and self-esteem trainings. In addition, Webster-Stratton and Hammond conducted observational measures of peer interactions, whereas Webster-Stratton et al. conducted school classroom observations. Compared with a wait-listed control group, children in the treatment group showed decreased problem behaviors and improved conflict management skills and social problem-solving skills, especially in their ability to generate multiple positive solutions to hypothetical problems (Webster-Stratton & Hammond; Webster-Stratton et al.). In addition, mothers of children in the treatment group showed fewer total criticisms and commands in their interactions with their children as compared with the control group; however, these differences were not found for fathers (Webster-Stratton & Hammond; Webster-Stratton et al.).

Two studies have explicitly compared multiple components of the training series. In the first study, participants were randomly assigned to one of four conditions: a parent training only group, a child training only group, a combined parent and child training group, or a wait-list control group (Webster-Stratton & Hammond, 1997). In the second replication, participants were randomly assigned to a parent training only, child training only, parent training plus teacher training, child training plus teacher training, child plus parent plus teacher training, or a wait-list control group (Webster-Stratton et al., 2004).

In the first study, Webster-Stratton and Hammond (1997) reported that participants who received both child training and parent training had lower mother reports of total child problem behaviors than those who received only child training. In addition, mothers who received parent training alone reported fewer child problem behaviors than mothers of children in the child training only group (Webster-Stratton & Hammond). However, fathers and teachers reported no group differences in behavior problems. Participants in the child training or combined child and parent training groups produced more positive solutions to hypothetical conflicts than children whose parents received parent training alone. In addition, children who were in the child training alone group showed a greater ratio of positive to negative solutions than children in the parent training alone group (Webster-Stratton & Hammond).

With regard to parenting behaviors, mothers were observed to give greater praise to their children if they were in one of the groups that received parent training compared with the group that received child training only (Webster-Stratton & Hammond, 1997). There were no group differences in observed child behavior during interactions with parents (Webster-Stratton & Hammond). At 1-year follow-up, all groups continued to show decreases in total child behavior problems, greater prosocial behaviors, greater positive solutions to conflict, lower child deviance at home, higher positive effect between parents and children, and increased positive parenting behaviors, compared with baseline measures. In addition, there were no significant differences between posttreatment results and follow-up results, indicating maintenance of these effects (Webster-Stratton & Hammond). In fact, there was evidence of continued improvement in mother-reported deviant behavior at home from posttreatment to follow-up. For child training only participants, there was no decrease in parenting stress from pretreatment to follow-up, although both of the groups that received parent training showed a decrease in stress over this period (Webster-Stratton & Hammond).

In the second study, Webster-Stratton et al. (2004) reported that parent plus teacher training led to greater decreases in negative parenting than parent training. Similarly, the group that received all three forms of training (parent, teacher, and child) showed decreases in negative parenting as well as increases in positive parenting compared with the group that received only child and teacher training (Webster-Stratton et al.). For maternal reports of negative or positive parenting there were no group differences. Relatedly, there were no group differences in parental reports of child conduct at home or in child conduct at school and with peers. At the 1-year follow-up, there were no significant differences between posttest results and follow-up scores, indicating maintenance of the major outcomes, with just one exception: children in the group who received all three types of training showed a slight deterioration in their school behavior after the conclusion of the training sessions (Webster-Stratton et al.). Effect sizes reported by Webster-Stratton et al. indicated moderate to large effects (Cohen's d ranged from .29 to .91).

Critical Analysis of Treatment Characteristics   IYS is based on the coercive family process theory developed by Patterson et al. (1992) and is designed to educate parents and teachers in effective parenting and classroom management skills, respectively. The program also aims to reduce negative peer affiliations that may lead to subsequent behavior problems. In addition, IYS is extremely comprehensive, given its focus on three areas of the child's environment: home, school, and peers. The program clearly states that its major goals are to prevent or reduce the occurrence of four specific risk factors that have been associated with later substance use: associations with peers who are deviant, harsh and inconsistent parenting, lack of monitoring, and academic difficulties (Webster-Stratton & Taylor, 2001). It is implemented using a wide variety of teaching methods (e.g., individual training, parent–teacher meetings), which is a key characteristic of effective prevention programs.

Another component of effective programs is the development of positive and supportive relationships. For the parent–child relationship, the BASIC program teaches parents to be more sensitive and attuned to the needs of their children and also teaches nonviolent discipline, problem-solving skills, and ways to respond to their children in consistent and appropriate ways (Webster-Stratton et al., 2001). The SCHOOL program builds connections between the multiple environments in which the children are involved—in particular the home and the school. Finally, the ADVANCE program aims to teach parents problem solving, cognitive self-control strategies, communication skills, and ways of giving and receiving support (Webster-Stratton et al.). In addition, the ADVANCE program helps parents build social support networks by offering group training and assigning each parent a buddy within the group to provide support.

The IYS has been implemented with children who are at risk in Head Start, inner-city Hispanic families in New York, and a low-income African American sample in Chicago. All of the replications showed improvements in target behaviors, including increased marital problem-solving strategies, decreased child aggression and destructive behavior, and increased prosocial behavior and social competence (Webster-Stratton, 1994; Webster-Stratton & Hammond, 1997; Webster-Stratton & Reid, 1999a). Thus, adapted versions of the program appear to be influential across multiple sociocultural groups, making it possible to generalize the results of this program to multiple groups in different locations. This is important for researchers who wish to use the program in future research.

Critical Analysis of Procedural Characteristics   Outcome evaluations show improved parenting skills, increased communication between parents and teachers, increased school readiness and social problem solving in children, decreased marital negativity, decreased classroom negativity, decreased corporal punishment, and increased social competence in children. For replications of the BASIC and ADVANCE programs, results were compared with wait-listed control groups. Also, the videotape series portion of these two programs has been adapted to allow parents to self-administer the trainings to provide another comparison group. The SCHOOL program results were compared with results from classrooms in which the teacher was not trained in the IYS program. It is also important to note that evaluations of the programs were made using multiple methodologies, including parent and teacher reports, home observations, and school observations.

Critical Analysis of Design Characteristics   Replications of the program have been conducted with several different cultural groups and also with children who have been previously identified as at risk for behavior problems. The program is aimed at children ages 2–10 years and their families. Although the program certainly begins early enough to prevent behaviors that may lead to substance abuse, it does not continue into the late middle school and high school years. For evaluation of adequate dosage levels, it is important for researchers to demonstrate that participants are, in fact, continuing to use these strategies. Booster sessions and follow-up evaluations for parents, teachers, and children would be useful for assessing whether the program has continued effects.

To promote treatment fidelity, therapists, teachers, and school personnel must attend an extensive training workshop to learn how to implement the program. This ensures that the participants are receiving all of the necessary components of the program and that they are committed to the proper implementation of the program. In addition, parents and teachers in the program fill out weekly evaluations of the program and of their own ability to implement the skills to monitor how well the program is being delivered. These evaluations allow the researchers to determine whether the instructors are adhering to the program and also assess the parents' ability to use the skills they are learning and generalize these skills across multiple situations.

MODEL PROGRAM FOR PREVENTION OF ADOLESCENT SUBSTANCE ABUSE

There is no one, single most effective program designed to prevent substance abuse for every individual or family; however, the inclusion of key characteristics may contribute to program effectiveness. Table 6.2 highlights some of the characteristics that are recommended for a model program on the prevention of substance abuse.

Characteristics of a Successful Substance Abuse Prevention Program

Programs are recommended that intervene at multiple ecological levels; that is, the program should include parents, children, teachers, and the broader commu-

Table 6.2. Components of a model substance abuse prevention program

Targets of intervention	Early to middle childhood
	Males and females
	Children, parents, and teachers
	General and at-risk populations
Content of intervention	Social competency and communication skill building through discussions and activities with peers, parents, and teachers
	Emotional understanding and self-regulation skills
	Innovative teaching techniques (e.g., role playing)
	Community involvement
Targeted outcomes of intervention	Increased use of problem-solving behaviors
	Decreased externalizing and internalizing behaviors
	Improved parent–child, parent–teacher, and child–teacher communication
	Increased emotional understanding and self-regulation
	Improved planning skills
	Delayed onset of alcohol and/or drug initiation
	Decreased use of substances
Duration	Intervention beginning as early as kindergarten and continuing through middle school
	Booster sessions in middle and high school

nity. These programs ideally would begin as early as preschool to provide children with the skills necessary to avoid substance abuse problems before they are presented an opportunity to engage in these behaviors. In particular, the programs should be aimed at reducing the specific risk factors that contribute to later alcohol and drug use. A comprehensive program would not be limited solely to in-school instruction and at-home interactions but be integrated into the community to change the broader social norms toward substance use. The programs also should continue through middle and high school to provide continued support for the youth as they begin to encounter opportunities to experiment with alcohol and drugs. Outcome evaluations should be conducted throughout middle and high school to determine the ongoing efficacy of the programs.

A successful program should target both general and at-risk populations. Specific program content should focus on teaching children to become more socially competent and to help build communication skills through discussions and activities that include peers, parents, and teachers. Teaching skills such as emotional understanding and self-regulation also are important for prevention of substance abuse. Participants of successful prevention programs should show increased use of problem-solving behaviors, as well as improved communication skills at home and in school. Students should show improved planning skills and decreases in externalizing and internalizing behaviors. Most important, students should show delayed onset and lower use of alcohol and other drugs compared with students who have not participated in the prevention program.

Finally, programs should make use of innovative teaching techniques, such as role play, videos, and interactive activities. Programs also should help parents and children build more effective social support systems. Community involvement and community support also are crucial components for making a program work. For instance, business sponsorship of programs, through rewards and incentives for participants and their families, would provide an important link between the prevention program and the community. The key to successful prevention is having a comprehensive focus that targets as many aspects of the participants' lives as possible.

❖

A Program for Kevin Taylor

The Taylor family has been going through a particularly rough time. Ten-year-old Kevin has been acting aggressively at school and his grades have been steadily declining since his older sister Allison had a baby. He's frustrated and angry because he is no longer the youngest child and no one pays any attention to him. He has started hanging out with an older group of kids at school, and some of them have been pressuring him to smoke and drink with them. Kevin knows that he shouldn't do these things, especially because he's seen the problems that drinking can cause (his father, Tom, is a recovering alcoholic). Kevin doesn't want to make his friends mad, though, and they seem to have a lot of fun, especially when they're drinking. Plus, he knows that his parents probably won't find out because they're too busy arguing with each other and worrying about Allison's baby. Even if he is caught, Kevin thinks the attention from his family might be nice.

It is evident from Kevin's aggressive behavior at school, his declining grades, and his association with older, deviant friends that he is not getting the structure or supervision a 10-year-old needs. He craves attention and a sense of belonging, which he gets from his new friends. Kevin's teacher notices that he is having problems and refers him to the school counselor. The counselor sets up a meeting with Kevin's parents and his teacher to discuss the troubles Kevin is having. Worried about their son, Kevin's parents, Tom and Cassie, start attending group training sessions recommended by the counselor. The sessions teach them more effective ways to deal with their marital conflict and better ways of talking to and managing their children. In addition, the group leaders and other parents talk about how they can be more aware of what their children are doing and with whom they are associating. They meet a lot of other parents who are going through similar situations and take comfort in the fact that they aren't the only ones feeling this way. It really helps to have other people to talk to about parenting difficulties and personal problems that make it difficult to be a good parent.

Kevin's teacher, aware that Kevin is having trouble getting along with his peers, begins to pay special attention to him. She focuses on dealing with possible behavior problems in the classroom before the situation escalates. A couple of days a week Kevin goes to a special class where he is taught how to better express himself without becoming angry or upset. At first he is embarrassed to be talking about his feelings around other kids, but he eventually becomes comfortable around his peers and stops hanging out with the older boys. Kevin and the other kids in the program watch videos and have discussions about the dangers of smoking, drinking, and doing drugs. They are given accurate information about substance abuse, and no one tries to scare them into avoiding these behaviors. Throughout the program, Kevin's parents and teacher meet regularly to discuss how things are going in the classroom and at home, and Kevin's grades begin to improve.

It is evident from Kevin's experience that successful programs for preventing substance abuse must focus on multiple areas in the life of a child or adolescent. The program must incorporate the child, his or her parents, teachers, and peers. Parents and teachers need to be taught effective home and classroom management skills. Parents should receive support from the program directors and other parents in similar situations. Parents and teachers should be encouraged to develop relationships so that they are aware of important things that are happening in their child's life. The children or adolescents must be taught social, behavioral, and cognitive skills, and they must be given plenty of opportunities to practice, develop, and integrate these new skills into their daily lives. The programs should be tailored to the needs of the individual child, and ideally they should begin before the child has been exposed to pressure to engage in risky behaviors. However, some kids such as Kevin will be exposed to these situations, and by identifying and implementing the appropriate program, interested adults (parents, teachers, community members) can help these children overcome risks for substance abuse problems and direct them toward more positive developmental outcomes.

FUTURE DIRECTIONS: IMPROVING PROGRAMS FOR PREVENTING ADOLESCENT SUBSTANCE ABUSE

The rigor and innovation characteristic of the programs described in this chapter offer an encouraging glimpse of the future of prevention science in the area of substance abuse. Some scientific yardsticks exist for developing, selecting, and implementing programs; it is essential to make preventive interventions available and manageable at the community level. Coalitions and other grass roots organizations exist because local leaders have identified problems and committed themselves to the problems' solutions. Community members possess expert knowledge of their constituencies and environments. Knowledge of the day-to-day lives of the target audience may offer solutions and insights into some of the problems that have thwarted the successful dissemination and adoption of research-based programs (e.g., Fox, Gottfredson, Kumpfer, & Beatty, 2004). Consulting services, such as CTC, may provide needed research expertise in selecting, planning for, implementing, and evaluating programs.

Collaboration between communities and universities represents another important path to bridging the gap between prevention research and application. An important trend has emerged: University-based researchers are focusing their scientific expertise and concerns in ways that contribute to the larger community, creating relationships of mutual benefit to parents, practitioners, and society at large (Spoth, Guyll, Trudeau, & Goldberg-Lillehoj, 2002; Spoth & Redmond,

2002). Communities profit from researchers' skills in understanding the relevant literature as well as their ability to develop, implement, and evaluate programs. Researchers benefit from the wealth of interesting and important problems that communities face, providing ample opportunities to test theory in applied settings. Community involvement and university collaboration offer a promising avenue for protecting and supporting youth at risk for substance use and abuse.

REFERENCES

Achenbach, T.M. (1991). *Manual for the youth self-report and 1991 profile.* Burlington: University of Vermont, Department of Psychiatry.

Bandura, A. (1977). *Social learning theory.* Oxford, England: Prentice Hall.

Biglan, A., Flay, B., & Foster, S. (2003). The prevention of drug abuse. In A. Biglan, M. Wang, & H. Walberg (Eds.), *Preventing youth problems* (pp. 87–111). New York: Kluwer Academic/Plenum Publishers.

Borkowski, J.G., & Weaver, C.M. (2006). *Prevention: Using science and art to promote healthy development.* Baltimore: Paul H. Brookes Publishing Co.

Botvin, G.J. (1986). Substance abuse prevention research: Recent developments and future directions. *Journal of School Health, 56,* 369–374.

Botvin, G.J., Baker, E., Dusenbury, L., Botvin, E., & Diaz, T. (1995). Long-term follow-up results of a randomized drug abuse prevention trial in a white, middle-class population. *Journal of the American Medical Association, 273,* 1106–1113.

Botvin, G.J., & Griffin, K.W. (2004). Life Skills Training: Empirical findings and future directions. *Journal of Primary Prevention, 25,* 211–232.

Botvin, G.J., Griffin, K.W., Diaz, T., & Ifill-Williams, M. (2001). Drug abuse prevention among minority adolescents: Posttest and one-year follow-up of a school-based preventive intervention. *Prevention Science, 2,* 1–13.

Botvin, G.J., Griffin, K.W., Diaz, T., Scheier, L.M., William, C., & Epstein, J.A. (2000). Preventing illicit drug use in adolescents: Long-term follow-up data from a randomized control trial of a school population. *Addictive Behaviors, 25,* 769–774.

Botvin, G.J., Mihalic, S.F., & Grotpeter, J.K. (1998). *Blueprints for violence prevention, book five: Life Skills Training.* Boulder, CO: Center for the Study and Prevention of Violence.

Center for Substance Abuse Prevention. (1999). *Understanding substance abuse prevention: Toward the 21st century: A primer on effective programs.* Washington, DC: U.S. Department of Health & Human Services, Substance Abuse and Mental Health Services Administration.

Communities That Care. (2003). *Investing in your community's youth: An introduction to the Communities That Care system* (Item 501968B). South Deerfield, MA: Channing Bete.

Community Anti-Drug Coalitions of America. (n.d.). *Frequently asked questions: What is CADCA?* Retrieved December 2, 2003, from http://www.cadca.org/CoalitionResources/FAQ.asp

Community Anti-Drug Coalitions of America. (2003, Summer). Moving the field forward: A look at CADCA's institute. *Coalitions, 11,* 1, 6–7.

Conduct Problems Prevention Research Group. (1999a). Initial impact of the Fast Track prevention trial for conduct problems: I. The high-risk sample. *Journal of Consulting and Clinical Psychology, 67,* 631–647.

Conduct Problems Prevention Research Group. (1999b). Initial impact of the Fast Track prevention trial for conduct problems: I. Classroom effects. *Journal of Consulting and Clinical Psychology, 67,* 648–657.

Crano, W.D., & Burgoon, M. (Eds.). (2002). *Mass media and drug prevention: Classic and contemporary theories and research.* Mahwah, NJ: Lawrence Erlbaum Associates.

DeMarsh, J., & Kumpfer, K.L. (1985). Family-oriented interventions for the prevention of chemical dependency in children and adolescents. *Journal of Children in Contemporary Society, 18,* 117–151.

Department of Health Promotion and Education: University of Utah. (n.d.) *Strengthening Families Program.* Retrieved December 1, 2003, from http://www.strengtheningfamilies program.org

Dishion, T.J., & Loeber, R. (1985). Adolescent marijuana and alcohol use: The role of parents and peers revisited. *American Journal of Drug and Alcohol Abuse, 11,* 11–25.

Domitrovich, C.E., Cortes, R., & Greenberg, M.T. (2004). *Improving young children's social and emotional competence: A randomized trial of the Preschool PATHS curriculum.* Unpublished manuscript, Prevention Research Center, Pennsylvania State University.

Domitrovich, C.E., Greenberg, M.T., Kusché, C.A., & Cortes, R. (2004). *Preschool PATHS.* South Deerfield, MA: Channing Bete.

Ellis, T.M., & Lenczner, S.J. (2000, September). *Lessons from the field community anti-drug coalitions as catalysts for change: A report to the Annie E. Casey Foundation from Community Anti-Drug Coalitions of America.* Alexandria, VA: Community Anti-Drug Coalitions of America.

Emery, R.E. (1982). Interparental conflict and the children of discord and divorce. *Psychological Bulletin, 92,* 310–330.

Ennet, S.T., Tobler, N.S., Ringwalt, C.L., & Flewelling, R.L. (1994). How effective is Drug Abuse Resistance Education? A meta-analysis of Project DARE outcome evaluations. *American Journal of Public Health, 84,* 1394–1401.

Fox, D.P., Gottfredson, D.C., Kumpfer, K.K., & Beatty, P.D. (2004). Challenges in disseminating model programs: A qualitative analysis of the Strengthening Washington DC Families Program. *Clinical Child and Family Psychology Review, 7,* 165–176.

Foxcroft, D.R., Ireland, D., Lister-Sharp, D.J., Lowe, G., & Breen, R. (2003). Longer-term primary prevention for alcohol misuse in young people: A systematic review. *Addiction, 98,* 397–411.

Goleman, D.P. (1995). *Emotional intelligence: Why it can matter more than IQ for character, health and lifelong achievement.* New York: Bantam Books.

Gondoli, D.M., & Silverberg, S.B. (1997). Maternal emotional distress and diminished responsiveness: The mediating role of parenting efficacy and parental perspective taking. *Developmental Psychology, 33,* 861–868.

Gorman, D.M. (2002). The "science" of drug and alcohol prevention: The case of the randomized trial of the Life Skills Training program. *International Journal of Drug Policy, 13,* 21–26.

Greenberg, M.T., & Kusché, C.A. (1998). Preventive intervention for school-aged deaf children: The PATHS curriculum. *Journal of Deaf Studies and Deaf Education, 3,* 49–63.

Greenberg, M.T., & Kusché, C.A. (2003). *The PATHS curriculum: Follow-up effects and mediational processes.* Unpublished manuscript, Prevention Research Center, Pennsylvania State University.

Greenberg, M.T., Kusché, C.A., & Mihalic, S. (1998). Promoting Alternative Thinking Strategies (PATHS). In D.S. Elliot (Ed.), *Blueprints for violence prevention.* Boulder: Center for the Study and Prevention of Violence, University of Colorado.

Gross, D., Fogg, L., & Tucker, S. (1995). The efficacy of parent training for promoting positive parent–toddler relationships. *Research in Nursing and Health, 18,* 489–499.

Gross, D., Fogg, L. Webster-Stratton, C., Garvey, C., Julion, W., & Grady, J. (2003). Parent training with families of toddlers in day care in low-income urban communities. *Journal of Consulting and Clinical Psychology, 71,* 261–278.

Hawkins, J.D., Catalano, R.F., & Arthur, M.W. (2002). Promoting science-based prevention in communities. *Addictive Behaviors, 27,* 951–976.

Jessor, R., & Jessor, G.L. (1977). *Problem behavior and psychosocial development: A longitudinal study of youth.* New York: Academic Press.

Johnston, L.D., O'Malley, P.M., & Bachman, J.G. (2003). *Monitoring the future national results on adolescent drug use: Overview of key findings, 2002* (NIH Publication No. 03-5374). Bethesda, MD: National Institute on Drug Abuse.

Kam, C.M., Greenberg, M.T., & Kusché, C.A. (2004). Sustained effects of the PATHS curriculum on the social and psychological adjustment of children in special education. *Journal of Emotional and Behavioral Disorders, 12,* 66–78.

Kam, C.M., Greenberg, M.T., & Walls, C.T. (2003). Examining the role of implementation quality in school-based prevention using the PATHS curriculum. *Prevention Science, 4,* 55–63.

Kosterman, R., Hawkins, D., Spoth, R., Haggerty, K.P., & Zhu, K. (1997). Effects of a preventive parent-training intervention on observed family interactions: Proximal outcomes from preparing for the drug free years. *Journal of Community Psychology, 25,* 337–352.

Kumpfer, K.L. (n.d.). *Identification of drug abuse prevention programs: Literature review.* Retrieved December 6, 2003, from http://www.drugabuse.gov/about/organization/hsr/da-pre/KumpferLitReview.html

Kumpfer, K.L., & Alder, S. (2003). Dissemination of research-based family interventions for the prevention of substance abuse. In Z. Sloboda & W.J. Bukoski (Eds.), *Handbook of drug abuse prevention* (pp. 75–119). New York: Kluwer Academic/Plenum.

Kumpfer, K.L., & Alvarado, R. (2003). Family strengthening approaches for the prevention of youth problem behaviors. *American Psychologist, 58,* 457–465.

Kumpfer, K.L., Alvarado, R., Smith, P., & Bellamy, N. (2002). Cultural sensitivity and adaptation in family-based prevention interventions. *Prevention Science, 3,* 241–246.

Kumpfer, K.L., Alvarado, R., Tait, C., & Turner, C. (2002). Effectiveness of school-based family and children's skills training for substance abuse prevention among 6–8-year-old rural children. *Psychology of Addictive Behaviors, 16,* S65–S71.

Kumpfer, K.L., Molgaard, V.K., & Spoth, R.L. (1996). The "Strengthening Families Program" for the prevention of delinquency and drug use. In R. Peters & R. McMahon (Eds.), *Preventing childhood disorders, substance abuse and delinquency* (pp. 241–267). Thousand Oaks, CA: Sage Publications.

Kumpfer, K.L., Trunnel, E.P., & Whiteside, A.O. (1990). The biopsychosocial model: Application to the addictions field. In R. Engs (Ed.), *Controversy in the addiction field* (pp. 55–66). Dubuque, IA: Kendall/Hunt Publishing Co.

Kumpfer, K.L., Turner, C., Hopkins, R., & Librett, J. (1993). Leadership and team effectiveness in community coalitions for the prevention of alcohol and other drug abuse. *Health Education Research, 8*, 359–374.

Kusché, C.A., & Greenberg, M.T. (1994). *The PATHS curriculum.* Seattle: Developmental Research and Programs.

Mayer, J.D., & Salovey, P. (1997). What is emotional intelligence? In P. Salovey & D. Sluyter (Eds.), *Emotional development and emotional intelligence: Implications for educators* (pp. 3–31). New York: Basic Books.

Miller, L.S., & Rojas-Flores, L. (1999). *Preventing conduct problems in urban, Latino preschoolers through parent training: A pilot study.* New York: New York University Child Study Center.

Molgaard, V., & Spoth, R. (2001). The Strengthening Families Program for young adolescents: Overview and outcomes. *Residential Treatment for Children and Youth, 18,* 15–29.

Office of Juvenile Justice and Delinquency Prevention. (1999). *Strengthening Families Program.* Retrieved December 2, 2003, from http://www.strengtheningfamilies.org/html/programs_1999/06_SFP.html

Office of National Drug Control Policy. (2000). *The national drug control strategy: 2000 annual report.* Washington, DC: Executive Office of the President.

Patterson, T.J., Reid, J.B., & Dishion, T.J. (1992). *Antisocial boys.* Eugene, OR: Castalia.

RAND. (2002). *What are the true benefits of school-based drug prevention programs?* (Research Brief No. 6009-RWJ). Retrieved December 11, 2003, from http://www.rand.org/publications/RB/RB6009/

Robin, A., Schneider, M., & Dolnick, M. (1976). The Turtle Technique: An extended case study of self-control in the classroom. *Psychology in the Schools, 13,* 449–453.

Roe, S., & Becker, J. (2005). Drug prevention with vulnerable young people: A review. *Drugs: Education, Prevention, and Policy, 12,* 85–99.

Rutter, M., Tizard, J., Yule, W., Graham, P., & Whitmore, K. (1976). Isle of Wight studies, 1964–1974. *Psychological Medicine, 6,* 313–332.

Schinke, S., Brounstein, P., & Gardner, S. (2002). *Science based prevention programs and principles, 2002* (DHHS Publication No. 03-3764). Rockville, MD: Center for Substance Abuse Prevention, Substance Abuse and Mental Health Services Administration.

Schinke, S., Cole, K., Diaz, T., & Botvin, G.J. (1997). Developing and implementing interventions in community settings. *Journal of Child and Adolescent Substance Abuse, 6,* 49–67.

Scott, S., Spender, Q., Doolan, M., Jacobs, B., & Aspland, H. (2001). Multicentre controlled trial of parenting groups for child antisocial behaviour in clinical practice. *British Medical Journal, 323,* 1–7.

Simons-Morton, B.G., & Haynie, D.L. (2003). Growing up drug free: A developmental challenge. In M.H. Bornstein, L. Davidson, C.L.M. Keyes, & K.A. Moore (Eds.), *Wellbeing: Positive development across the life course. Crosscurrents in contemporary psychology* (pp. 109–122). Mahwah, NJ: Lawrence Erlbaum Associates.

Smith, E.A., Swisher, J.D., Vicary, J.R., Bechtel, L.J., Minner, D., Henry, K.L., & Palmer, R. (2004). Evaluation of Life Skills Training and Infused-Life Skills Training in a rural setting: Outcomes at two years. *Journal of Alcohol and Drug Education, 48,* 51–70.

Spaccarelli, S., Cotler, S., & Penman, D. (1992). Problem-solving skills training as a supplement to behavioral parent training. *Cognitive Therapy and Research, 16,* 1–18.

Spoth, R.L., Guyll, M., Chao, W., & Molgaard, V. (2003). Exploratory study of a preventive intervention with general population African American families. *Journal of Early Adolescence, 23,* 435–468.

Spoth, R.L., Guyll, M., & Day, S.X. (2002). Universal family-focused interventions in alcohol-use disorder prevention: Cost-effectiveness and cost–benefit analyses for two interventions. *Journal of Studies on Alcohol, 63,* 219–228.

Spoth, R.L., Guyll, M., Trudeau, L., & Goldberg-Lillehoj, C. (2002). Two studies of proximal outcomes and implementation quality of universal preventive interventions in a community–university collaboration context. *Journal of Community Psychology, 30,* 499–518.

Spoth, R.L., Kavanagh, K.A., & Dishion, T.J. (2002). Family-centered preventive intervention science: Toward benefits for larger populations of children, youth, and families. *Prevention Science, 3,* 145–152.

Spoth, R.L., & Redmond, C. (2002). Project Family prevention trials based in community–university partnerships: Toward scaled-up preventive interventions. *Prevention Science, 3,* 203–221.

Spoth, R., Redmond, C., & Lepper, H. (1999). Alcohol initiation outcomes of universal family-focused preventive interventions: One- and two-year follow-ups of a controlled study. *Journal of Studies on Alcohol, 13,* 103–111.

Spoth, R., Redmond, C., & Shin, C. (1998). Direct and indirect latent-variable parenting outcomes of two universal family-focused preventive interventions: Extending a public health-oriented research base. *Journal of Consulting and Clinical Psychology, 66,* 385–399.

Spoth, R., Redmond, C., & Shin, C. (2001). Randomized trial of brief family interventions for general populations of adolescent substance use outcomes 4 years following baseline. *Journal of Consulting and Clinical Psychology, 69,* 1–15.

Spoth, R., Redmond, C., Shin, C., & Azevedo, K. (2004). Brief family intervention effects on adolescent substance initiation: School-level growth curve analyses 6 years following baseline. *Journal of Consulting and Clinical Psychology, 72,* 535–542.

Spoth, R., Redmond, C., Trudeau, L., & Shin, C. (2002). Longitudinal substance initiation outcomes for a universal preventive intervention combining family and school programs. *Psychology of Addictive Behaviors, 16,* 129–134.

Spoth, R., Reyes, M., Redmond, C., & Shin, C. (1999). Assessing a public health approach to delay onset and progression of adolescent substance use: Latent transition and log-linear analyses of longitudinal family preventive intervention outcomes. *Journal of Consulting and Clinical Psychology, 67,* 619–630.

Swisher, J.D., Smith, E.A., Vicary, J.R., Bechtel, L.J., & Hopkins, A.M. (2004). A cost-effectiveness comparison of two approaches to Life Skills Training. *Journal of Alcohol and Drug Education, 48,* 71–87.

Taylor, T.K., Schmidt, F., Pepler, D., & Hodgins, H. (1998). A comparison of eclectic treatment with Webster-Stratton's Parents and Children Series in a Children's Mental Health Center: A randomized controlled trial. *Behavior Therapy, 29,* 221–240.

Trudeau, L., Spoth, R., Lillehoj, C., Redmond, C., & Wickrama, K.A.S. (2003). Effects of a preventive intervention on adolescent substance use initiation, expectancies and refusal intentions. *Prevention Science, 4,* 109–122.

Vicary, J.R., Henry, K.L., Bechtel, L.J., Swisher, J.D., Smith, E.A., Wylie, R., & Hopkins, A.M. (2004). Life Skills Training effects for high and low risk rural junior high school females. *Journal of Primary Prevention, 25,* 399–416.

Walker, D. (1995). *Violence in schools: How to build a prevention program from the ground up* (OSSC Bulletin Series). Eugene: Oregon School Study Council.

Webster-Stratton, C. (1981). Modification of mothers' behaviors and attitudes through videotape modeling group discussion program. *Behavior Therapy, 12,* 634–642.

Webster-Stratton, C. (1982a). The long-term effects of a videotape modeling parent training program: Comparison of immediate and 1 year follow-up results. *Behavior Therapy, 13,* 702–714.

Webster-Stratton, C. (1982b). Teaching mothers through videotape modeling to change their children's behaviors. *Journal of Pediatric Psychology, 7,* 279–294.

Webster-Stratton, C. (1984). A randomized trial of two parent training programs for families with conduct-disordered children. *Journal of Consulting and Clinical Psychology, 52,* 666–678.

Webster-Stratton, C. (1994). Advancing videotape parent training: A comparison study. *Journal of Consulting and Clinical Psychology, 62,* 583–593.

Webster-Stratton, C. (1998). Preventing conduct problems in Head Start children: Strengthening parent competencies. *Journal of Consulting and Clinical Psychology, 66,* 715–730.

Webster-Stratton, C., & Hammond, M.A. (1997). Treating children with early-onset conduct problems: A comparison of child and parent training interventions. *Journal of Consulting and Clinical Psychology, 65,* 93–109.

Webster-Stratton, C., Kolpacoff, M., & Hollinsworth, T. (1988). Self-administered videotape therapy for families with conduct-problem children: Comparison with two cost-effective treatments and a control group. *Journal of Consulting and Clinical Psychology, 56,* 558–566.

Webster-Stratton, C., Mihalic, S., Fagan, A., Arnold, D., Taylor, T., & Tingley, C. (2001). *Blueprints for violence prevention, book eleven: The Incredible Years: Parent, teacher and child training series.* Boulder, CO: Center for the Study and Prevention of Violence.

Webster-Stratton, C., & Reid, J. (June, 1999a). *Effects of teacher training in Head Start classrooms: Results of a randomized controlled evaluation.* Paper presented at the Society for Prevention Research, New Orleans, LA.

Webster-Stratton, C., & Reid, J. (November, 1999b). *Treating children with early-onset conduct problems: The importance of teacher training.* Paper presented at the Association for the Advancement of Behavior Therapy, Toronto, Canada.

Webster-Stratton, C., Reid, J., & Hammond, M. (2001). Social skills and problem-solving training for children with early-onset conduct problems: Who benefits? *Journal of Child Psychology and Psychiatry, 42,* 943–952.

Webster-Stratton, C., Reid, J., & Hammond, M. (2004). Treating children with early-onset conduct problems: Intervention outcomes for parent, child, and teacher training. *Journal of Clinical Child and Adolescent Psychology, 33,* 105–124.

Webster-Stratton, C., & Taylor, T. (2001). Nipping early risk factors in the bud: Preventing substance abuse, delinquency, and violence in adolescence through interventions targeted at young children (0 to 8 Years). *Prevention Science, 2,* 165–192.

Wechsler, D. (1974). *Wechsler Intelligence Scale for Children–Revised.* New York: The Psychological Corporation.

Zickler, P. (2003). *Few middle schools use proven prevention programs.* Bethesda, MD: U.S. Department of Health and Human Services, National Institutes of Health, National Institute on Drug Abuse.

7

PREVENTING RISKY
SEXUAL BEHAVIOR

Chelsea M. Weaver, Elizabeth H. Blodgett,
and Shannon S. Carothers

Epidemic levels of Acquired Immune Deficiency Syndrome (AIDS), sexually transmitted diseases (STDs), and early unwanted pregnancies place many teenagers at risk for problematic physical and emotional development. According to the Centers for Disease Control and Prevention (CDC) Youth Risk Behavior Surveillance (2004), 7.4% of adolescents have engaged in sexual intercourse prior to age 13. By ninth grade, one third of adolescents are already sexually active; this rate jumps more than 25% in the next 3 years. Specifically, 33% of youth in the ninth grade had sexual intercourse, 44% in the tenth grade, 53% in the eleventh grade, and 61.5% in the twelfth grade. Similar trends have been reported regarding increasing pregnancy rates and decreasing condom use for adolescents during their high school years (CDC, 2004). Contradictory evidence suggests that teenage pregnancy and birth rates have been steadily declining (Martin et al., 2005), indicating that adolescents' overall knowledge of sexuality may be increasing. Teenagers who do not have an accurate understanding of the risks related to early sexual activity may be more likely to experience negative outcomes. Unintended consequences, such as unwanted pregnancy and disease contraction, often have a long-term, damaging impact on the lives of young people, especially on their physical and emotional health.

Risky sexual behavior places the physical health of adolescents in jeopardy. Among females 10–44 years of age, those between ages of 15–19 showed the highest rate of gonorrhea in 2002 (Centers for Disease Control and Prevention [CDC], 2002). Although many STDs can easily be treated with antibiotics if detected early, infections such as human immunodeficiency virus (HIV) have no cure. According to the CDC (2001), there were 998 identified adolescents between ages 13–19 in the United States living with HIV and 1,967 adolescents of the same ages living with AIDS in 2001. Due to the devastating health and mortality risks associated with potentially life-altering decisions about sexuality, risky behaviors must be considered a matter of public health safety.

Similarly, unplanned pregnancies are another significant consequence of sexual risk taking during adolescence. Despite recent reported declines in the adolescent pregnancy and birth rates, teenage parenthood remains a serious social problem. In 2000, there were 84.5 pregnancies per 1,000 teenagers ages 15–19 years (Martin et al., 2005). Moreover, 41.6 per 1,000 teenage women between the same ages became mothers in 2003 (Martin et al.). Early pregnancies place adolescents at increased risk for experiencing personal and social adversity, particularly if the pregnancy results in parenthood.

Previous research has consistently found both adolescent mothers and their children to be at increased risk for experiencing social and emotional problems such as poverty, maladaptive parenting, and depression (Furstenburg, Levine, & Brooks-Gunn, 1990; Whitman, Borkowski, Keogh, & Weed, 2001). In turn, problems related to adolescent pregnancy cost taxpayers more than $7 billion per year (Maynard, 1997). Domino effects on each individual's ecological systems, including personal, family, community, and societal domains, highlight the importance of identifying the causes and correlates of adolescents' risky sexual behaviors, allowing for the design of effective prevention programs.

FACTORS RELATED TO RISKY SEXUAL BEHAVIOR

Sexual risk taking in adolescence is associated with multiple social factors, such as parenting practices and substance use. For example, adolescents who were closely monitored by a parent demonstrated fewer risky sexual behaviors than peers who were less supervised (Huebner & Howell, 2003). Parental permissiveness has been linked to risk-taking behaviors, such as having sex while using drugs or alcohol and having sex without a condom (Donenberg, Wilson, Emersom, & Bryant, 2002). Relatedly, drug and alcohol use during adolescence has been related to having more sexual partners as well as to a lack of consistent condom use in early adulthood (Guo et al., 2002). Overall, positive parenting including monitoring has been found to protect against the effects of negative peer influences (Bogenschneider, Wu, Raffaelli, & Tsay, 1998). This is important in light of recent research findings indicating that reports of sexual risk taking among friends are positively related to sexual behavior during adolescence (Bachanas et al., 2002). In short, parents may play an important role in preventing sexual risk taking.

In addition to heightened risks for HIV, STDs, and early pregnancy, unsafe sexual practices place young people in danger of victimization. For example, Howard and Wang (2003a) found that high school girls who were involved in dating violence were more likely than nonvictims to engage in risky sexual behaviors. Furthermore, in a representative sample of high school males, those who had multiple sex partners and those who had sex without a condom were more likely to be victims of physical dating violence (Howard & Wang, 2003b). Risky sexual behavior may be one symptom of a greater problem placing teenagers at physical and emotional risk.

Social competence may mediate the relationship between precipitating factors and the outcomes of risky sexual behavior among adolescents. Waters and Sroufe (1983) have found that a competent person has the ability to use environmental and personal resources to achieve a positive developmental outcome; therefore, personal competence is defined, in part, by social context. According to a model developed by Spence (2003), social competence is the result of socially skilled responding, which is defined by multiple constructs including interpersonal problem-solving skills, affect regulation, and self-regulation/self-monitoring skills. In the context of adolescent risky sexual behavior, this framework suggests that the teenagers must be equipped with tools to make positive decisions regarding sexual health under potentially stressful situations. Relatedly, Horwitz, Klerman, Kuo, and Jekel (1991) asserted that most adolescent pregnancies result from impulsivity, difficulty in modulating behavior, and a sense of invulnerability, underscoring the importance of targeting mechanisms such as adolescent social competency in conjunction with regulatory abilities in the prevention of risky sexual behaviors.

PREVENTION PROGRAMS: DESIGN AND IMPLEMENTATION ISSUES

An important component in the development and implementation of risky sexual behavior programs is the identification, and prior specification, of important targeted outcome(s). In focused, narrow prevention programs, information is often simply provided to participants in hopes that knowledge will lead to changes in attitudes and behaviors. It has been documented that knowledge alone does not decrease sexual risk-taking behaviors (Wayment & Aronson, 2002), suggesting that programs encompassing domains such as competency enhancement will be more effective in changing targeted outcomes. Programs targeting mechanisms of change are by definition more comprehensive and address skill-building in order to not only increase adolescents' knowledge but also to arm them with the tools necessary to make positive decisions and avoid engaging in risky behaviors within their actual social contexts.

Prevention programs sometimes target similar outcomes while differing in the general message conveyed to participants. At the extremes, some programs underscore the importance of having safe, protected sex, whereas others advocate abstinence from sexual activity. Even though these messages are very different, the goal of both is to prevent adolescents from engaging in risky sexual behaviors. It is important to note that in general, there have been few methodologically rigorous abstinence-only programs, and most have found either inconclusive or no evidence of behavioral change (e.g., Kirby, Korpi, Barth, & Cagampang, 1995; St. Pierre, Mark, Kaltreider, & Aikin, 1995). However, due to their design limitations, conclusions about abstinence programs must be drawn with caution (Kirby, 2002; Moore & Sugland, 1997). However, regardless of content, consistency in the message being sent to participants is an essential component of successful efforts to prevent risky adolescent sexual behaviors (Kirby, 2002).

Scientific evaluation is crucial in accurately assessing the impact of prevention programming. Assessments are typically conducted with respect to three types of outcomes: knowledge and attitude change, behavioral change, and the maintenance of change. First, enhancement of knowledge about and attitudes toward targeted outcomes (e.g., the methods of disease transmission) are often thought to impact the manifested behaviors (e.g., delayed initiation of sex, condom/contraception use), which are the most important gauge of program effectiveness. Behavioral changes must be maintained for participants to reap the benefits of program participation throughout adolescence and into adulthood. Multiple programs have shown immediate and even short-term impacts, but few have provided evidence of long-term effectiveness (Kirby, 2002). It is imperative that prevention efforts be designed to develop and build on process-oriented skills among participants to promote deep cognitive processing of programming content and, in turn, facilitate long-term maintenance of behavioral change.

The timing of implementation is another critical element of programs designed to prevent risky sexual behaviors in adolescence. As discussed earlier, self-reports of risk-taking behaviors reveal alarming rates of unsafe sexual activity among high school students (Centers for Disease Control and Prevention [CDC], 2001). More important, risky sexual behaviors increase dramatically with each consecutive grade level, indicating a pattern of escalating risk with each passing year. These disturbing statistics illustrate the importance of early program participation to prevent an upsurge of dangerous sexual behaviors among youth, particularly if a treatment goal is to delay the initiation of sex.

Evidence has shown that sexual risk taking in adolescence may lead to devastating physical and emotional consequences. In response, many prevention programs have been implemented and evaluated in an effort to decrease the precarious and often dangerous activities of youth (Coyle et al., 2001; Kirby, Barth, Leland, & Fetro, 1991; Philliber & Allen, 1992; Philliber, Kaye, Herrling, & West, 2000); however, evidence of long-term, comprehensive program effectiveness is scarce (Kirby, 2002).

PREVENTION PROGRAMS AND THEIR EVALUATIONS

This chapter evaluates and critiques three exemplar programs in terms of their design and efficacy: 1) Safer Choices (Coyle et al., 1996), 2) Teen Outreach Program (Philliber & Allen, 1992), and 3) Children's Aid Society Carrera Program (Philliber et al., 2000). The essential characteristics of these programs are summarized in Table 7.1. They are presented in terms of their increasing individualization and comprehensiveness, with the Children's Aid Society Carrera Program being closest to what is advocated as a model program to prevent risky sexual behaviors.

Safer Choices

Safer Choices is a theory-driven, 2-year, multicomponent HIV, STD, and pregnancy prevention program (Coyle et al., 1996). The primary goals of Safer Choices are 1) to decrease the number of students engaging in unprotected sex by delaying initiation of sexual intercourse and 2) to increase the use of condoms by those who are sexually active. A unique aspect of this program is its focus on levels of decision making regarding sexuality. Participants are taught the basic message that engaging in sexual intercourse before one is ready and/or unprotected is an unsafe choice; using protection against diseases and pregnancy while engaging in sexual intercourse is a safer choice; and abstaining from sex is the safest choice of all (Basen-Engquist et al., 2001; Coyle et al., 1996). Through the varying levels of protection from the consequences of risky sexual behaviors conveyed by the program, the Safer Choices message may be relevant to all students regardless of sexual experience and values.

Based on social cognitive theory (Bandura, 1986), social influences models (McGuire & Papageoris, 1961), and models of school change, Safer Choices focuses on the influence of school environments on behavioral change (Basen-Engquist et al., 2001). Specifically, changes within schools are achieved not only from direct effects of programming but also from indirect effects of information diffusion by students with higher levels of program exposure.

Safer Choices is implemented in schools and targets the decision-making skills of adolescents in grades 9 through 12. Five components make up the

Table 7.1. Three sexual behavior programs and their defining characteristics

	Safer Choices	Teen Outreach Program (TOP)	Children's Aid Society (CAS) Carrera
Targets of intervention	Males and females Grades 9–12 Parents of participants School and community environments	Males and females Middle school and high school students Volunteers and teenagers at risk for maladjustment	Males and females Ages 13–15 Ethnic minorities Impoverished urban areas Families of participants
Content of intervention	Teacher and peer modeling Direct skill training Skill practice in large and small groups Group discussion Drama productions Student–parent homework activities Building school, family, and community links	Supervised involvement in community volunteer services (1 hour per week) Classroom-based discussions Social and communication skill training Role plays	Job club (e.g., banking assistance, career awareness) Academic assistance Family life and sexuality education Art activities Sports involvement Mental health services Medical care Summer maintenance
Outcomes of intervention	Behavioral changes 31 months postbaseline: Increased use of condoms Increased use of pregnancy protection Psychosocial changes 31 months post-baseline: More positive attitude toward condom use Higher self-efficacy in condom use Increased communication with parents Fewer barriers to condom use	Reduced rates of: Pregnancy School suspension Course failure School dropout Arrest Truancy Increased contraception use Increased academic achievement	Increased knowledge of sexual health Increased receipt of good health care Decreased likelihood of sexual initiation (for females) Increased resistance to pressure to have sex (for females) Increased use of dual contraception methods (for females) Lower rates of pregnancy and birth for females at 3-year follow-up
Costs and/or duration	Grades 9–12	$500–$700 per student; 9-month school year	5 days a week during school year and summer booster sessions

prevention package: school organization, curriculum and staff development, peer resources, school environment, and school–community relationships. The curriculum consists of 20 sessions implemented by teachers and/or peer leaders for individuals in ninth and tenth grades (10 per grade; Coyle et al., 1996). The sessions are based on the Reducing the Risk: Building to Prevent Teen Pregnancy curriculum, which targets knowledge, attitudes and beliefs, social competency, peer norms, and parent–child communication (see Kirby et al., 1991). Specific activities include teacher and peer modeling of skills (e.g., role playing), explicit teaching of small tasks that comprise targeted skills, skill practice in small and large groups, small-group discussions, and drama productions targeting HIV- and AIDS-related issues (Coyle et al.).

Safer Choices incorporates multiple individuals who come into daily contact with students, including parental, school, and community figures. At each school, there is a School Health Promotion Council whose members include parents, teachers, administrators, students, and community representatives (Coyle et al., 1996). The council plans, implements, and monitors activities in four domains: curriculum and staff development (e.g., faculty in-service activities), peer resources and school environment (e.g., anonymous peer role model stories), parent education (e.g., parent night featuring student plays), and school–community linkages (e.g., youth service resource guide). Parents are also encouraged to participate in Safer Choices by completing student–parent homework activities designed to facilitate positive communication. In addition, project newsletters containing information about STDs, HIV/AIDS, and pregnancy as well as parenting information are sent to participants' parents. The Safer Choices program involves the community through providing students with lists of resources for HIV-, STD-, and pregnancy-related services as well as by assigning homework to students, requiring further investigation of local services available within the area. In addition, a lecture by an individual who is HIV positive and who lives within the community is included in the curriculum.

Program Evaluation   The Safer Choices program conducted a randomized clinical trial in 20 ethnically and socioeconomically diverse high schools at two urban sites (N=8,319); 10 schools in northern California and 10 schools in southeastern Texas (Basen-Engquist et al., 2001). Five schools at each site were randomly assigned to receive either the Safer Choices program or a knowledge-based curriculum on HIV and STDs (five 50-minute sessions addressing information regarding contraception, STDs, HIV, and the consequences of unsafe sex). Students in grades 9 and 10 were exposed to one of the two intervention conditions, whereas students in grades 11 and 12 were either exposed to Safer Choices' schoolwide activities if they attended an intervention school or no activities if they attended a comparison school. Program efficacy was measured in terms of behavioral and psychosocial change at 7, 19, and 31 months postbaseline (Basen-Engquist et al., 2001).

At the end of the first year of intervention (7 months postbaseline), a cohort sample (N = 3,677) was used to test the short-term effects of Safer Choices. Among behavioral variables, multilevel analyses revealed that the intervention group had a significantly lower frequency of recent sexual intercourse without a condom ($p = .03$) and fewer recent sexual partners without a condom ($p = .07$) than the comparison group (Coyle et al., 1999). The experimental group was also more likely to have used condoms ($p = .02$) and to have used pregnancy protection ($p = .03$) at last intercourse than the control group. No other behavioral differences were found ($p = .35$ to .88; Coyle et al., 1999). Psychosocial change included increased HIV and STD knowledge ($p = .00$ and $p = .00$, respectively) and risk perception ($p = .00$ and $p = .02$, respectively) of intervention schools compared with control schools. Also, students in intervention schools had more positive attitudes toward condom use ($p = .00$), self-efficacy in condom use ($p = .00$), communication with parents ($p = .03$), and fewer barriers to condom use ($p = .00$) than comparison schools. No other psychosocial differences were found. Multilevel analyses assessing long-term change in a cohort of students (N = 3,869) 12 months after the second year of intervention (31 months postbaseline) yielded similar results (Coyle et al., 2001). All behavioral effects were maintained; psychosocial effects were maintained with the exception of normative beliefs about condom use and communication with parents, both of which were marginally nonsignificant.

In addition to cohort analyses, researchers conducted cross-sectional analyses using three samples of ninth- through twelfth-grade students: preintervention (baseline), following year 2 of intervention (19 months postbaseline), and 1 year following year 2 of intervention (31 months after baseline). At the 19-month follow-up, multilevel analyses within schools of behavioral variables revealed that students at Safer Choices schools had less frequent recent sex without a condom than students at comparison schools ($p = .03$); no other within-school behavioral variables were significant ($p = .06$ to .91; Basen-Engquist et al., 2001). An analysis of the significant behavioral finding within grades revealed that ninth-grade students who received intervention had less frequent recent sex without a condom than comparison ninth-grade students ($p = .01$). There were no differences in tenth, eleventh, or twelfth grades, with effect sizes decreasing as grade level increased.

Psychosocial changes within schools among intervention students 19 months postbaseline included increased HIV and STD knowledge ($p < .01$ and $p < .01$, respectively), normative beliefs about condom use ($p = .02$), self-efficacy in refusing sex ($p < .01$), self-efficacy in condom use ($p < .01$), and communication with parents ($p = .02$) as compared with control students. No other within-school psychosocial variables were significant. Within grade level, HIV knowledge in intervention schools was higher across all grades as compared with control schools, whereas STD knowledge was only higher for students who received intervention in ninth grade. Condom use self-efficacy and communication with parents was higher only for ninth- and tenth-grade intervention students as compared with control students (Basen-Engquist et al., 2001).

At the 31-month assessment, within-school analyses of behavioral variables revealed that ninth- through twelfth-grade students at Safer Choices schools had fewer recent sexual partners without using a condom ($p < .01$). There was no difference, however, in the number of students who engaged in recent sexual intercourse ($p = .45$; Basen-Engquist et al., 2001). Within grades, only ninth- and eleventh-grade students in Safer Choices schools had significantly fewer partners with whom they had unprotected sex than comparison students ($p = .03$ and $p = .05$, respectively). Within-school analysis of psychosocial variables at the 31-month assessment revealed that HIV knowledge and self-efficacy in condom use were significantly higher for students who received intervention than comparison students ($p < .01$ and $p = .02$, respectively). Furthermore, the effect of HIV knowledge was significant at all grade levels; however, condom use self-efficacy was greater only for tenth- and eleventh-grade students at Safer Choices schools than at comparison schools (Basen-Engquist et al., 2001).

Safer Choices is a cost-effective prevention program (Wang et al., 2000). More specifically, behavioral changes at 7-month follow-up were used to calculate costs averted through prevented AIDS, STD, and pregnancy cases, assuming that intervention effects lasted for 1 year. For every dollar invested in Safer Choices (total cost = $105,243), $2.65 was saved (Wang et al.), yielding a total savings of $278,894 in medical and social costs.

Critical Analysis of Treatment Characteristics   Safer Choices incorporates multiple treatment characteristics, including a basis in theory and comprehensive programming. In addition, the program characteristics overlap to fulfill several goals of effective programming. Consequently, Safer Choices addresses personal, environmental, and behavioral domains through components such as knowledge training, resource availability, and modeling (Coyle et al., 1996). Social networks are used to tackle topics such as resisting negative social pressures.

Intervention components such as the School Health Promotion Council do more than promote organizational change within the school. Elements that incorporate multiple social systems, such as family, peer, and community networks, are necessary in facilitating the development and maintenance of behavioral change (Bronfenbrenner, 1977). Other program strategies that tap various social domains include teacher and peer role plays, drama productions, parent–child homework activities, and speakers who are HIV positive (Coyle et al., 1996). These components serve other critical functions of successful intervention programs, such as incorporating varied teaching methods in implementation as well as facilitating positive relationships among program participants, their families, schools, and program staff. The fact that the program components are intertwined and overlapping in meeting multiple goals indicates a well-planned, developed, and executed school-based intervention program that is theory driven and comprehensive.

Critical Analysis of Procedural Characteristics   The Safer Choices program included comprehensive staff training techniques in order to promote competence in curriculum implementation. In addition to program staff, school staff and peer leaders underwent extensive training prior to the implementation of the program. For instance, teachers received 30 hours of training, site coordinators received 10 hours of training, and peer leaders received 3 hours of training. Safer Choices had adequate dosage levels in order to produce desired change; however, increased exposure across domains (e.g., school, family, community) would have likely produced even greater effects, especially in terms of their long-term maintenance. Relatedly, summer booster sessions with school staff, participants, and their families also may have benefited adolescents, principally due to the decreased amount of structure and increased peer socialization opportunities experienced during summer months.

The timing of implementation is a crucial aspect of prevention programs, particularly in the area of sexual risk behavior (Kirby, 2002). This factor may be related to the fact that Safer Choices was not effective in achieving the program's primary goal of delaying initiation of sexual intercourse. In particular, initiation of sexual intercourse was not delayed at the 7-month (Coyle et al., 1999), 19-month, or 31-month time points (Basen-Engquist et al., 2001; Coyle et al., 2001). This lack of significant findings may have been related to poor timing of program implementation; specifically, the ninth grade (about 14–15 years of age) may be too late to prevent the onset of sexual initiation in adolescents. It is imperative that prevention programs begin before risky behaviors are developed and become accepted.

Critical Analysis of Design Characteristics   Methodologically, Safer Choices is one of the most scientifically rigorous school-based prevention programs evaluated to date. First, a randomized block design was employed to assign schools to treatment and control conditions within each of the two study sites utilizing a restricted randomization procedure (Basen-Engquist et al., 1997). Specifically, investigators created an index of possible confounding variables such as socioeconomic status, number of students, and dropout rates, which were then tested for their potential influence on program outcomes using principal components analysis. The most influential components were identified for each site (accounting for approximately 90% of the variance at each location) and weighed in order of importance; composite scores were then created for each school (with higher scores indicating greater expected success due to the intervention). Schools were ranked and paired; one school from each pair was randomly assigned to either the treatment or control condition (Basen-Engquist et al., 1997).

Another methodological strength of Safer Choices is the testing of the concurrent validity of the Sexual Risk Behavior Beliefs and Self-Efficacy Scales, which measured psychosocial determinants of behavior (Basen-Engquist et al., 1999). Specifically, multivariate analysis revealed that intercourse involvement scales (norms about sexual intercourse, attitudes about sexual intercourse, and self-efficacy in refusing sex) differentiated students who were sexually experienced from those who were not as well as those who were sexually active in the last 3 months and those who were not. Similarly, among recently sexually active students (n = 1,855), norms about condom use, attitudes about condom use, self-efficacy in communication, self- efficacy in using condoms, and barriers to condom use differentiated between consistent and nonconsistent condom users. All relationships were in the expected direction—for example, consistent condom users had higher self-efficacy in condom use and competence in communicating with partners about condom use.

Other design strengths of the Safer Choices program include the use of an active control condition as well as a statement of clear goals related to outcome evaluation. Students who attended a comparison school were exposed to a standard knowledge-based HIV prevention curriculum (Coyle et al., 1999), thereby increasing their ability to attribute change to the actual intervention rather than to mere attention or knowledge provision. In terms of outcome evaluation, investigators clearly stated its primary goals as "to reduce the number of students engaging in unprotected sexual intercourse by reducing the number of students who begin or have sexual intercourse during their high school years, and by increasing condom use among those students who have sex" (Coyle et al., 1996, p. 89). Secondary goals were to reduce the number of students who had multiple sex partners; reduce drug use (particularly intravenous); and to increase the number of students who seek HIV/STD counseling, testing, and consultation. To assess progress toward program goals, investigators systematically investigated behavioral and psychosocial change in respect to relevant variables associated with outcome constructs using both cohort and cross-sectional designs (Basen-Engquist et al., 2001; Coyle et al., 1999; Coyle et al., 2001; Parcel et al., 1999).

An important methodological concern of the Safer Choices program was the attention paid to attrition. Students who dropped out of the school cohort as well as students who did not complete the follow-up survey were less likely to live with both parents and more likely to be older, to have received lower grades, to have engaged in more risk behaviors, to have had poorer scores on many psychosocial scales (Coyle et al., 1999), and to be males (Coyle et al., 2001). Due to the elevated level of risk of these children, they potentially could have benefited most from the Safer Choices program. It is important to note that the level of attrition compromises the extent to which findings can be generalized to the population. However, Safer Choices maintained a large heterogeneous sample of high school students in the program, thereby increasing external validity despite selective attrition.

Teen Outreach Program

The Teen Outreach Program (TOP) is a 1-year, school-based youth development program with the goals of preventing pregnancy and encouraging school success through classroom education, group discussions, and community volunteer services. Participation in TOP has been growing steadily since the program's beginning in the late 1970s. There are more than 130 sites across the United States and Canada providing services to thousands of adolescents in middle schools, junior high schools, and senior high schools (Allen, Kuperminc, Philliber, & Herre, 1994; Allen & Philliber, 2001; Dryfoos, 1990; Kirby, 1997). The classroom size for each of these sites ranges from 5 to 25, with an average of 15 students in a single section (Philliber & Allen, 1992). Participants enlist in TOP in several ways. In some schools, students volunteer by responding to advertisements, whereas students in other schools are referred due to at-risk status (e.g., prior pregnancy, low academic achievement). For example, 41% of teenagers in the program came from families that were not intact, 40% had failed a course, 20% had parents with less than a high school education, 17% had been suspended from school, and 4% had already been pregnant (Philliber & Allen).

TOP has three main components: supervised involvement in community volunteer service, classroom-based discussion of service experience, and classroom-based discussion and activities related to key social-developmental tasks of adolescents (Allen, Philliber, Herrling, & Kuperminc, 1997; Philliber & Allen, 1992). TOP is usually offered after school, but programs also have been offered during school hours and for course credit, either as part of general health curricula or as an academic elective (Allen et al., 1994; Philliber & Allen).

TOP participants meet for 1 hour once a week throughout the 9-month school year, starting in August or September and ending in May or June (Allen et al., 1997; Allen & Philliber, 2001; Philliber & Allen, 1992). They participate in discussions involving topics such as understanding the self, values, communication skills, decision making, human growth and development, life options, parenting, family relationships, and community resources (Kirby, 1997; Philliber & Allen). An important characteristic of TOP is that it aims to enhance students' competence in social-developmental skills instead of specifically targeting the problem behaviors it seeks to prevent (Allen et al., 1997). The program includes traditional sex education information, but this is not the main emphasis. In fact, material about sexuality is less than 15% of the curriculum (Allen, Philliber, & Hoggson, 1990; Allen et al.; Allen & Philliber, 2001). TOP is a youth development program that works from an empowerment perspective by enhancing participants' autonomy and relatedness with others (Allen et al., 1994; Allen & Philliber).

TOP's curriculum is student centered, meaning that group discussions and activities are facilitated rather than taught. Facilitators create supportive environments that encourage sharing and openness among students through structured discussion, group exercises, and role plays. Volunteer activities vary in their settings and responsibilities, reflecting different community needs and student interests (Philliber & Allen, 1992). Activities are selected by participants under the supervision of facilitators and include work in hospitals, participation in walkathons, and tutoring (Allen et al., 1990). TOP requires that students perform at least 1 hour a week of volunteer service, with a minimum community service commitment of 20 hours; however, the average student's volunteer time is more than 40 hours (Allen et al., 1997; Kirby, 2002). Cost analyses of TOP show that the program can be offered for $500–$700 per student for a year (Allen et al., 1997). When facilitator costs are provided by outside sources, the program cost falls to less than $100 per student.

Program Evaluation

TOP targets a wide range of individuals. More than 75% of the students enrolled in the program were females (Philliber & Allen, 1992). The overall age range for all participants was 11–19 years, with an average age of 14.9 (Kirby, 1997; Philliber & Allen). Students from 5th to 12th grades participated, with most students in ninth or tenth grades. In nationwide Teen Outreach Programs, the distribution of race was 40% African American; 40% Caucasian; 13% Hispanic; and 7% Asian, Native American, or other (Philliber & Allen). Evaluation of TOP first began by comparing school suspension and course failures as well as dropout and pregnancy rates for both TOP participants and the control groups. As the program has developed and expanded, data also has been collected on arrests, truancy, illegal substance use, sexual activity, contraceptive use, involvement in after-school activities, academic achievements, and educational aspirations. Evaluations of TOP sites have shown that attrition has been fairly low, not exceeding 10.2% (Philliber & Allen).

Evaluations of TOP have shown that the risk of pregnancy, school suspension, course failure, and school dropout among students in the program is less than half the risk in comparison groups (Allen et al., 1997; Allen & Philliber, 2001; Kirby, 2002; Philliber & Allen, 1992). In addition, TOP participants were less likely to drop out of school, even when controlling for grade and pregnancy. Participation in TOP was related to fewer arrests, higher rates of school attendance, more regular use of contraception, and a higher rate of achieving academic awards and honor roll status (Philliber & Allen). Participation was not significantly associated with illegal substance use or aspirations to finish high school.

Analyses of TOP have indicated under which conditions and for which kinds of participants this program is most successful. For example, participants in programs involving older, high school students had fewer problem behaviors at the program's termination (Allen et al., 1990; Allen et al., 1994; Philliber & Allen, 1992). Similarly, students who perceived the program as promoting their autonomy and relatedness with others and who viewed their volunteer work as important had better outcomes than students who did not maintain a similar outlook (Allen et al., 1994). Programs that most fully implemented services had higher success rates (Philliber & Allen). In particular, TOP students who performed more volunteer work were at lower risk for course failure during the program and had fewer overall problems at program exit (Allen et al., 1990; Allen et al., 1997). TOP appeared to be especially effective for adolescents who were most at risk for the targeted behaviors. For example, the program had a sizable impact in reducing future pregnancies among those who had already given birth (Allen & Philliber, 2001). TOP was more effective for teenagers who had previously been suspended or failed a course (Allen & Philliber). Gender, minority status, parent education, classroom hours, credit for participation, and after versus during school hours were not related to program success (Allen et al., 1990; Philliber & Allen, 1992).

Critical Analysis of Treatment Characteristics   TOP addresses noticeable gaps in prior research by targeting broad developmental tasks instead of individual behaviors and microskills (Allen et al., 1997). Its developmental focus helps participants understand and evaluate their future life options, including relationship and career decisions. Because of its broader goals, TOP distances itself from the social stigma that often surrounds many pregnancy prevention programs. In addition, TOP has produced reliable changes, thereby lending support to the efficacy of the program. The curriculum is comprehensive and incorporates volunteer service, which can provide students with new perspectives on school and adult responsibilities. Volunteer service has been linked to positive outcomes in youth, providing theoretical justification for inclusion of this component (Allen et al., 1990; Allen et al., 1997).

TOP utilizes a variety of teaching methods, including supervised community service as well as classroom-based activities dealing with key social-developmental tasks. Activities include discussions, group exercises, role plays, guest speakers, films, and informational presentations (Allen et al., 1990; Allen et al., 1997). The program involves mentoring from a caring and supportive facilitator, work experience in the community that offers the opportunity to develop skills and a sense of purpose, and a supportive peer environment (Philliber & Allen, 1992). Also, the curriculum focuses on developing life skills related to coping, assertiveness, decision making, and communication. Nationwide sites promote student autonomy and competence, allowing students to become connected to others in the school and community. This provides TOP participants with the opportunity to be viewed positively by program facilitators and other adults in the community as well as by their peers. In addition, it allows students the opportunity to feel pride and a sense of belonging with the program (Philliber & Allen). In short, TOP is a comprehensive prevention program that focuses on promoting strong and positive relationships between students, their peers, and the community.

Critical Analysis of Procedural Characteristics   TOP emphasizes the use of activities in which students are facilitated but not taught. Facilitators receive formal training in order to successfully lead students. They attend the annual national Teen Outreach Program conference, which offers workshops dealing with the program structure, curriculum, and its desired facilitator style (Philliber & Allen, 1992). In addition, they are encouraged to become mentors and friends to their students and are taught the skills necessary for creating a trusting environment that ensures confidentiality.

TOP mainly targets adolescents in grades 7 through 12. Because appropriate timing is important in prevention programs on risky sexual behaviors, seventh grade may not be early enough. TOP has attempted to address this concern, however, by starting some children in the program as early as the fifth grade. Programs targeting younger students are likely to be successful if classroom components are more intensive (Allen et al., 1990). Although TOP has demonstrated success with males and females as well as those of different racial groups (Philliber & Allen, 1992), most participants to date have been female. Thus, the program should specifically target males in their future recruitment strategies. In addition, members of racial minorities should be actively recruited because TOP is more effective for minority students who are at risk for academic difficulty (Allen & Philliber, 2001).

Although a limited number of 1-year follow-up data have been collected, maintenance of effects has not been evaluated (Philliber & Allen, 1992). Therefore, it is not known if the program provides sufficient dosage to produce lasting change. Booster sessions should be implemented to provide students with the opportunity to maintain learned skills, and long-term follow-up data should be obtained.

Critical Analysis of Design Characteristics   TOP uses a rigorous experimental approach and has been replicated in many locations nationwide and throughout Canada, involving thousands of teenagers. The program includes multiple sites within multiple cities, random assignment procedures, control groups, large sample sizes, and rigorous evaluation procedures. Although self-report measures have typically been used in TOP, most students were found to be accurate reporters of course failure and school suspension when compared with school data (Allen et al., 1997).

The goals of TOP are very clear: prevent early pregnancy and encourage school success in adolescents. The program is systematically organized often with a randomly assigned control group and a matched experimental group to allow researchers to adequately assess the program's impact on participants' rates of pregnancy, school suspension, course failure, and school dropout. When randomization was not used in the early years of the program, comparison students were selected by participants who identified them as similar (Philliber & Allen, 1992). Randomly and nonrandomly assigned groups had similar treatment effect sizes (Allen & Philliber, 2001); however, randomization has been used consistently. Regardless of the participant selection method, entry differences between treatment and control groups were discovered, indicating the importance of collecting data before students know about their group membership (Allen et al., 1994, 1997).

Findings indicated that the program was successful in significantly reducing the frequency of all four targeted outcomes: pregnancy, school suspension, course failure, and school dropout (Allen & Philliber, 2001). Research also has indicated that TOP was successful for both high- and low-risk individuals; however, the program was most effective for those teenagers at the highest risk for the specific problem behavior being addressed (Allen & Philliber). Because these significant changes were seen, TOP can be thought of as a clinically and socially significant program for young adolescents during a time in which obtaining the skills necessary to prevent pregnancy and succeed academically is crucial.

Children's Aid Society Carrera Program

The Children's Aid Society (CAS) Carrera Program is a sex education, pregnancy prevention, and youth development program for urban minority youth ages 13–15 who are considered to be at high risk because of poverty (Alford, 2003). Using a family-systems structure, the program promotes a stable and nurturing home environment. The key element of this program is that staff believe in adolescents, continually supporting their dreams and encouraging their creativity. The comprehensive intervention rests on six principles: 1) staff treats participants as if they were family; 2) staff views each person as pure potential; 3) the program offers holistic services and comprehensive, integrated case management; 4) the program includes continuous, long-term contact with participants; 5) the program involves parents and families; and 6) all services are available under one roof in a nonpunitive environment. The overall philosophy of this approach is based on the belief that those participating in the program are not *at risk* but rather *at promise* (Children's Aid Society, 2002).

Throughout the school year, program activities run 5 days a week, generally for about 3 hours per day (Alford, 2003). Participants are divided into groups that rotate among five major activities: 1) job club—offering stipends, help with bank accounts, employment experience, and career awareness; 2) academics—including individual assessment, tutoring, PSAT and SAT preparation, and assistance with applying to colleges; 3) comprehensive family life and sexuality education; 4) arts—including weekly music, dance, writing, or drama workshops; and 5) individual sports activities that emphasize impulse control, such as golf and swimming. In addition, two service components are offered: mental health and medical care, including reproductive health care, primary care, and dental care. Over the summer, program activities include maintenance meetings to reinforce youth's sex education, academic skills, job assistance, social events, recreational activities, and cultural trips. For females, the program expresses clear norms about abstinence and contraceptive use by encouraging them to avoid sex or to use contraceptives, by providing role-playing in sex education classes, and by helping those who are sexually active obtain contraceptives from a health clinic (Kirby, 2001).

Each program site is staffed by part-time employees who implement the various components and by a full-time coordinator who oversees the program (Philliber et al., 2000). In addition, a full-time community organizer handles day-to-day logistics and maintains continuous contact with participants and their parents. Community organizers are community members selected because of their good rapport with residents.

Over a 3-year time span, adolescents in the CAS Carrera Program were compared with those recruited as a control condition from six other service agencies throughout New York City (Advocates for Youth, 2003). Adolescents were not eligible to participate if they were enrolled in an ongoing structured after-school program that had a regular meeting schedule (Philliber, Kaye, & Herrling, 2001). Programs used a variety of recruitment strategies including practicing outreach in the schools, distributing fliers throughout the neighborhood, contacting families on the agency's mailing list, and recruiting teenagers involved in general recreation activities at the agency. Participants were randomly assigned to the CAS Carrera Program or to an alternative program. At most sites, the alternative was the agency's regular program for youth. Each site recruited approximately 100 students who, following baseline data collection by the evaluation team, drew envelopes out of a bag to determine if they would be in the Carrera program or the alternative (Philliber et al.). Parents of prospective program and control teenagers were given an extensive orientation about these programs prior to data collection. Participants (N = 484; 50% male) ranged in age from 13 to 15 years. Among females, 54% of participants were African American and 46% were Hispanic; among males, 47% were African American and 53% were Hispanic. The majority of the youth (55%) lived in single parent homes.

To facilitate tracking, especially of the control group, students were contacted several times a year, sent birthday cards, and received cash and other incentives at each assessment phase (Philliber et al., 2001). A part-time tracker helped maintain the sample through home visits, telephone calls, and visits to the program sites to find and survey participants who did not appear for the regular data collection time points. At sites outside of the New York City areas, local evaluators helped with this process. Initiatives resulted in retaining 484 out of 600 participants over the course of the study.

Program Evaluation   The program's effectiveness was assessed using pre- and posttests of knowledge related to sexuality topics, attendance data, and participant follow-up data (e.g., delayed initiation of sexual intercourse, increased resistance to sexual pressures, increased use of dual methods of good health care, rates of teenage pregnancy). Information was provided by program staff, participant contact information documented by the mental health counselors, a data base maintained by the central CAS office to document the medical component, and interviews conducted by the research team with program staff (Philliber et al., 2001). Participants' knowledge of sexual health issues rose by 22%, compared with 11% among control youth. Male participants showed greater sexual health knowledge gains than did control males (18% and 6%, respectively). Females in the program were significantly less likely than control females to have ever had sex (46% versus 34%). Females in the program were significantly more likely than those in the control group to say they had successfully resisted pressure to have sex (75% and 36%, respectively). Sexually experienced program females were significantly more likely than control females to have used a condom along with a highly effective method of contraception (i.e., the pill, the injection, the implant) at most recent sex (36% and 20%, respectively). Both male and female participants were more likely than controls to receive good health care. Among sexually experienced males, those in the treatment group were significantly more likely to visit reproductive health care facilities than those in the control group (74% and 46%, respectively). Furthermore, at the 3-year follow-up, females in the Carrera Program had significantly lower rates of pregnancy and births than did control females.

In short, the CAS Carrera Program has been shown to delay initiation of female sexual intercourse, increase resistance to sexual pressure (females only), increase female use of dual methods of contraception, and reduce rates of teenage pregnancy (Advocates for Youth, 2003). However, data on males in the program showed no positive, significant behavioral differences except increased receipt of good health care. Program males were less likely than control males to report use of dual methods of contraception at most recent sex. The data suggested that reaching young men sooner may strengthen outcomes, and, as a result, the Children's Aid Society has begun implementing programs with 11- and 12-year-old youth (Children's Aid Society, 2002).

Critical Analysis of Treatment Characteristics The CAS Carrera Program was implemented in an effort to address four concerns regarding teenage pregnancy: 1) 4 out of 10 girls get pregnant at least once before age 20, 2) teenagers are having sex earlier, 3) teenagers use contraceptives inconsistently, and 4) there are enormous costs associated with teenage pregnancy. By addressing gaps evident in previous efforts (e.g., single intervention programs), the CAS Carrera Program is based on the theory that cognitive approaches alone are insufficient in addressing teenage childbirth. The program founders set out to address these concerns by developing a sex education, pregnancy prevention, and youth development program for urban youth considered to be at high risk. The program has great sociocultural relevance when considering that these individuals see little employment opportunities and will probably face a life of low economic status, ever-present racism, and inadequate opportunities for quality education (Children's Aid Society, 2002).

The CAS Carrera Program is a holistic approach that aims to empower youth (Children's Aid Society, 2002). Through varied teaching methods, the program helps young people develop personal goals and the desire for a productive future, as well as help them realize that early pregnancy may interfere with these goals. The program includes youth development, daily after-school activities, summer programs, health care, family involvement, interpersonal skill development, and access to social services. In addition to promoting sexual literacy and educating teens about the consequences of sexual activity, the program also emphasizes the importance of education and employment (Children's Aid Society).

A critical component of the CAS Carrera Program is the conscious effort by staff to form close relationships with teenagers. In some cases, staff members were characterized as surrogate parents for youth participating in the program (Kirby, 2001). As such, in addition to its philosophy and structure, staff roles may contribute to the successful long-term relationships that a large proportion of the participants formed with the program and its staff (Philliber et al., 2000). In short, the comprehensiveness of the CAS Carrera Program addresses multiple domains that have been suggested by Ivry and Doolittle (2003) as necessary in improving the economic and life outcomes of youth who are at risk, particularly in home, school, and community settings. Most important is the program's ability to foster relationships with adults who are concerned about participant well-being.

Critical Analysis of Procedural Characteristics   The CAS Carrera Program is an example of a program that has sufficient dosage, well-trained staff, and treatment fidelity. In particular, a critical aspect of the curriculum that sets it apart from other programs is that activities are offered 5 days a week throughout the school year. In addition, summer programs (booster sessions) were offered that reinforced sex education, academic skills, and job assistance. Moreover, extensive training of staff was highly enforced throughout each site. Specifically, the program has established a four-part training system: 1) initial training on the philosophy of the program and its organizing principles, duration, and intensity; 2) a 5-day training session lasting from 9 A.M. to 5 P.M. where staff are given copies of the curriculum and protocol and lessons focus on the objectives and techniques for each of the seven components of the model; 3) mandatory maintenance training to be held once a month each year for all staff by their individual components (educators, social workers, sex education); and 4) annual visits by Dr. Carrera to each program site to reinforce the philosophy of the program and discuss problem-solving techniques (M.A. Carrera, personal communication, March 16, 2004).

The CAS Carrera Program generally focused on both males and female, ages 13–15. Appropriate timing is of most importance for any program geared toward reducing risky sexual behavior. Consequently, it may be the case that many youth recruited to participate in the CAS Carrera Program have already engaged in sexual intercourse prior to entry into the program. This reality directly contradicts efforts to teach the importance of delaying sexual intercourse. In fact, the program developers have recognized this drawback and are implementing the program with 11- and 12-year-old participants. Overall, the procedural aspects of the CAS Carrera Program set it apart from other sex prevention programs; however, improvement is needed in the area of appropriate timing.

Critical Analysis of Design Characteristics   The CAS Carrera Program is rigorous and includes multiple sites, random assignment, control groups, a large sample size, long-term measurement, measurement of behavior, and rigorous statistical analyses (Kirby, 2002). The social significance of the CAS Carrera Program is evident in that, particularly for girls, studies have shown that after 3 years of participation, the program significantly delayed the onset of sexual intercourse, increased the use of condoms as a secondary method with another highly effective method of contraception (e.g., Depo-Provera shots), reduced pregnancy rates, and reduced birth rates (Kirby). However, participation in the program created no significant impact on males' sexual and reproductive behavior outcomes (Philliber et al., 2000).

Despite possessing the above-mentioned design characteristics, the program has encountered several limitations. First, in relation to internal validation, the program did not have significant positive behavioral effects for males, but the study did have one unexpected finding: Males in the programs were significantly less likely to report using both condoms and another highly effective contraception method at last sex than boys in the control group (Kirby, 2002). As stated earlier, this may be due to the high percentage of males who had initiated sexual activity prior to the onset of the program (Kirby), suggesting the need to begin the program earlier. Second, it should also be recognized that the CAS Carrera Program requires complex implementation, utilizing significant financial and staff resources, such that sites not able to implement all program components cannot expect to achieve positive results (Kirby). Third, in reference to the control groups, program and control teenagers sometimes attended different programs located at the same site, suggesting that some exchange of information, or contamination of the control group, might have occurred (Philliber et al., 2000). Fourth, analyses were conducted for 3 years; however, the observed advantages among program students might dissipate over a longer period of time (Philliber et al.). Fifth, due to the fact that the participants were minority teenagers living in New York City, findings regarding the study's effectiveness may not be generalizable (Philliber et al.). Sixth, Philliber and colleagues mentioned that their sites benefited from the extensive training and support provided by Children's Aid Society staff. Sites that lack intensive support may find implementing the program to be challenging.

MODEL PROGRAM FOR
THE PREVENTION OF RISKY SEXUAL BEHAVIORS

A model program designed to prevent risky sexual behaviors should be comprehensive, individualized, person-oriented, and based on a multisystemic perspective, joining together several domains of each young person's life. Table 7.2 presents the recommended components of a model prevention program in terms of the targeted individuals, curriculum content, targeted outcomes, and program duration. Specifically, programming must be integrated into each individual's ecological system, which includes school settings, family life, and community resources (Bronfenbrenner, 1977). For example, children and their families must be encouraged to be highly involved in one another's lives as well as within the community

Table 7.2. Components of a model risky sexual behavior prevention program

Targets of intervention	Preadolescent males and females
	Participants' families
	Community environment
	Both general and high-risk populations
Content of intervention	Social competency and communication skill building through discussions and activities with peers, parents, teachers, and community figures
	Innovative teaching techniques (e.g., role playing)
	Sexual health education
	Community involvement
	Academic assistance (e.g., peer tutoring)
Targeted outcomes of intervention	Reduce incidence of sexual initiation
	Increase use of disease and pregnancy protection
	Increase social competency, self-efficacy, and communication skills
	Increase school achievement
	Improve family relationships as well as school and community atmospheres
Duration	2 years of intense intervention in grades 6 and 7 with summer booster sessions; booster sessions in grades 8–12

as demonstrated by the Teen Outreach (Philliber & Allen, 1992) and CAS Carrera (Philliber et al., 2000) programs. Education and training regarding specific skills that apply across environmental contexts, such as effective communication, problem solving, and parenting, should be implemented with individuals as well as their peers and families in risky sexual behavior prevention programs. Curricula should intervene with numerous areas of life to transform entire systems, such as the ways in which school, family, and community settings interact with one another to influence individual behavior, thereby promoting lasting change.

Within comprehensive programs, staff members must be salient figures who are not only trusted and respected by participants, but also equally important, they must respect and believe in participants. Relatedly, project staff must wholeheartedly support the basic tenets of the program for which they are advocating (Kirby, 2002). This ideology is at the heart of the CAS Carrera Program and is believed to be crucial to the program's success (Philliber, Kaye, & Herrling, 2002). Both of these characteristics work together to build positive, supportive relationships among those involved in the program, thereby facilitating successful outcomes targeted by the curriculum.

Prevention curricula must incorporate multiple facets and be dictated by each individual's needs. First, straightforward, clear information regarding sexual risk-taking behaviors, their consequences, methods of refusing sex, and methods of protecting oneself must be provided (Kirby, 2002). Clear program goals of behavioral change should be identified and targeted. In addition, participants should be taught underlying skills of social competency that will assist them in negotiating multiple social pressures and potentially risky situations. All of the exemplar programs included in this chapter have demonstrated this essential attribute (Coyle et al., 1996; Kirby et al., 1991; Philliber & Allen, 1992; Philliber et al., 2000). Participants also should have safe, nonjudgmental environments in which to practice their newly developing skills.

In summary, a model program to prevent the development of sexual risk-taking behaviors among adolescents should be comprehensive and multifaceted. Within this multisystemic framework, investigators must not lose sight of the individual. Participants should be monitored and their particular needs explicitly addressed by the program implementers or by referrals to appropriate community services. Because children are at the heart of prevention programming, this model program is adapted to address the needs of Kathy Taylor.

❖

A Program for Kathy Taylor

The Taylor family has experienced several adversities that have placed strains on their personal relationships as well as on their emotional well-being. In particular, Kathy, age 12, has found it difficult to be the middle child, especially when her dad has been drinking. Kathy feels that her position in the family has become obsolete, especially now that her older sister Allison has given birth to an baby girl. It was hard enough before the birth of the baby for Kathy to feel equally included in her family because of her younger brother's behavior problems.

Kathy, currently in seventh grade, feels as though she must gain her friends' approval and maintain their acceptance. She has started dating one of the most popular ninth-grade boys in her school, and recently he has been hinting that he wants to take their relationship "to the next level." She loves the way she feels when she and her boyfriend are kissing; in fact, they came close to having sex, but she changed her mind at the last minute. This on-again off-again behavior has caused a strain in their relationship. He constantly tells her that "everybody's doing it" and that he could be with any other person, but he has chosen to be with her. Kathy can just imagine how good having sex would feel, but the thought also frightens her. Even though she knows she's not ready, Kathy is starting to think that the only way she can keep her new boyfriend and maintain her popularity is to have sex. On the bright side, Kathy loves the time that she spends with her new niece. When the baby looks at her and smiles, Kathy feels as though the baby is the only one who truly accepts Kathy for who she is. Kathy notices all the attention her sister gets from having such a wonderful baby, and she wonders what it would be like if she had a child of her own who loved her unconditionally. Kathy's boyfriend has already said that he would love her more if she had sex with him; how much more would he love her if she gave him a child, she wonders.

It is obvious from the case study that Kathy is searching for love and a sense of being valued. She is about to consent to sexual intercourse for the wrong reasons. In effect, Kathy may be looking at sex as a way to cope with her problems at home: having a father who is a recovering alcoholic, mounting financial concerns, and feeling left out among her family members. It is important that she realize that sex will not solve her problems; in fact, it will likely worsen her situation with her family and boyfriend, especially if she were to get pregnant or contract an STD. As for wanting to get pregnant, Kathy needs to discuss with her sister the *true* experiences and feelings about being a teenage mother.

❖

On the first day of school, Kathy learns about a required health course and discovers that she will be attending classes twice a week, discussing issues at home with her family, and becoming involved with her community. At the first session, Kathy feels comfortable. She is surrounded by her peers and instructed by two enthusiastic leaders, one male and one female. They open the session by making introductions and assuring students that this is a safe environment because "what is said in the classroom stays in the classroom." The leaders describe the program, including the activities in which students and their parents will be involved, and their goals for helping students make sound decisions regarding topics such as sexuality and academic success. For example, Kathy learns that she will be participating with her friends in role plays that tackle issues such as peer pressure to practice how to make good choices. Also, at the end of the year, the class will put on a play for the whole school to demonstrate what they have learned. The instructors encourage group discussion and participation and are clearly excited and knowledgeable about the program.

As part of the course requirements, Kathy chooses to volunteer at a local hospital in the pediatrics unit because of her recent fascination with infants. She is immediately struck by how difficult it is to care for young children, especially when they are sick. Upon returning to class, Kathy shares her experiences at the hospital with her peers. Many students offer similar accounts, one sharing his experience working in an AIDS-prevention clinic. The class launches into a discussion about sexuality and how it is important to postpone sex until one is absolutely ready. In addition, the instructors facilitate a discussion on the importance of using contraception in preventing STDs for those who choose to be sexually active, specifically stressing the importance of maintaining personal health and safety.

The class also acknowledges the pressures that exist in society today; after all, it seems that "everybody's doing it," they say. Kathy specifically recalls the many conversations she had with her boyfriend about this and wonders what she should do. She feels comfortable and safe in the classroom, so she asks how to deal with this type of pressure. This leads the class into a role-playing activity designed to promote social competence and self-esteem by demonstrating how to say no when pressured. For the first time, Kathy begins to feel confident that she can tell her boyfriend that she is not comfortable having sex with him yet.

Throughout the remaining weeks of class, Kathy is exposed to guest speakers (e.g., single mothers with children, individuals who are HIV positive) and offered advice on where to find free clinics and how to obtain contraception, and is engaging in group discussions and role-play activities. In addition, she has discussed these topics at home with her family as part of homework assignments, and she has noticed that she is better able to talk with them about her concerns. She feels more comfortable approaching her sister, and Allison shares how difficult it is being a single, teenage mother with very little money. Kathy's family enjoys having a daughter who feels more comfortable speaking with them about such serious issues, and they commend her intelligence and sophistication with regard to the subject matter.

Kathy has made a wonderful group of friends in this program, having established positive relationships with her peers, instructors, and family members. To Kathy, it seems as though this program was made just for her and the issues she has been dealing with. Her friends in the class have told her that they feel the same way, even though they are in different situations. Based on what she has learned from her friends in the program, her teachers, her family, and her mentors in the community, Kathy expressed to her boyfriend that no one should be coerced into having sex before he or she is ready. There are times, however, when she feels as though she wants to give in, and it's a struggle to do what she knows is right.

It is evident from this example that Kathy has benefited from her experience in this model prevention program. She continues to struggle with the issues regarding sexuality that seem to permeate her relationship with her boyfriend. This highlights the need to continue providing booster sessions to help teenagers deal with the long-term difficulties that arise in their intimate relationships. Kathy's success is a reminder of how the science and art of prevention programming combine to promote positive change in the lives of individuals and their families.

FUTURE DIRECTIONS: IMPROVING
PROGRAMS FOR PREVENTING RISKY SEXUAL BEHAVIORS

Researchers aiming to prevent the development of sexual risk-taking behaviors among adolescents have made great strides in advancing the field; however, important limitations remain, especially in the adequacy of the theoretical frameworks and the timing and duration of specific programs.

Ideally, prevention programs are built on evidence-based psychological theory; however, the quality of underlying empirical research must be considered. Although research has been conducted on the causes and correlates of risky sexual behavior, many studies do not have optimal methodological designs. To develop an effective prevention program that is based on extant literature, causal predictions must be made more confidently. For example, research on risky sexual behaviors has generally been conducted concurrently with adolescents, and there is a lack of prospective longitudinal research that begins early in children's lives (see Kotchick, Shaffer, Forehand, & Miller, 2001), which can better capture the directionality of effects among constructs such as social competency and effective parenting as well as elucidate how individuals change over time. Furthermore, these factors must be measured before the onset of the risky behaviors, making causal assumptions more plausible. With the ability to make more accurate claims about how and why early factors lead to risky sexual behaviors during adolescence, more precisely defined prevention programs can be developed.

The timing and duration of prevention programs should be given more consideration. For the most part, the onset of programs designed to prevent sexual risk taking occurs too late in adolescence (Kirby, 2002). Statistics show that 33% of adolescents are already sexually active by the time they reach high school (CDC, 2004), which is when many of the most exemplar prevention programs have just begun (e.g., Coyle et al., 1996; Philliber et al., 2000). Children must become involved in prevention programming before they become sexually active in order to develop the skills necessary for effectively delaying the onset of sexual activity as well as sexual risk-taking behaviors.

In addition to early implementation, programs must extend the duration of children's involvement in prevention programs to reinforce the skills and values that are taught, especially as youth become exposed to real-world intimate situations. This can be achieved in a cost-effective manner through decreasing the intensity of programming over time or by integrating periodical booster sessions into prevention curricula. By incorporating sufficient dosage levels of program curricula, long-term maintenance of psychosocial and behavioral change will be facilitated.

In short, preventing the development of risky sexual behaviors among adolescents depends on the ability of researchers to design and implement effective, theoretically based programs. Comprehensive programs must be initiated with preadolescent children and continued throughout adolescence to prevent the onset of sexual initiation and risky sexual behaviors as well as to promote lasting changes in their overall social competence, thereby positively impacting their interpersonal relationships and emotional adjustment.

REFERENCES

Advocates for Youth. (2003). *Advocates for Youth: Rights. Respect. Responsibility.* Retrieved December 15, 2003, from http://www.advocatesforyouth.org

Alford, S. (2003). *Science and success: Sex education and other programs that work to prevent teen pregnancy, HIV and sexually transmitted infections.* Washington, DC: Advocates for Youth.

Allen, J.P., Kuperminc, G., Philliber, S., & Herre, K. (1994). Programmatic prevention of adolescent behaviors: The role of autonomy, relatedness, and volunteer service in the Teen Outreach program. *American Journal of Community Psychology, 22,* 617–638.

Allen, J.P., & Philliber, S. (2001). Who benefits most from a broadly targeted prevention program? Differential efficacy across populations in the Teen Outreach Program. *Journal of Community Psychology, 29,* 637–655.

Allen, J.P., Philliber, S., Herrling, S., & Kuperminc, G.P. (1997). Preventing teen pregnancy and academic failure: Experimental evaluation of a developmentally based approach. *Child Development, 64,* 729–742.

Allen, J.P., Philliber, S., & Hoggson, N. (1990). School-based prevention of teenage pregnancy and school dropout: Process evaluation of the national replication of the Teen Outreach program. *American Journal of Community Psychology, 18,* 505–524.

Bachanas, P.J., Morris, M.K., Lewis-Gess, J.K., Sarrett-Cuasay, E.J., Sirl, K., Ries, J.K., et. al. (2002). Predictors of risky sexual behavior in African American adolescent girls: Implications for prevention interventions. *Journal of Pediatric Psychology, 27,* 519–530.

Bandura A. (1986) *Social foundations of thought and action: A social cognitive theory.* Englewood Cliffs, NJ: Prentice Hall.

Basen-Engquist K., Coyle, K.K., Parcel, G.S., Kirby, D., Banspach, S.W., Carvajal, S.C., et. al. (2001). Schoolwide effects of a multicomponent HIV, STD, and pregnancy prevention program for high school students. *Health Education & Behavior, 28,* 166–185.

Basen-Engquist K., Masse, L.C., Coyle, K.K., Kirby, D., Parcel, G.S., Banspach, S., & Nodora, J. (1999). Validity of scales measuring the psychosocial determinants of HIV/STD-related risk behavior in adolescents. *Health Education Research, 14,* 25–38.

Basen-Engquist, K., Parcel, G., Harrist, R., Kirby, D., Coyle, K., Banspach, S., et al. (1997). Methodological issues in school-based health promotion intervention research: The Safer Choices Project. *Journal of School Health, 67,* 365–371.

Bogenschneider, K., Wu, M., Raffaelli, M., & Tsay, J.C. (1998). Parent influences on adolescent peer orientation and substance use: The interface of parenting practices and values. *Child Development, 69,* 1672–1688.

Bronfenbrenner, U. (1977). Toward an experimental ecology of human development. *American Psychologist, 32,* 513–531.

Centers for Disease Control and Prevention (CDC). (2001). *HIV/AIDS Surveillance Supplemental Report, 9.* Atlanta, GA: Author.

Centers for Disease Control and Prevention (CDC). (2002). *National Profile: STD Surveillance 2002.* Atlanta, GA: U.S. Department of Health and Human Services.

Centers for Disease Control and Prevention (CDC). (2004). *Surveillance summaries: Morbidity and Mortality Weekly Report.* Atlanta, GA: U.S. Department of Health and Human Services.

Children's Aid Society. (2002). *Carrera Adolescent Pregnancy Prevention Program.* Retrieved December 15, 2003, from http://www.stopteenpregnancy.com

Coyle, K.K., Basen-Engquist, K.M., Kirby, D.B., Parcel, G.S., Banspach, S.W., Collins, J.L., et al. (2001). Safer Choices: Long-term impact of a multi-component school-based HIV, STD, and pregnancy prevention program. *Public Health Reports, 116* (Suppl. 1), 82–93.

Coyle, K., Basen-Engquist, K., Kirby, D., Parcel, G., Banspach, S.W., Harrist, R., et al. (1999). Short-term impact of Safer Choices: A multi-component, school-based HIV, other STD, and pregnancy prevention program. *Journal of School Health, 69,* 181–188.

Coyle, K.K., Kirby, D.B., Parcel, G.S., Basen-Engquist, K.M., Banspach, S.W., Collins, J.L., et al. (1996). A multicomponent school-based HIV/STD and pregnancy prevention program for adolescents: The Safer Choices project. *Journal of School Health, 66,* 89–94.

Donenberg, G.R. Wilson, H.W. Emersom, E., & Bryant, F.B. (2002). Holding the line with a watchful eye: The impact of perceived parental monitoring on risky sexual behavior among adolescents in psychiatric care. *AIDS Education and Prevention, 14,* 138–157.

Dryfoos, J.G. (1990). *Adolescents at risk: Prevalence and prevention.* New York: Oxford University Press.

Furstenburg, F.F., Levine, J.A., & Brooks-Gunn, J. (1990). The children of teenage mothers: Patterns of early childbearing in two generations. *Family Planning Perspectives, 22,* 54–61.

Guo, J., Chung, I.J., Hill, K.G., Hawkins, J.D. Catalano, R.F., & Abbott, R.D. (2002). Developmental relationships between adolescent substance use and risky sexual behavior in young adulthood. *Journal of Adolescent Health, 31,* 354–362.

Horwitz, S.M., Klerman, L.V., Kuo, H.S., & Jekel, J.F. (1991). Intergenerational transmission of school-age parenthood. *Family Planning Perspectives, 23,* 168–172.

Howard, D.E., & Wang, Q.W. (2003a). Risk procedures of adolescent girls who were victims of dating violence. *Adolescence, 38,* 1–14.

Howard, D.E., & Wang, Q.W. (2003b). Psychosocial factors associated with adolescent boys' reports of dating violence. *Adolescence, 38,* 519–533.

Huebner, A.J., & Howell, L.W. (2003). Examining the relationship between adolescent sexual risk taking and perceptions of monitoring, communication, and parenting styles. *Journal of Adolescent Health, 33,* 71–78.

Ivry, R., & Doolittle, F. (2003, Spring). *Improving the economic and life outcomes of at-risk youth.* New York: MDRC.

Kirby, D. (1997). *No easy answers: Research findings on programs to reduce teen pregnancy.* Washington DC: The National Campaign to Prevent Teen Pregnancy.

Kirby, D. (2002). Effective approaches to reducing adolescent unprotected sex, pregnancy, and childbearing. *The Journal of Sex Research, 39,* 51–57.

Kirby, D., Barth, R.P., Leland, N., & Fetro, J.V. (1991). Reducing the risk: Impact of a new curriculum on sexual risk taking. *Family Planning Perspectives, 23,* 253–263.

Kirby, D., Korpi, M., Barth, R.P., & Cagampang, H.H. (1995). *Evaluation of education now and babies later (ENABL): Final report.* Berkeley, CA: University of California, School of Welfare, Family Welfare Research Group.

Kotchick, B.A., Shaffer, A., Forehand, R., & Miller, K.S. (2001). Adolescent sexual risk behavior: A multi-system perspective. *Clinical Psychology Review, 21,* 493–519.

Martin, J.A., Hamilton, B.E., Sutton, P.D., Ventura, S.J., Menacker, F., & Munson, M.S. (2005, September). Births: Final data for 2003. *National Vital Statistics Report* (Vol. 53, No. 2). Hyattsville, MD: National Center for Health Statistics.

Maynard, R.A. (1997). The costs of adolescent childbearing. In R.A. Maynard (Ed.), *Kids having kids: Economic costs and social consequences of teen pregnancy* (pp. 285–338). Washington, DC: The Urban Institute Press.

McGuire, W., & Papageoris, D. (1961). The relative efficacy of various types of prior belief-defense in producing immunity to persuasion. *Journal of Abnormal Social Psychology, 62,* 237–337.

Moore, K.A., & Sugland, B.W. (1997). Using behavioral theories to design abstinence programs. *Children and Youth Services Review, 19,* 485–500.

Parcel, G., Basen-Enquist, K., Banspach, S.W., Coyle, K., & Kirby, D. (1999). Psychosocial predictors of delay of first sexual intercourse of adolescents. *Health Psychology, 18,* 1–10.

Philliber, S., & Allen, S.J. (1992). Life options and community service: Teen Outreach Program. In B.C. Miller, J.J. Card, R.L. Paikoff, & J.L. Peterson (Eds.), *Preventing adolescent pregnancy* (pp. 139–155). Thousand Oaks, CA: Sage Publications.

Philliber, S., Kaye, J., & Herrling, S. (2001). *The national evaluation of the Children's Aid Society Career-Model Program to Prevent Teen Pregnancy.* New York: Philliber Research Associates.

Philliber, S., Kaye, J.W., Herrling, S.W., & West, E. (2000). *Preventing teen pregnancy: An evaluation of the Children's Aid Society Carrera Program.* New York: Philliber Research Associates.

Philliber, S., Kaye, J.W., & Herrling, S. (2002). Preventing pregnancy and improving health care access among teenagers: An evaluation of the Children's Aid Society Carrera Program. *Perspectives on Sexual & Reproductive Health, 34,* 244–251.

Spence, S.H. (2003). Social skills training with children and young people: Theory, evidence and practice. *Child and Adolescent Mental Health, 8,* 84–96.

St. Pierre, T.L., Mark, M.M., Kaltreider, D., & Aikin, K.J. (1995). A 27-month evaluation of a sexual activity prevention program in boys & girls clubs across the nation. *Family Relations: Journal of Applied Family and Child Studies, 44,* 69–77.

Wang, L.Y., Davis, M., Robin, L., Collins, J., Coyle, K., & Baumler, E. (2000). Economic evaluation of Safer Choices: A school-based Human Immunodeficiency Virus, other sexually transmitted diseases, and pregnancy prevention program. *Archives of Pediatrics and Adolescent Medicine, 154,* 1017–1024.

Waters, E., & Sroufe, L.A. (1983). Social competence as a developmental construct. *Developmental Review, 3,* 79–97.

Wayment, H.A., & Aronson, B. (2002). Risky sexual behavior in American white college women: The role of sex guilt and sexual abuse. *Journal of Health Psychology, 7,* 23–733.

Whitman, T.L., Borkowski, J.G., Keogh, D.A., & Weed, K. (2001). *Interwoven lives: Adolescent mothers and their children.* Mahwah, NJ: Lawrence Erlbaum Associates.

8

PREVENTING DATING VIOLENCE

Kimberly S. Howard

Dating violence among teenagers is a significant social and public health problem in the United States. Although estimates of the prevalence of dating violence among high school students range from 1 in 10 (Centers for Disease Control and Prevention, 2000) to 1 in 5 students who report being the recipient of abusive behavior such as physical or sexual abuse (Silverman, Raj, Mucci, & Hathaway, 2001), the actual prevalence of dating violence may be much higher. Dating violence is often underreported to authorities, and police records rarely include information about whether the perpetrator was the victim's boyfriend or girlfriend, thus obscuring whether incidents of teenage violence actually constitute dating violence (Irwin & Rickert, 2005). In addition, dating violence includes not only physical and sexual abuse, but emotional abuse as well (SafeYouth, 2005). Aside from the fact that emotional abuse is not recorded in police records, many teenagers are not even aware that their relationships may be emotionally abusive because they interpret jealous and controlling behaviors as signs of love (Lavoie, Robitaille, & Herbert, 2000). Finally, because there appears to be no standard way of defining dating violence, researchers may choose to use a broader or narrower definition, further confusing the actual prevalence among teenagers (O'Keefe, 2005). Despite the inherent difficulties in quantifying rates of dating violence among teenagers, it is still obvious that the rates of both violence perpetration and victimization are quite high (O'Keefe).

It is generally believed that rates of physical violence perpetration in dating relationships are similar for both boys and girls (Irwin & Rickert, 2005). However, the meanings associated with violence perpetrated by males versus females are often quite different. Although anger is a commonly reported reason for engaging in domestic violence for both genders, boys also tend to report using violence as a means of controlling their partners, whereas girls often report engaging in violence as a means of self-defense (SafeYouth, 2005). Typically, it is also the case that the consequences of male on female violence are more severe, as boys often have the potential to cause more bodily harm than girls, and girls are more likely than boys to sustain injuries that require medical treatment as a result of dating violence (Makepeace, 1987). The rates of sexual violence perpetration, however, reveal a much different pattern with females being significantly more likely to be the victim of sexual violence than males (Bennett & Fineran, 1998; Foshee, 1996).

FACTORS RELATED TO DATING VIOLENCE

There are many predictors of dating violence among teenagers. For example, urban residence (Makepeace, 1987), use of alcohol and drugs (Silverman et al., 2001), low self-esteem (O'Keefe & Treister, 1998), depression, and suicidal tendencies (Howard & Wang, 2003) have all been found to be related to dating violence, although sometimes in different ways. Specifically, dating violence victimization is predicted by depression and suicidal tendencies, as well as low self-esteem in girls. Alcohol and drug consumption and urban residence are related to increased rates of both perpetration and victimization of dating violence. Because it is related to so many teenage problems, dating violence is an issue of great importance in terms of prevention.

Family origin factors such as history of child maltreatment (Wolfe, Wekerle, Scott, Straatman, & Grasley, 2004) and witnessing domestic violence (O'Keefe & Treister, 1998) also are related to dating violence. Wolfe and colleagues (2004) examined the relationships between child maltreatment and adolescent dating violence over 1 year in a sample of students from 10 high schools in urban, rural, and semirural communities. They found that boys with maltreatment histories were more likely to have attitudes supporting dating violence, and girls with maltreatment histories were more likely to have deficits in relationship empathy and self-efficacy. For both boys and girls, trauma-related symptoms mediated the relationship between early maltreatment and adolescent dating violence (Wolfe et al., 2004). That is, maltreatment history did not impact dating violence on its own, rather, the traumatic symptoms that resulted from early maltreatment led to a heightened risk for dating violence. Thus, those adolescents who had experienced child maltreatment were not at an increased risk for dating violence unless they continued to manifest trauma symptomatology. In light of these findings, it is important to design and implement intervention programs to meet the needs of both special populations (i.e., youth with maltreatment histories) as well as more typically developing adolescents.

PREVENTION PROGRAMS: DESIGN AND IMPLEMENTATION ISSUES

In recent years, federal, state, and local agencies have begun to develop programs aimed at preventing domestic violence; however, little systematic research has been conducted assessing the effectiveness of these programs. Because many programs do not share common themes, the results of these studies are difficult to compare (Kruttschnitt, McLaughlin, & Petrie, 2004). For example, some programs aim to change adolescents' beliefs or attitudes (MacGowan, 1997), and other programs are geared toward changing actual behaviors (Foshee et al., 1996; Wolfe et al., 1996). Still others are simply focused on presenting information to students and do not evaluate any outcomes associated with the program (e.g., Sex Offense Services, 2003). The result is a large and somewhat disunified body of literature with very little in the way of solid findings and a set of *violence prevention* programs that lack any evidence that they actually prevent dating violence. The following is an effort to organize past and present models of domestic violence prevention in order to suggest best practices for future research.

Programs aimed at preventing domestic violence are extremely varied in their focus and the method by which efforts are mounted. There are four main categories of programs: 1) system effectiveness, 2) victim advocacy, 3) batterer intervention, and 4) teenage dating violence prevention. The first category of programs is aimed at making the criminal justice system more effective at addressing domestic violence crimes to decrease their prevalence in the future (Farrell, Buck, & Pease, 1993). The second category of programs focuses on providing specific services to victims—for example, advocates and other professionals who offer support and guidance regarding ending violent relationships and developing safety plans to promote healthy relationships in the future (Bybee & Sullivan, 2002). The third category aims to prevent recidivism among people with histories of domestic abuse; *participants* are typically convicted offenders who have been court ordered to receive treatment (Davis, Taylor, & Maxwell, 2000; Feder & Forde, 2000; Jackson et al., 2003; Shepard, Falk, & Elliott, 2002). The fourth category, dating violence prevention programs, is designed to be used in schools with younger children to empower them with tools to make healthy choices in relationships (Avery-Leaf, Cascardi, O'Leary, & Cano, 1997; Foshee, 1998; Weisz & Black, 2001; Wolfe et al., 2003). This last category of programs, dealing with preventing dating violence and sexual assault, will be the primary focus of this chapter because it represents the area that is most relevant to adolescents.

PREVENTION PROGRAMS AND THEIR EVALUATIONS

A review of the literature on dating violence prevention programs for school-aged children revealed a dearth of research in this area (Whitaker et al., 2004). Fourteen studies were identified with published results, and these represented 11 dating violence prevention programs. Of these, only 9 programs reported any positive outcomes (Whitaker et al., 2004). The three most exemplar programs are evaluated and critiqued in this chapter: 1) Safe Dates (Foshee, 1998; Foshee et al., 1996; Foshee et al., 1998; Foshee et al., 2000), 2) Youth Relationships Project (YRP; Wolfe et al., 1996; Wolfe et al., 2003), and 3) Reaching and Teaching Teens to Stop Violence (RTTSV; Weisz & Black, 2001). The essential characteristics of these programs are summarized in Table 8.1. The Safe Dates program was geared toward all students in the target county. In contrast, YRP focused on youth with histories of maltreatment, and RTTSV began early, with seventh-grade students as the target of the intervention.

Table 8.1. Characteristics of model programs for dating violence prevention

	Safe Dates	Youth Relationships Project (YRP)	Reaching and Teaching Teens to Stop Violence (RTTSV)
Target of intervention	Eighth- and ninth-graders in a rural North Carolina County (N = 1886)	Child Protective Services (CPS) referred 14- to 16-year-olds from seven communities (N = 158)	Seventh graders in an urban midwestern public charter school (N = 46)
Outcomes of intervention	Less initiation of psychological abuse and sexual violence

Less acceptance of beliefs that promote dating violence | Decrease in reports of abuse perpetration or victimization and fewer symptoms of emotional distress | Increase in knowledge and attitudes about sexual assault and dating violence |
| Follow-up outcomes | Less physical and sexual dating violence perpetration

Less physical abuse victimization

No effects from booster | All outcomes evident for at least 16 months after treatment ended | Greater knowledge and more positive attitudes than comparison group |

Safe Dates

The most extensively tested program in the literature for preventing dating violence among youth is Foshee and colleagues' Safe Dates program (Foshee, 1998; Foshee et al., 1996; Foshee et al., 1998; Foshee et al., 2000; Foshee et al., 2004). The program was developed in collaboration with 33 community agencies (including schools, police departments, and other community service providers) for use in a rural county in North Carolina. The 14 schools in the county were randomly assigned to either a treatment (school and community activities, n = 7) or control (community activities only, n = 7) condition. The Safe Dates program was designed to serve as both primary and secondary prevention of dating violence. That is, for students who had not yet been either a victim or a perpetrator of violence in a dating relationship, the program served as primary prevention, but for those who had been a victim or perpetrator, the program served as secondary prevention with the goal of decreasing the occurrence of such behaviors in the future (Foshee, 1998).

Schools assigned to the treatment condition implemented a series of activities for eighth- and ninth-grade students including 1) a theater production performed by high school students, 2) a 10-session curriculum during required health class, and 3) a poster contest. The theatrical production was presented in the beginning of the fall semester, 2 months before the start of the 10-session classroom curriculum. The 45-minute play about an adolescent victim of dating violence seeking help with her violent relationship was designed to address beliefs and attitudes related to help-seeking behaviors (Foshee et al., 1996).

The curriculum was presented by 16 teachers who taught the required health courses in which Safe Dates was implemented. Each received 20 hours of training from Safe Dates staff regarding teenage dating violence and the specifics of the curriculum before delivering it to students. In addition, during the implementation of the curriculum, classrooms were randomly monitored by Safe Dates staff to ensure that the material was being presented correctly (Foshee et al., 1996).

The curriculum included a number of topics related to relationships and dating violence. In the first three sessions, the emphasis was on sharing information relevant to understanding dating violence. The first session involved defining caring relationships. During this session, students were asked to consider the qualities that were most important to them in dating relationships and discuss ways that people act to show that they care. They also were asked to consider how they want to treat a dating partner as well as how they would want to be treated in a dating relationship, emphasizing the fact that they are able to choose their behavior and how they are treated in relationships. In the second session, which focused on defining dating abuse, students were asked to describe potentially harmful behaviors in dating relationships and to then differentiate between harmful and abusive behaviors and between physically and emotionally abusive behaviors. They were also presented with a number of facts about dating violence. In the third session, students were asked to consider the question "Why do people abuse?" They were asked to discuss reasons why people abuse others and ways in which manipulation, power, and control are at work in abusive relationships. Students also were challenged to question the notion that violence resulting from jealousy indicates love and to consider the warning signs of an abusive relationship.

The fourth through seventh sessions emphasized topics related to providing support, seeking help, and communicating effectively. The fourth and fifth sessions dealt with how to help friends who were in abusive relationships. The difficulties associated with seeking help as a victim of dating violence also were addressed. More specifically, during the fourth session, students were given information about resources that were available in the community. In the fifth session, students discussed *red flags* for being a perpetrator or a victim of dating abuse, and practiced talking to a friend who was either violent toward a dating partner or being abused by a dating partner. The sixth session was designed to promote discussion regarding students' images of what relationships are like by increasing awareness that images concerning relationships influence the way people act within relationships. Students also were asked to consider the effects of gender stereotypes on dating interactions and dating abuse. In the seventh session, students identified eight communication skills that are helpful in resolving conflict, and they were given the opportunity to practice their skills and consider nonviolent strategies for interacting with dating partners who do not communicate effectively.

The final three sessions addressed issues related to dating violence such as anger and sexual assault. The eighth session dealt with the importance of acknowledging feelings and discussed methods of dealing with anger. The ninth session focused on defining sexual assault and teaching students strategies for reducing the risk of sexual violence in a dating situation. The tenth and final session provided a summary of the entire curriculum and also obtained student feedback and gave instructions for the poster contest.

In addition to the theater production and the curriculum that was integrated into health classes, students had the opportunity to participate in a poster competition that addressed the themes in the Safe Dates curriculum. Although not every student designed a poster for the contest, all had the opportunity to view the posters and vote on them. In this way, the poster competition provided another mechanism for exposing students to positive messages regarding dating relationships (Foshee et al., 1996).

In addition to the school curriculum, a number of supports were included within the broader community to strengthen the response to dating violence among adolescents. All schools in the treatment and control conditions were given access to community supports. First, service providers who interacted with adolescents as part of their professional activities were eligible to participate in a 3-hour training session involving the cognitive experiences of individuals who provide help to victims of dating violence (Foshee et al., 1996). Approximately 63% of service providers who were eligible to receive the training actually did so (Foshee et al., 1998). Second, volunteers at the local crisis line received specific training regarding how to work with adolescent victims of dating violence. Third, materials were developed to assist parents of children who had experienced abusive dating relationships. Finally, support groups were offered for adolescents who had already been victims of dating violence (Foshee et al., 1996).

Program Evaluation   Results of the Safe Dates project were evaluated at a 1-month follow-up and yearly for the next 4 years. In addition, a booster session was administered to a randomly selected half of the students who had been in the original treatment group between the 2- and 3-year follow-ups (Foshee et al., 2004). It has been found that adolescents in the treatment condition reported initiating significantly less psychological, physical, and sexual abuse perpetration than students in the control condition ($p < .05$; Foshee et al., 1998). These students also were less likely to endorse the notion that dating violence is sometimes acceptable and more likely to report that it is wrong in any situation ($p < .05$). They also perceived fewer positive consequences from using dating violence, used more constructive communication skills and responses to anger, were less likely to engage in gender stereotyping, and were more aware of services available in the community than students in the control condition ($p < .05$ for all; Foshee et al., 1998).

The 1-year follow-up revealed no differences between students in the treatment and control conditions on any of the behavioral outcomes such as violence perpetration. However, students in the treatment group were still less accepting of dating violence, perceived more negative consequences from engaging in dating violence, reported using less destructive responses to anger, and had higher awareness of victim and perpetrator services available in the community than students in the control condition (Foshee et al., 2000).

Booster sessions were administered to a randomly selected half of the initial sample between 2 and 3 years posttreatment. The booster consisted of an 11-page newsletter with information and worksheets based on the content of the Safe Dates curriculum. Approximately 4 weeks after the newsletter was sent, health educators followed up with a telephone call to answer any questions and determine if the newsletter activities had been completed. Although 82% of adolescents assigned to the booster condition actually read the newsletter and completed the activities, there were no significant advantages associated with those in the booster condition compared with the nonbooster condition in terms of dating violence perpetration or victimization (Foshee et al., 2004).

Data collected at the 4-year follow-up assessed only the behavioral outcomes of perpetration and victimization and did not examine whether the cognitive outcomes that were evident at the 1-year follow-up were still manifest. However, 4 years after the conclusion of the program, adolescents who had participated in the treatment condition reported perpetrating significantly less physical and sexual violence than their counterparts in the control condition. They also reported less physical abuse victimization (Foshee et al., 2004).

Critical Analysis of Treatment Characteristics   Safe Dates was rooted within a strong theoretical framework that emphasized how changes in beliefs would promote help-seeking behavior, which was a key to secondary prevention (Foshee et al., 1996). With goals of both primary and secondary prevention (i.e., to prevent dating violence from ever occurring, to prevent repeat occurrences), Safe Dates involved a number of community- and school-based services to meet these goals. Their theoretical model illustrated that varied school activities were designed to alter dating abuse norms, gender stereotypes, and conflict management skills, all of which are helpful in preventing dating violence. In addition, school activities were intended to alter students' beliefs in both the need for help (i.e., perceptions of the seriousness of dating violence) and the belief that both school and community resources will help deal with problems relating to dating violence. The model also showed that community services were aimed at enhancing dating violence services, thereby providing secondary prevention. Training community service providers was aimed at altering beliefs of individuals in the community about the severity of dating violence to increase their willingness to help, thereby enhancing dating violence services in the community (Foshee et al., 1996).

The theoretical model of the Safe Dates program elucidates other positive characteristics of the treatment. The program was comprehensive in that it had multiple components based in both the school and the community. Additional community resources for parents allowed families to be involved in the prevention of dating violence. The program implemented varied teaching methods by sharing information first through a theatrical production, then in a health class curriculum, and finally through a poster contest to give students the opportunity to express their views about dating violence to one another. By engaging 33 organizations in the development of the program within a rural southern community, Safe Dates was specifically tailored to the needs of students in that community and was likely high in sociocultural relevance, another key component in effective programs (Nation et al., 2003). The only weakness in the treatment characteristic of the Safe Dates program was that it did not promote building positive relationships that may have hindered the students' ability to make personal connections based on the health class curriculum. The addition of small groups led by mentors may have brought about a more lasting change in the lives of the young people who participated in the program.

Critical Analysis of Procedural Characteristics The methodology employed in the administration of the Safe Dates program had several positive features. First, the teachers who were responsible for administering the material each received 20 hours of training to prepare them for disseminating the curriculum. Second, to promote treatment fidelity, 35% of the curriculum classes were monitored by Safe Dates staff (Foshee et al., 1996). In addition, approximately 20 workshops were offered to community service providers by Safe Dates staff to increase the awareness of dating violence within the community and to bolster the effectiveness of existing community resources (Foshee et al.).

Although Safe Dates is one of the most effective dating violence programs that has been evaluated to date, a standing criticism is that the 10-session curriculum was likely too short to truly effect lasting change for those who received the treatment (Meyer & Stein, 2000). Despite this criticism, 4-year follow-up outcomes revealed continued differences between treatment and control groups in terms of dating violence perpetration and victimization (Foshee et al., 2004). The timing of the program, aimed at eighth- and ninth-grade students was also likely appropriate. It was early enough to be at a time when many adolescents had not yet experienced dating violence, thus providing primary prevention. It also was relevant to students who had already experienced dating violence and reached out to those students with school and community resources aimed at secondary prevention of dating violence (Foshee et al., 1996).

The implementation of the booster sessions between 2 and 3 years posttreatment demonstrated an important component of effective prevention programs (Nation et al., 2003), but the project demonstrated that it did not have any further effect beyond that of the original intervention. It is possible, however, that a more intensive booster session would have yielded significant results. That is, the newsletter and telephone follow-up format of the Safe Dates booster may not have been as effective as additional sessions related to the original curriculum.

Critical Analysis of Design Characteristics Methodologically, Safe Dates is one of the most scientifically rigorous dating violence prevention programs evaluated to date. The 14 schools in the county were matched based on school size, and one school from each pair was randomly assigned to treatment or control (Foshee et al., 1996). By randomly assigning entire schools to groups, students who attended treatment schools were able to fully experience the range of activities that were implemented. In addition, students who attended control schools were much less likely to interact with students in the treatment group than they would have been if they were randomly assigned to groups within schools—thereby increasing the likelihood that the treatment would not also be shared with students in the control group. In addition, random assignment strengthened the design of the overall study by providing internal validation and ensuring that the positive effects of the treatment were not due to preexisting differences between schools.

Evaluations of the program were thorough and well done. Baseline data was collected in all schools, and follow-up data were collected 1 month postintervention and each year after the intervention for 4 years. Attrition was minimized by making attempts to collect follow-up data from students who dropped out of school or moved to another school system. This was done to ensure that the data were representative of all the students who participated in the intervention (Foshee et al., 1996). Outcome variables pertaining to dating violence victimization and perpetration were obtained. In addition, data were collected on hypothesized mediating variables such as acceptance of norms, perceived consequences of dating violence, and conflict management to identify the process by which the intervention affected the outcomes of violence perpetration and victimization (Foshee et al., 1998). One area in which the Safe Dates evaluation could have been strengthened would have been the inclusion of additional variables such as students' attendance and progress during the implementation of the program to account for differing effectiveness of the program across different students. Furthermore, including measures of adolescents' personal characteristics that may contribute to the effectiveness of the intervention (i.e., social competence, maltreatment history) would be helpful for understanding any differential impact of the intervention on adolescents' behaviors.

In contrast to previous dating violence programs that found no effects (Levy, 1984), the Safe Dates program has demonstrated effectiveness in both short-term and longer-term follow-ups. One year after the intervention, cognitive effects were maintained, and 4 years after the intervention, students from the treatment group reported significantly lower levels of dating violence perpetration and victimization than students from the control group (Foshee et al., 2004). These outcomes represented socially important effects that were obtained as a result of the Safe Dates program.

Youth Relationships Project

The Youth Relationships Project (YRP) is an 18-session program that aims to prevent violence in relationships by promoting positive alternatives to aggression-based problem solving and gender-based role expectations (Wolfe et al., 2003).

The curriculum has three components: 1) education of abuse and power dynamics in relationships, 2) skill development, and 3) social action (Wolfe et al., 1996).

Education and awareness sessions were focused on identifying abusive behaviors and understanding power dynamics within male–female relationships. Information on dating violence was presented by guest speakers, video presentations, and group discussions. Skill development sessions helped participants solve conflict peacefully and avoid abusive situations. Communication skills and assertive problem solving also were presented. The purposes of the social action activities were to provide information about resources that were available in the community and to help participants overcome their fears regarding community service providers such as police officers, welfare workers, and counselors (Wolfe et al., 1996).

The program took place in a community center with adolescent participants who had histories of child maltreatment and were referred for participation by Child Protective Services (CPS) agencies from seven urban, rural, and semirural communities. Eligible participants were randomly assigned to either a preventive–intervention group or a no-treatment control group. The 158 participants in the project were interviewed at baseline and again 4 months later. They also were contacted bimonthly to obtain information regarding whether they were currently involved in healthy dating relationships. Additional face-to-face interviews were scheduled at 6-month intervals. Participants in the control condition completed all assessments and also continued to receive standard CPS services such as caseworker visits (Wolfe et al., 2003).

The prevention program was administered by trained social workers and other community professionals who had past histories of experience with youth and/or victims of domestic violence. All facilitators participated in a 10-hour training seminar over 2 days in which they were presented with the YRP curriculum. Fifteen coeducational intervention groups were conducted. Each of the 2-hour sessions was led by male and female cofacilitators who modeled positive relationship skills such as sharing power and assertiveness (Wolfe et al., 2003).

To ensure high treatment fidelity, all group sessions were audiotaped to be reviewed for adherence to the program protocol. In addition, research assistants rated the extent to which the goals for each session were met across groups to modify the presentation of the material if necessary. It was found that on average, 88% of goals were met in a given session.

Program Evaluation   Analyses of YRP revealed that over time, there was a significant decrease in physical ($p < .01$) and emotional ($p < .05$) abuse perpetration against a dating partner. There also were trends indicating decreases in the amount of threatening behaviors used toward a dating partner. The changes were more marked for boys than for girls (Wolfe et al., 2003). By the end of the follow-up period, rates of physical abuse perpetration in this sample of youth referred by CPS was similar to rates in a normative sample, with 21% of girls and 11% of boys reporting abuse perpetration. In contrast, the comparison group reported much higher rates of perpetration (41% of girls and 19% of boys; Wolfe et al.).

The YRP also had an important impact on reducing the likelihood that participants would become victims of dating violence in the future. There were significant reductions in all forms of victimization (physical and emotional abuse and threatening behaviors; $p < .01$, respectively). Although all participants experienced this decrease in victimization, girls reported higher levels of initial victimization and had steeper declines over time in experiencing threats from dating partners ($p < .05$). Finally, the intervention also positively affected a number of characteristics of youth's emotional well-being. For example, participants reported significant decreases over time in interpersonal hostility ($p < .05$) and trauma symptoms ($p < .01$).

Markers of adolescents' progress within the program, such as attendance and facilitator ratings of responsiveness during treatment sessions, were identified to help explain the effects of the treatment. Not surprisingly, these variables helped to explain the results. For example, youth who had higher levels of attendance and better listening skills during sessions exhibited steeper reductions in physical abuse perpetration than those with lower ratings ($p < .01$) and were less likely to be victimized over time ($p < .05$). Facilitator ratings of listening skills also were related to greater decreases in trauma symptoms over time ($p < .05$; Wolfe et al., 2003).

Critical Analysis of Treatment Characteristics   Building on previous scientific evidence that young people with maltreatment histories are at an increased risk for relationship violence (Bank & Burraston, 2001), YRP was intended to prevent dating violence among a group of adolescents referred by local CPS agencies who had histories of child maltreatment by implementing a curriculum that emphasized a health-promotion approach. The program was steeped in feminist theories regarding societal values that maintain inequality and promote gender-based violence (Wolfe et al., 2003). In addition, varied teaching methods were implemented; guest speakers, videos, role playing, visits to community organizations, and social action projects all provided variability to the group format, thereby allowing the nonviolence messages to reach the participants via multiple avenues.

The group format that was implemented also fostered positive relationships. Specifically, groups were led by a man and a woman who modeled positive relationship skills. This gave participants the opportunity to build relationships with individuals of both genders who provided positive examples of interactions within relationships. Because the program was specifically designed for use with previously maltreated youth, relevance was likely high. However, the combination of rural, semirural, and urban adolescents may have introduced challenges for the sociocultural relevance of the program to all participants.

The program was not comprehensive in the sense that it did not include multiple domains of influence, instead focusing only on curriculum content that was disseminated in the context of intervention groups at a community center. However, to recruit participants for the project, the researchers collaborated with existing community agencies, thus building on existing service-providing organizations within the community.

Critical Analysis of Procedural Characteristics   To ensure treatment fidelity, a number of precautions were taken. First, a manual was used for training facilitators that specifically outlined all of the information that was to be presented during the course of the intervention (Wolfe et al., 1996). Second, facilitators were social workers or other community professionals who received 10 hours of training over the course of 2 days in which they were prepared to administer the intervention material. Third, sessions were audiotaped and reviewed for adherence to protocol. Independent ratings done by research assistants revealed that 88% of the objectives were typically met in any given session, indicating strong fidelity in the program delivery across groups (Wolfe et al., 2003).

No booster sessions were administered, but multiple teaching settings were used during the implementation of the curriculum to help participants generalize their new skills in different settings. The program consisted of 18 2-hour sessions, which provided extensive information and support regarding dating violence. The implementation of the program with 14–16-year-olds also represents an appropriate time to administer dating violence intervention before patterns of adult domestic violence have begun (Wekerle & Wolfe, 1999).

Critical Analysis of Design Characteristics   One of the most methodologically strong aspects of the YRP was its use of a true experimental design. Eligible adolescents were randomly assigned to either a treatment or control group, making the interpretation of the findings much more straightforward (Wolfe et al., 2003). The outcome evaluation also was strong. The analysis of program effects involved growth curve modeling of behavioral and socioemotional changes over time of individuals in the treatment and control conditions. Use of advanced analytical strategies allowed for investigation of more complex questions such as the effects of the interaction between the intervention and the participant's gender over time.

The program demonstrated positive changes such as decreased dating violence victimization and perpetration over time—a socially significant outcome. The examination of variables such as the number of sessions attended and the facilitator's rating of the adolescents listening and paying attention during the sessions further helped to strengthen the explanation of the results of the intervention. Specifically, it was determined that treatment youth who attended more sessions and listened more attentively achieved positive outcomes at a faster rate than those who attended fewer sessions or did not pay attention during the sessions (Wolfe et al., 2003).

Reaching and Teaching Teens to Stop Violence

The Nebraska Domestic Violence Sexual Assault Coalition (NDVSAC; 1995) developed a curriculum called Reaching and Teaching Teens to Stop Violence (RTTSV) that was culturally sensitive and adaptable for either high school or junior high students. The curriculum included information on sexual harassment, gender roles, and physical violence dynamics. It also emphasized consequences associated with using violence in interpersonal relationships. A broad conceptualization of dating was used to include any interactions between youth who are attracted to each other and are spending time together to make the program more relevant to younger students (Weisz & Black, 2001). Program goals included 1) increasing knowledge about the prevalence and causes of teenage dating violence, 2) promoting intolerance of sexual assault and teenage dating violence, and 3) increasing appropriate behavior for preventing or responding to sexual assault and dating violence (Weisz & Black).

The program was administered as an option offered to students during the school's mandatory after-school program and included 12 1.5-hour sessions. In the spring, the entire program was completed in 6 weeks, but because this format seemed rushed, during the following fall, the sessions were administered over a 12-week period. The curriculum was administered separately to boys and girls by trained facilitators. The female facilitators were from a local rape counseling center, and the male facilitators were university students. In each group, at least one facilitator was a master's-level social worker or a social work student who was working toward a master's degree. The facilitators met weekly to discuss the outcomes of the group sessions and to monitor the consistency of the intervention (Weisz & Black, 2001).

Program Evaluation   The evaluation of the RTTSV took place in an urban midwestern public charter middle school that had approximately 400 students. Recruitment information was sent home with 250 seventh graders, and 46 students volunteered to participate as part of their mandatory after-school activities. An additional 20 students who did not participate in the program were selected to serve as a comparison group. The mean age of students across both the treatment group and the comparison group was 12.84 (SD = .54). Students did not give their names, so student scores on knowledge and attitude questionnaires could not be analyzed based on the number of sessions they attended (Weisz & Black, 2001).

Only 37% of students in the intervention group completed both the pretest and the follow-up knowledge measures, and 43.5% completed both the attitude measures. Forty-five percent of the comparison group completed all of the instruments. Attrition was attributed to joining other after-school activities, absence during testing dates, or avoiding the sessions altogether (Weisz & Black).

To assess the effects of the program on students' knowledge and attitudes about sexual assault and dating violence, pretest and posttest scores were compared in order to examine immediate effects. In addition, 6-month follow-up scores were used to compare intervention and comparison groups. Between pretest and posttest, there were significant increases in students' knowledge ($p = .005$) and attitudes ($p = .004$) about dating violence (Weisz & Black, 2001). Similarly, from pretest to follow-up, the intervention group performed better than the comparison group on both knowledge ($p < .01$) and attitudes ($p < .05$). Overall, the RTTSV program was effective in increasing knowledge and improving attitudes, and effects were maintained for 6 months after the completion of the intervention (Weisz & Black).

Critical Analysis of Treatment Characteristics One of the main strengths of the RTTSV program was its sociocultural relevance, which was stressed as being an integral part of the curriculum (NDVSAC; 1995). The adaptability of the program to younger or older students with varying levels of dating experience also reflected a high degree of relevance to a diverse group of students. The program leaders were all either African American or had considerable experience in working with African American youth, further providing opportunities for both sociocultural relevance and building positive relationships between African American youth and adult role models.

Varied teaching methods also were employed because the curriculum included modeling, role plays, experiential exercises, and discussions. Another strength was the potential for students to build positive relationships. The small-group, single gender format allowed for building positive relationships. For young African American boys especially, the opportunity to interact with African American male university students was likely beneficial in promoting the positive outcomes of the program (Weisz & Black, 2001).

The RTTSV program was weak in the area of comprehensiveness. Because it took place as an optional activity during a mandatory after-school program, it likely was only a peripheral part of the students' lives at best. In contrast, programs that involve families, communities, and schools have a much greater likelihood of effecting change among students (see Foshee et al., 2000). There also was little information given regarding the theoretical framework from which the curriculum was derived. Because the program was developed by the NDVSAC (1995), it may or may not have been built on a strong theoretical foundation.

Critical Analysis of Procedural Characteristics   The fact that the RTTSV program was administered by master's-level social workers emphasizes the importance of using well-trained staff. In addition, the trainers had weekly audiotaped meetings to discuss the outcome of the group sessions and to monitor the consistency of the interventions, thereby ensuring treatment fidelity across groups. The dosage of the 12-session treatment was comparable to other successful dating violence prevention programs in the literature (Foshee et al., 1998; MacGowan, 1997) and likely contributed to the success of the program.

The timing of the program with seventh-grade students was different from many other dating violence programs that target high school students (Avery-Leaf et al., 1997; Wolfe et al., 2003), but special efforts were made to make the curriculum content applicable for younger students (Weisz & Black, 2001). The problems with attrition and skipping sessions could probably be explained primarily in terms of the students' young ages. For example, some students "hid in hallways or bathrooms to avoid the program and testing sessions" (Weisz & Black, p. 94). Although the content of the curriculum was designed to be age appropriate for seventh graders, perhaps more varied activities were needed to maintain the interest of young students after they had already been in school for the entire day. In addition, the program may have been more effective if multiple teaching sessions were used, or if the group leaders administered booster sessions a few months after the end of the treatment to ensure that the participants were still thinking about and applying the things they had learned.

Critical Analysis of Design Characteristics   Although there was a control group, its members were not randomly selected; therefore, students in the control group may have differed in significant ways from students who volunteered to participate in the intervention program. The evaluation procedure was straightforward, with pre- and posttests and a 6-month follow-up. The main problem was the small sample size because several students who participated in the program did not fill out the assessment packets. An additional problem with the data collection was that no process variables were obtained. For example, there were students who were part of the treatment but often skipped sessions in favor of lingering in the halls (Weisz & Black, 2001), and if those students were present on assessment days, results could have been skewed.

Results of the program revealed that students in the treatment group evidenced increases in knowledge about dating violence and intention to engage in help seeking and decreases in attitudes supporting dating violence and the use of conflict behaviors. There were no changes in scores for the control group. Further follow-up actually examining the effects of the program on decreasing students' dating violence victimization and perpetration would have strengthened the social significance of the project. Although attitude changes were maintained for 6 months, without evidence for behavioral change, it is unclear that the RTTSV program actually prevents dating violence.

MODEL PROGRAM FOR THE PREVENTION OF DATING VIOLENCE

A model program aimed at preventing dating violence should be comprehensive, theory driven, and socioculturally relevant to the students for which the program is designed (see Table 8.2). The need for comprehensive programs aimed at reducing dating violence among teenagers cannot be overemphasized. It is imperative to involve not only schools and service providers, but also to mount a response to the problem of dating violence that incorporates the entire community, including individual families. Similar to the Safe Dates program (Foshee et al., 1996),

Table 8.2. Components of a model dating violence prevention program

Targets of intervention	Young adolescents (around eighth or ninth grade)
	Parents
	School environment
	Community environment
	Both general and high-risk populations
Content of intervention	Information regarding what constitutes dating violence
	Strategies for maintaining healthy relationships
	Information on helping friends
	Knowledge of community resources
	Varied teaching techniques (e.g., group discussions, role playing, community events)
	Community involvement
	Emphasis on nonviolent principles
	Parent training and information dissemination in the community
Targeted outcomes of intervention	Reduce dating violence perpetration and victimization
	Increase knowledge about dating violence
	Increase skills that support healthy relationships (e.g., gender equality, open communication)
	Decrease the use of conflict behaviors to solve interpersonal problems
	Increase family cohesiveness and decrease family violence
Duration	School emphasizes nonviolent principles in multiple classes for the entire year
	Specific information regarding dating violence is shared in 12–15 sessions during health class
	Each year, students are reminded of principles of nonviolence within their school and community

school programs should integrate information regarding community services, and community service providers should be well-trained in terms of their abilities to respond to the specific needs of teenagers who are in violent dating relationships. The provision of information and resources to parents from both school and community resources would be another way to involve more aspects of the adolescent's world in the solution for decreasing the prevalence of dating violence. In addition, a model program would encourage parent participation in more active ways. For example, community organizations could offer programs to parents who are either dealing with issues of family violence or who are simply concerned about preventing dating violence in their children's relationships.

It is important that dating violence prevention programs are socioculturally relevant and promote building positive relationships to increase program effectiveness. A sensitive topic such as dating violence should be approached by staff who are well-trained and knowledgeable in the area and able to maintain a high level of relevance to students' lives. In addition, it is important that the program provide students with the opportunity to develop positive relationships in which they will feel comfortable sharing their experiences and concerns about dating violence. For programs that are conducted within the context of a regular school curriculum, building relationships may be a difficult aspect, but efforts should be made—for example, incorporating small groups led by older high school or university students that help students process the information they receive in the classroom. If intervention programs fail to promote positive relationships, it is less likely that the program material will genuinely impact students.

One of the main critiques of the prevention programs to date is that they are limited in duration (e.g., 10–18 sessions; Foshee et al., 1996; Wolfe et al., 2003) and fail to adequately address the issue of dating violence (Meyer & Stein, 2000). One alternative is to integrate nonviolence principles into the entire curriculum so that information regarding domestic violence is shared directly and indirectly throughout the entire semester. For example, the Choosing Non-Violence Program (CNV; Matthews, 2000) is a curriculum for adults who work with children to help them integrate violence-free principles into their everyday interactions with young people. Teaching nonviolent principles to teachers, service providers, and parents will help to change the norms about what sort of behavior is acceptable in interpersonal relationships. Integrating such messages throughout the curriculum and other areas of teenager's lives, along with specific education regarding dating violence, will likely maximize the impact of the nonviolence message among teenagers and help them apply what they have learned to their own dating relationships.

A dating violence prevention program that includes all of the features just described will likely make a significant impact on young people who are exposed to it. In addition, by providing the program to students who are in the early stages of dating relationships (eighth or ninth grade), there will be a greater likelihood that the program could provide primary prevention in addition to secondary prevention. To provide a more concrete example of what such a program would look like for a young person, the experience of Keisha Smith will now be considered.

❖

A Program for Keisha Smith

The Smith family had a history of domestic violence that finally resulted in Gary and Debra getting a divorce. Although Gary has joined a batterer intervention program in hopes of dealing with his problems, the family is still in turmoil. Keisha has witnessed a great deal of violence, and her mother is concerned that her daughter will end up like her when she gets older. Keisha is unhappy in the new school she has to attend because she and her mother have moved to a different part of town, and her recent school problems and failing grades have caused further friction within the family. Her mother really started to worry when Keisha started dating a 17-year-old high school student named Brian.

Keisha enjoys spending time with Brian because it means that she is able to get her mind off of the difficulties she is experiencing at home. In addition, Brian is in high school, which makes the other eighth-grade girls jealous. Sometimes Brian gets upset if he can't reach Keisha when he tries to call her, or if she wants to spend time with her friends on weekends when he wants to spend time with her. His behavior frustrates her a bit, but she believes that he's only acting that way because he really cares about her. He always makes up for his outbursts by being really sweet later, so she doesn't think much about it when he gets upset.

It is clear that Keisha is at risk for a violent dating relationship. Not only has she witnessed violence in the past within her family, but she also is involved with an older boy whose jealousy and desire to control her she interprets as love.

At her new school, Keisha is exposed to nonviolent messages throughout the day. There are posters on the walls about violence being wrong, and many of her teachers stress the importance of communication skills and handling conflict in constructive ways. Several weeks into the semester, her health class curriculum begins to cover the topic of dating violence. She is learning about what dating violence is and about some of the resources in the community that help people who are in abusive relationships. Her friends in class ask questions about her relationship with Brian because they've seen him yell at her for being late to meet him after school. Keisha wonders why they are being so nosy.

One day during a role-play exercise, Keisha realizes that the jealous behaviors remind her of Brian. She wonders why the health teacher would include something like that in the examples of what dating violence might look like. She knows that Brain would never hurt her, and he is only posses-sive because he really cares about her. It upsets her that her friends ask so many questions about her relationship, and she begins to withdraw from them and does even worse in her classes at school.

Debra is more and more concerned about Keisha's behavior and her per-formance at school. She notices that Keisha is spending less time with her friends and more time with Brian. Desperate to try something to help her daughter, and because of her own previous history in an abusive relationship, Debra joins a parent's group at a local community center where she learns nonviolent ways to express her emotions. At the parent's group, she hears about an after-school program for 13- to 15-year-old students that stresses nonviolence and gender equality. Although she forgot to write down informa-tion about the group, she noticed a public service announcement on a local television channel with statistics about teenage dating violence and an adver-tisement for the after-school program. She decides to enroll Keisha in the pro-gram, hoping that the college students who lead the groups will be good role models and that Keisha will enjoy the program as much as Debra enjoyed her parent's group.

Keisha is not happy about having to go to an after-school program, and Brian is not happy about it either. He tells Keisha that she needs to grow up and tell her mom that she should be able to do what she wants. He is so mad at her that he doesn't talk to her for a week, and this really upsets Keisha. As she is walking to the community center after school for her after-school pro-gram, she thinks she sees Brian coming toward her. He is carrying flowers and she is really happy to see him, but before he gets to her, she sees another girl join him. He gives the flowers to the girl, not noticing that Keisha is nearby. Kesiha is heartbroken. She skips the after-school program and goes home because she is so upset. The next day, she can't pay attention in class.

A couple of days later as she is on her way to her after-school program, Brian catches up with her. He tells her that he is sorry for getting upset and that he was wrong. He tells her that he loves her and misses her and wants to spend time with her again. He doesn't realize that she had seen him cheating on her. She is very angry. She tells him that she has to go. He grabs her arm to try to get her to stay. It hurts her a little bit, but she doesn't want to let him know that. She pulls her arm away from him and goes inside the community center.

Elizabeth, her group leader, sees Keisha come in and goes over to talk to her. Because they have begun to develop a relationship, Keisha feels comfortable talking to Elizabeth, and she tells her what happened with Brian. Elizabeth uses the opportunity to remind Keisha that Brian's behaviors are not right and that she deserves to be respected in her relationships. It finally occurs to Keisha that Brian's behavior hasn't been loving; in fact, he has been trying to control her all of this time. With help from Elizabeth, her mom, and her school, Keisha begins to work on having positive relationships. Although her friends are still upset that she sees Brian from time to time, they are happy that she now makes a connection between what she has learned in health class and what is going on in her life.

It is evident from this example that dating violence prevention is not necessarily a straightforward endeavor, and it may take efforts from parents, school, and the community to reach troubled youth. Even when information is presented directly to students, they may have difficulties seeing the connection between what they are learning and their own experiences. Therefore, it is important for nonviolent messages to be presented in multiple contexts and in settings that promote positive relationships so that wherever a student is when the information sinks in, he or she will be ready and able to receive help.

FUTURE DIRECTIONS: IMPROVING PROGRAMS FOR PREVENTING DATING VIOLENCE

Since the 1990s, researchers have begun to address the need for theoretically based and methodologically rigorous programs aimed at preventing adolescent dating violence (Foshee et al., 1996; Wolfe et al., 2003). Although programs often report positive attitudinal changes as a result of intervention, many fail to truly document changes in behavior. For example, Building Relationships in Greater Harmony Together (BRIGHT; Avery-Leaf et al., 1997) was a five-session dating violence prevention program based in high school health classes. Results indicated that there were significant decreases in attitudes justifying the use of dating violence among those students who participated in the treatment (Avery-Leaf et al., 1997); however, no information was collected regarding the effect of the program on reducing actual instances of dating violence. Similarly, in the RTTSV (Weisz & Black, 2001) program, results showed that the intervention had an impact on students' knowledge and attitudes, but with no data on rates of dating violence, it remains uncertain whether the intervention had an impact on students' behaviors. In contrast, more methodologically rigorous programs such as Safe Dates (Foshee et al., 2000) included a change in attitude as a process-oriented measure to help explain the mechanisms by which the intervention resulted in behavioral change for students in the treatment group. Such an approach was recommended by Cicchetti and Hinshaw (2002), who advocated including process variables to highlight mediators and moderators of positive intervention outcomes.

Overall, there needs to be a shift in the field of dating violence prevention so that more programs aim to actually prevent violent behaviors and victimization rather than simply alter beliefs and attitudes. In addition, the field would benefit significantly from more consistent programs with clear goals and objectives, as well as high-quality research examining changes in both attitudes and behaviors for extended periods of time after the completion of the study (Meyer & Stein, 2000).

Preventing dating violence among adolescents will take comprehensive, communitywide efforts. By implementing programs in schools and community centers that advocate nonviolent approaches to resolving conflict and gender equality, young people will more likely be exposed to positive messages that will encourage them to seek healthy relationships. Further research also must be conducted on the types of programs that have positive effects on adolescent outcomes. Many communities use curricula designed to prevent dating violence among teenagers, but few of these are actually evaluated for their effectiveness. For example, the RTTSV program was developed by a community agency in Nebraska in 1995, and the evaluation of the program's effectiveness took place in Michigan but was not published until 2001 (Weisz & Black, 2001). An effort to encourage program evaluation and publication of other community-based dating violence prevention programs would promote an increase in the quality of programs to which adolescents are exposed.

To decrease the rates of dating violence among teenagers, current research must not only continue but also expand to include programs that are more comprehensive and that apply more rigorous methodologies involving thorough measurement of both process and outcome variables and extended follow-ups to demonstrate lasting effects of the intervention. Finally, collaboration between scientists and service providers is essential to effectively meet the needs of young people in the community. Effective collaborations would combine the rigors of developmental science with the practical experience of community agencies, close the gap that has long existed between researchers and practitioners (Cicchetti & Hinshaw, 2002), and result in higher-quality programs to promote healthy relationships for youth.

REFERENCES

Avery-Leaf, S., Cascardi, M., O'Leary, K.D., & Cano, A. (1997). Efficacy of a dating violence prevention program on attitudes justifying aggression. *Journal of Adolescent Health, 21,* 11–17.

Bank, L., & Burraston, B. (2001). Abusive home environments as predictors of poor adjustment during adolescence and early childhood. *Journal of Community Psychology, 29,* 195–217.

Bennett, L., & Fineran, S. (1998). Sexual and severe physical violence among high school students: Power beliefs, gender, and relationship. *American Journal of Orthopsychiatry, 68,* 645–652.

Bybee, D.I., & Sullivan, C.M. (2002). The process through which an advocacy intervention resulted in positive change for battered women over time. *American Journal of Community Psychology, 30,* 103–132.

Centers for Disease Control and Prevention. (2000, June 9). Youth risk behavior surveillance—United States 1999. *Morbidity and Mortality Weekly Report, 49,* 1–96.

Cicchetti, D., & Hinshaw, S. P. (2002). Prevention and intervention science: Contributions to developmental theory. *Development and Psychopathology, 14,* 667–671.

Davis, R.C., Taylor, B.G., & Maxwell, C.D. (2000). *Does batterer treatment reduce violence?: A randomized experiment in Brooklyn.* Retrieved March 3, 2006, from http://www.ncjrs.gov/pdffiles1/nij/grants/180772.pdf

Farrell, G., Buck, W., & Pease, K. (1993). The Merseyside Domestic Violence Prevention Project: Some costs and benefits. *Studies on Crime and Prevention, 2,* 21–33.

Feder, L., & Forde, D.R. (2000). *A test of the efficacy of court-mandated counseling for domestic violence offenders: The Broward Experiment.* Retrieved March 3, 2006, from http://www.ncjrs.gov/pdffiles1/nij/grants/184752.pdf

Foshee, V.A. (1996). Gender differences in adolescent dating abuse prevalence, types, and injuries. *Health Education Research, 11,* 275–286.

Foshee, V.A. (1998) Involving schools and communities in preventing adolescent dating abuse. In X.B. Arriage & S. Oskamp (Eds.), *Addressing community problems: Psychological research and interventions* (pp. 104–132). Thousand Oaks, CA: Sage Publications.

Foshee, V.A., Bauman, K.E., Arriaga, X.B., Helms, R.W., Koch, G.G., & Linder, G.F. (1998). An evaluation of Safe Dates, an adolescent dating violence prevention program. *American Journal of Public Health, 88,* 45–50.

Foshee, V.A., Bauman, K.E., Ennett, S.T., Linder, G.F., Benefield, T., & Suchindram, C. (2004). Assessing the long-term effects of the Safe Dates program and a booster in preventing and reducing adolescent dating violence victimization and perpetration. *American Journal of Public Health, 94,* 619–624.

Foshee, V.A., Bauman, K.E., Greene, W.F., Koch, G.G., Linder, G.F., & MacDougall, J.E. (2000). The Safe Dates program: 1-year follow-up results. *American Journal of Public Health, 90,* 1619–1922.

Foshee, V.A., Linder, G.F., Bauman, K.E., Langwick, S.A., Arriaga, X.B., Heath, J.L., et al. (1996). The Safe Dates project: Theoretical basis, evaluation design, and selected baseline findings. *American Journal of Preventive Medicine, 12,* 39–47.

Howard, D.E., & Wang, M.Q. (2003). Psychosocial factors associated with adolescent boys' reports of dating violence. *Adolescence, 38,* 519–533.

Irwin, C.E., & Rickert, V.I. (2005). Coercive sexual experiences during adolescence and young adulthood: A public health problem. *Journal of Adolescent Health, 36,* 359–361.

Jackson, S., Feder, L., Forde, D.R., Davis, R.B., Maxwell, D.C., & Taylor, B.G. (2003). *Batterer intervention programs: Where do we go from here?* (Report No. NCJ195079). Rockville, MD: U.S. Department of Justice.

Kruttschnitt, C., McLaughlin, B.L., & Petrie, C.V. (2004). *Advancing the federal research agenda on violence against women.* Washington, DC: National Academies Press.

Lavoie, F., Robitaille, L., & Herbert, M. (2000). Teen dating relationships and aggression: An exploratory study. *Violence Against Women, 6,* 6–36.

Levy, B. (1984). *Skills for violence free relationships: Curriculum for young people ages 13–18.* St. Paul: Minnesota Coalition for Battered Women.

MacGowan, M.J. (1997). An evaluation of a dating violence prevention program for middle school students. *Violence and Victims, 12,* 223–235.

Makepeace, J.M. (1987). Social factors and victim offender differences in courtship violence. *Family Relations, 36,* 87–91.

Matthews, N.A. (2000). Generic violence prevention and gendered violence: Getting the message to mainstream audiences. *Violence Against Women, 6,* 311–331.

Meyer, H., & Stein, N. (2000). *Review of teen dating violence prevention.* National Violence Against Women Prevention Research Center. Retrieved March 25, 2005, from http://www.vawprevention.org/research/teendating.shtml

Nation, M., Crusto, C., Wandersman, A., Kumpfer, K.L., Seybolt, D., Morrissey-Kane, E., et al. (2003). What works in prevention: Principles of effective prevention programs. *American Psychologist, 58,* 449–456.

Nebraska Domestic Violence Sexual Assault Coalition. (1995). *Reaching and teaching teens to stop violence.* Lincoln: Author.

O'Keefe, M. (2005, April). *Teen dating violence: A review of risk factors and prevention efforts.* Retrieved March 3, 2006, from http://www.vawnet.org/DomesticViolence/Research/VAWnetDocs/AR_TeenDatingViolence.pdf National Electronic Network on Violence Against Women.

O'Keefe, M., & Treister, L. (1998). Victims of dating violence among high school students: Are the predictors different for males and females. *Violence Against Women, 4,* 195–223.

SafeYouth. (2005). *Facts for teens: Teen dating violence.* National Youth Violence Prevention Resource Center. Rockville, MD: Author.

Shepard, M.E., Falk, D.R., & Elliott, B.A. (2002). Enhancing coordinated community responses to reduce recidivism in cases of domestic violence. *Journal of Interpersonal Violence, 17,* 551–569.

Silverman, J.G., Raj, A., Mucci, L.A., & Hathaway, J.E. (2001). Dating violence against adolescent girls and associated substance use, unhealthy weight control, sexual risk behavior, pregnancy and suicidality. *Journal of the American Medical Association, 286,* 572–579.

Weisz, A.N., & Black, B.M. (2001). Evaluating a sexual assault and dating violence prevention program for urban youth. *Social Work Research, 25,* 89–100.

Wekerle, C., & Wolfe, D.A. (1999). Dating violence in mid-adolescence: Theory, significance, and emerging prevention initiatives. *Clinical Psychology Review, 19,* 435–456.

Whitaker, D., Williams, M., Morrison, S., Lindquist, C., Hawkins, S., O'Neill, J., et al. (2004, July). *Interventions to prevent dating violence.* Paper presented at the American Psychological Association National Convention, Honolulu, HI.

Wolfe, D.A., Wekerle, C., Gough, B., Reitzel-Jaffe, D., Grasley, C., Pittman, A., et al. (1996). *The youth relationships manual: A group approach with adolescents for the prevention of woman abuse and the promotion of healthy relationships.* Thousand Oaks, CA: Sage Publications.

Wolfe, D.A., Wekerle, C., Scott, K., Straatman, A., & Grasley, C. (2004). Predicting abuse in adolescent dating relationships over 1 year: The role of child maltreatment and trauma. *Journal of Abnormal Psychology, 113,* 406–415.

Wolfe, D.A., Wekerle, C., Scott, K., Straatman, A., Grasley, C., & Reitzel-Jaffe, D. (2003). Dating violence prevention with at-risk youth: A controlled outcome evaluation. *Journal of Consulting and Clinical Psychology, 2,* 279–291.

9

MARITAL CONFLICT
AND THE AFTERMATH OF DIVORCE

Prevention Programs for Families

Patricia M. Mitchell,
W. Brad Faircloth, and Peggy S. Keller

Conflict between couples is unavoidable simply because no two people can agree on everything. For some couples, however, conflict becomes an escalating cycle of anger and hurt that jeopardizes their families and may eventually lead to divorce. It is not surprising that the National Center for Health (2002) estimated that more than 50% of all marriages will end in divorce within the first 15 years, often because of high rates of conflict. Although the effects of conflict and divorce may be detrimental for the adults involved, the consequences for children can be even more severe.

INTERPARENTAL CONFLICT IN INTACT
AND DIVORCED FAMILIES

Children exposed to interparental conflict in intact families are at risk for internalizing problems such as depression and anxiety, and externalizing problems such as aggression and delinquency, poor academic performance, and poor peer and social functioning (Baruch & Wilcox, 1944; Gassner & Murray, 1969; Hubbard & Adams, 1936; Jouriles, Bourg, & Farris, 1991; Porter & O'Leary, 1980; Rutter, 1970; Towle, 1931; Wallace, 1935). Children of divorced parents are at increased risk for the same adjustment problems (Amato, 1993, 2000; Cherlin et al., 1991) often because of continued exposure to interparental conflict (Amato, 1993; Goodman, Bonds, Sandler, & Braver, 2004). Children of divorced parents show more behavior problems, have lower academic achievement compared with children of intact families (Cherlin et al., 1991), and have reduced self-esteem, social functioning, and physical health (Amato, 2000). Even in adulthood, children of divorced parents are at risk: They are less likely to attend or complete college and are more likely to experience divorce themselves (Amato, 1993). Therefore, exposure to interparental conflict is a major problem for children and families within society.

Constructive versus Destructive Conflict

Research shows that *how* parents disagree with each other plays a major role in whether disagreements are harmful to children (Cummings & Davies, 1994). Two distinct types of conflict—constructive conflict and destructive conflict— have been identified based on how children respond (Cummings & Davies, 1994; Goeke-Morey, 1999). Destructive conflict may be frequent, intense, unresolved, or child related. Destructive conflict behaviors, including physical aggression, verbal anger, or withdrawal, place children at heightened risk for a variety of adjustment problems (Cummings, 1997). These behaviors sensitize children to conflict, resulting in increased arousal to relatively mild disagreements. In intact families, destructive conflict decreases children's feelings of security about the family, causing them to worry about family stability, the availability of parents, and their own well-being. In divorced families, the effects of continued destructive conflict are compounded when children are involved in custody battles, become the sole means of communication between parents, or are asked to choose between parents (Hans & Fine, 2001).

In contrast to destructive conflict, constructive conflict is characterized by warmth, effective communication, and progress toward resolution. Constructive conflict tactics include humor, support, affection, calm discussion, listening, and problem solving (Cummings, 1998; Goeke-Morey, 1999). In intact families, constructive conflict may reduce the risk of adjustment problems and distress in children by modeling effective conflict strategies, promoting children's sense of well-being about the family, and allowing children to devote their energy to social and academic functioning rather than worry about the state of the family (Cummings, Ballard, El-Sheikh, & Lake, 1991; Cummings, Simpson, & Wilson, 1993). Constructive conflict can have similar positive effects within divorced families. Although divorced couples may not necessarily feel warmth or affection for each other, they can adopt effective and constructive communication strategies to better understand each other's perspectives. As in intact families, constructive inter-parental conflict may benefit children in divorced families by modeling appropri-ate conflict behaviors and by freeing up time to focus on developmental goals. It also may prevent children of divorce from feeling caught in the middle of their parents' arguments or from feeling responsible for the marital dissolution.

Preventing Negative Effects of Conflict on Children

A major issue for researchers is how to prevent the detrimental effects of destruc-tive conflict on children by promoting constructive conflict. Destructive inter-parental conflict plays a significant role in the development of childhood prob-lems. To the extent that divorce eliminates interparental conflict, children benefit. Unfortunately, couples who are unable to handle conflict well before divorce will not necessarily handle it well after divorce. In addition, many parents cannot dis-cern the differences between destructive and constructive conflict behaviors on their own and are unaware of the detrimental influences that negative discord may have on their children. It is therefore essential to develop prevention and intervention programs that educate parents on how to work toward adopting con-structive conflict practices in both intact and divorced families. Furthermore, pro-grams that focus on different stages of development are essential to help children who have been exposed to varying levels of conflict. These programs can teach children to cope with the feelings of insecurity and fear that arise from witness-ing destructive conflict between their parents and improve family relations.

Direct and Indirect Effects of Interparental Conflict on Children

In considering prevention programs, it is important to understand why destruc-tive interparental conflict is harmful to children. Several different but comple-mentary theories of direct relations between interparental conflict and children's adjustment have been proposed. Emotional security theory (EST; Davies & Cummings, 1994) maintains that children have a sense of family stability and safety called emotional security. Destructive conflict undermines children's emo-tional security, which is demonstrated by their intense negative emotional reac-tions to conflict, their behavioral strategies to reduce the threat of conflict (i.e., interrupting, intervening), and their cognitive representations of the family as unstable and conflicts as irresolvable. Over time, these emotional, behavioral, and cognitive reactions may lead to chronic anxiety or depression, tendencies to act out aggressively, and impairments in social and academic functioning. Alterna-tively, the cognitive–contextual framework (Grych & Fincham, 1990) claims that how children think and feel about interparental conflict affects their reactions to conflict and their long-term development. Grych and Fincham (1990, 1993) proposed that only children who perceive a threat or blame themselves for interparental conflict will be negatively affected by it.

In addition to the direct relationship between interparental conflict and child adjustment proposed by EST and the cognitive–contextual framework, interparental conflict can indirectly harm children by disrupting the parent–child relationship. In both intact and divorced families, conflict and hostility in the interparental relationship can spill over into the parent–child relationship (Cox, Paley, & Harter, 2001; Erel & Burman, 1995). Concern over spousal conflict may reduce parental warmth, sensitivity, consistent monitoring, and discipline. Furthermore, bitter conflicts may result in one parent withdrawing emotionally or physically from the child. In divorced families, parents may be overwhelmed with anger or sadness over the failure of their relationship, or they may be anxious about the changes divorce entails and have difficulty coping with these changes. As a result, they may monitor their children's behavior less and use less effective disciplinary strategies (Heatherington, Cox, & Cox, 1982; Simons, Beaman, Conger, & Chao, 1993; Simons, Lin, Gordon, Conger, & Lorenz, 1999).

Theories regarding the effects of interparental conflict on children's development have important implications for prevention programs. For example, children must learn that all people experience conflict, including parents, and that it is normal to be upset by it. At the same time, children should be taught that they are not to blame and are not responsible for conflict resolution. Adaptive, age-appropriate coping strategies to reduce the stress associated with marital conflict should be presented. Theory also suggests that programs should bolster parenting skills in the context of conflict and promote communication about parenting. Finally, programs targeting divorced families must teach methods of coping with the increased stress of postdivorce life and help establish an effective co-parenting relationship.

Few researchers and practitioners have attempted to develop theory-based programs focused on preventing the problems associated with marital conflict within intact or divorced families. Most programs, however, focus on either the children or the parents but not both, and on "fixing" problematic marriages without focusing on the potential long-term effects for children (Halford, Markman, Kline, Galena, & Stanley, 2003; Lindsay, Pedro-Carroll, & Davies, 2001). This chapter reviews a selection of current programs for intact and divorced families that meet criteria for effective prevention programs and makes suggestions for future improvements (see Table 9.1). Programs were selected for review if empirical evaluations of program effectiveness were available in peer-reviewed journals. Theoretically driven programs can prevent the detrimental effects of conflict on children in intact families by equipping them with the tools necessary to cope

Table 9.1. Summary of prevention programs for the effects of marital conflict and divorce

	Premarital Relationship Enhancement Program (PREP)	Family Conflict Intervention Program (FCIP)	New Beginnings (NB)	Children of Divorce Intervention Program (CODIP)
Targets	Engaged or newly married couples	Children from intact families Programs for second and third graders	Divorced mothers Custody of children ages 9–12 Divorced in past 2 years Mother only and mother and child versions	Children with divorced parents Programs for kindergarten through eighth grade Urban or suburban populations
Content	Main goals: Educate couples to manage negative communication and affect during conflict Enhance positive aspects of couples' relationships	Main goals: Establish supportive environment for children Help children identify and express conflict-related feelings Enhance coping skills and problem-solving skills Enhance positive self-perceptions	Main goals: Train parents on parental monitoring, reinforcing child behavior, listening, and effective discipline Practice anger-management training Promote father involvement	Main goals: Establish supportive environment Enhance coping with feelings Increase understanding of divorce Improve communication and problem solving Enhance family- and self-esteem
Outcomes	Improves: Positive communication skills Problem-solving strategies Relationship satisfaction Reduces: Communication negativity Relationship aggression	Improves: Expression of feelings Emotional reactivity Problem-solving skills Reduces: Involvement in arguments Fear of conflict	Improves: Mother–child relationship quality Maternal discipline Child mental health Reduces: Children's behavior problems, including internalizing problems, sexual activity, and substance abuse	Improves: Expression of feelings Communication skills Problem-solving skills Reduces: Anxiety Behavioral disruptions

with interparental conflict. Alternatively, if the marriage does end, programs can prepare families for the possible consequences of divorce on the couple and the children.

PREVENTION PROGRAMS AND THEIR EVALUATIONS

Although there are many relationship enhancement programs available through various service providers, the Premarital Relationship Enhancement Program (PREP) represents the most well-documented and thoroughly evaluated program for couples. The focus of PREP is to work with couples in an effort to raise awareness of the harmful effects of negative communication and conflict as well as to provide couples with skills for improving marital communication. In addition, the Family Conflict Intervention Program (FCIP) represents one of the most effective programs for preparing children to deal with conflict at home. FCIP focuses on educating children about different types of emotions and the situations that evoke those emotions. It also provides children with problem-solving and coping skills to appropriately handle exposure to conflict between parents.

For families facing divorce, the New Beginnings (NB) program and the Children of Divorce Intervention Program (CODIP) focus on providing parents with information about divorce (i.e., dual households, stepfamilies, interparental conflict) and skills to cope with it. NB represents a highly comprehensive program available for divorcing families. It provides mothers with information regarding parenting and conflict through multiple methods of presentation and has been shown to improve mothers' parenting practices and children's adjustment. CODIP is one of the most widely tested programs for children of divorce. Knowledge about emotions, problem-solving skills, self-esteem, and supportive relationships is developed with children as a means of providing the most effective ways of coping with divorce.

All of these programs, whether for intact or divorced families, work to raise awareness of parents and children regarding the effects of conflict and divorce on the family system and teach family members to better communicate with one another. The goal is to help families avoid the harmful consequences of conflict and divorce.

Prevention and Relationship Enhancement Programs

Despite the popularity of marriage enrichment programs, only about two dozen have been evaluated empirically (Bagarozzi & Rauen, 1981; Hawley & Olson, 1995; Sayers, Kohn, & Heavey, 1998). Typically, these relationship enhancement

programs consist of a combination of four components regarding marital communication: 1) awareness, 2) feedback, 3) cognitive change, and 4) skills training (Halford,
Markman, Kline, & Stanley, 2003). Sayers et al. (1998) found that only 2 of 13 studies indicated program effectiveness on some level beyond a 6-month follow-up. One
of these is a collection of studies by Halford and colleagues (1998) on Premarital
Relationship Enhancement Program (PREP) (Markman, Floyd, Stanley, & Storaasli,
1988; Markman, Jamieson, & Floyd, 1983), the most extensively researched, evaluated, and well-developed premarital program available to couples today.

PREP (Markman et al., 1983; Markman et al., 1988) is designed to help
couples make behavioral changes that will prevent marital problems before they
are established. Specific skills are taught to couples as a means of structuring communication in a more productive format. The underlying theoretical rationale for
PREP is that communication difficulties lead to distress in the marriage. That is,
marital distress may be prevented by teaching couples effective ways of speaking,
listening, and problem solving (Markman et al., 1983; Renick, Blumberg, &
Markman, 1992). Therefore, PREP targets the specific strategies that couples use
to handle conflicts and regulate their negative affects (Markman et al., 1988;
Stanley, Markman, St. Peters, & Leber, 1995). An additional goal is to enhance
the positive aspects of the relationship, including friendship, fun, and sensuality.

The program is currently offered in two versions, both of which are presented in a group format using lectures, discussion, and exercises intended to
strengthen program content. The extended version of the program consists of six
weekly group sessions with four to eight couples, whereas the weekend version is
offered over a weekend to approximately 20–40 couples. PREP material consists
of 12 different units, each focusing on productive and problematic aspects of couple communication. In both versions, each couple is paired with a coach who
helps them complete communication activities based on a method known as the
speaker–listener technique. Units one and two of PREP provide an overview of
the entire program. The couples are given information based on relevant research
findings, and instructors teach couples about theoretical concepts such as safety
and structure (Gottman, Notarius, Gonso, & Markman, 1976). The speaker–
listener technique is introduced and couples practice it with a coach. Units three,
four, and five provide further background information regarding negative and
positive styles of communicating. Couples are encouraged to examine their expectations for their relationship and how these expectations may be detrimental to
their marriage. Units six to eight focus on enhancing positive aspects of the marriage, such as having fun together, and finding solutions with which both partners can be happy. Lectures and homework encourage couples to incorporate the
material into their relationship. Units 9 and 10 of PREP are optional and depend
on the specific needs of each couple. In these units, the focus is on the connec-

tion between spiritual beliefs and the marital relationship. Concepts such as respecting your spouse, intimacy, and forgiveness are discussed. The final two units serve as a wrap-up of the program and are intended to synthesize the material previously presented.

PREP has been adapted for implementation with couples who are at high and low risk (Behrens & Halford, 1994; Schilling, Baucom, Burnett, Allen, & Ragland, 2003), for couples expecting their first child (Heavey, Larson, & Carpenter, 1997), and for German, Dutch, Christian, and community-based clergy-led samples (Markman & Hahlweg, 1993; Stanley, et al., 2001; Stanley & Trathen, 1994; Van Widenfelt, Hosman, Schaap, & van der Staak, 1996).

Program Evaluation   The majority of studies evaluating the program's effectiveness up to the 5-year mark are favorable. Markman and Floyd (1980), Markman and Hahlweg (1993), and Markman, Floyd, Stanley, and Storaasli (1988) have shown that in comparison with control couples, couples attending PREP showed improved positive communication skills and problem-solving strategies; fewer negative interactions; lower rates of relationship aggression 1, 2, and 3 years after the program; lower rates of breakup or divorce; and higher levels of relationship satisfaction at a 5-year follow-up (Markman et al., 1988; Markman, Renick, Floyd, Stanley, & Clements, 1993). Burnett (1994) found that couples participating in the weekend version of PREP learned communication skills at least as well as couples attending the original PREP, and Schilling (1999) demonstrated that the weekend PREP was as effective in preventing declines in marital satisfaction during the first 3 years of marriage as was the original version (Markman et al., 1988). Despite these positive findings, however, some independent studies have indicated that PREP may have adverse effects for women participants (Schilling et al., 2003) and for men and women from countries other than the United States, including Holland (Van Widenfelt et al., 1996).

Critical Analysis of Treatment Characteristics   PREP is considered an effective prevention program because it specifically targets engaged couples and newlyweds in the hopes of preventing maladaptive relationship patterns before they emerge. It also utilizes multiple methodologies and presentation modalities. Lectures presented by PREP leaders along with interactive coaching sessions serve to increase awareness of issues concerning marital communication. Skills training is provided as a concrete way for couples to take charge of their behavior and the progress of their relationship. By providing couples with useful information regarding communication, as well as specific behavioral techniques to improve their interactions early in marriage, PREP clearly targets negative communication as a risk factor.

Unfortunately, the PREP program has not been adequately tested among couples who may potentially be in the greatest need of such an intervention, including couples who are currently experiencing divorce. In addition, PREP does not address issues concerning the family system beyond that of the couple (i.e., parenting, parent–child attachment, child rearing) or provide intervention for children. Because the maladaptive consequences of destructive conflict reach beyond couples to children, it would be a great benefit to provide children with information regarding ways to cope with conflict. Finally, despite receiving PREP training, couples still have to navigate through both old and new disagreements. They may return to their previous styles of ineffective communication tactics without ongoing coaching and training.

Critical Analysis of Design Characteristics PREP represents one of the most effective models for helping newlyweds navigate the inherent difficulties of marriage. The program is multifaceted in its mode of presentation (i.e., leader presentation, coaching time, homework activities) and its specific target of intervention. It increases couples' awareness of communication difficulties and enhances communication skills. PREP also is offered in multiple formats, including a new take-home version of the program, which allows couples to select the version that best suits their needs and schedules.

However, further testing of PREP is needed to establish effectiveness beyond the specific measures tailored to the study. Assessing the broader impact of marital communication on the entire family, including children, will provide additional information regarding program effectiveness. For example, future tests of PREP training on various aspects of the marital, parental, and other family relationships could investigate whether PREP has a greater benefit for individuals based on their age, gender, or culture.

The Family Conflict Intervention Program

The Family Conflict Intervention Program (FCIP) focuses on preventing the negative effects of marital conflict on children (Lindsay, 2002; Lindsay et al., 2001). Based on the CODIP (Pedro-Carroll & Cowen, 1985), which is reviewed later in this chapter, FCIP teaches children of intact families to better deal with interparental conflict. This program stems from research on divorce that emphasizes the detrimental effects of interparental conflict (before, during, and after divorce) on children (Cummings & Davies, 1994; Lindsay, 2002). The primary goals of FCIP are to foster a safe and supportive group environment in which children can learn to identify and express conflict-related feelings and to help children learn to cope with stress by teaching problem-solving skills and enhancing positive self-perception (Lindsay et al., 2001, p. 98).

FCIP comprises eight after-school sessions, each of which lasts approximately 35 minutes. The program is designed for second- and third-grade children and is implemented in group format (approximately 40 children). Sessions are led by two group leaders: a mental health professional trained to work with children and a trained associate. Training for group leaders is conducted before the program begins, and leaders are supervised for the duration of the program.

The curriculum for FCIP is broken into three substantive blocks. The first block, which consists of the first three sessions, provides children with a safe and supportive group environment. During these sessions, children get to know and feel comfortable with their group leaders. Games such as the "Name Game" are played, and rules for the groups are established. Particularly, the first three sessions focus on a poster titled "Helpful Hints for a Fun and Safe Group" that includes tips such as 1) listen carefully to others and 2) please do not speak out of turn. It is during the first block that "Terry the Turtle," the puppet used to help children identify the emotions felt by themselves and others, is introduced. Terry the Turtle is a sand turtle who "retracts into her shell" when placed in compromising situations, such as witnessing conflict between her parents (Lindsay, 2002; Lindsay et al., 2001).

The second block, consisting of sessions four to six, teaches children social problem-solving skills for everyday situations and for interparental conflict. These skills are combined with coping techniques to offer children various solutions to social problems. In session four, leaders begin to discuss the topic of interparental conflict and the concept of children intervening in parental conflict. A "Point of View" exercise is adapted in which the leaders model a low-to-moderate conflict by taking different points of view concerning a particular topic. The leaders simulate an argument and then Terry the Turtle is used to explore different points of view. Session five helps children distinguish between helpful and unhelpful ways of dealing with problems. A "Social Problem-Solving" cartoon and exercise are used, and the children practice problem-solving skills by thinking up problems and consequences of and solutions to the problems (Lindsay, 2002; Lindsay et al., 2001). In session six, children are taught to distinguish between solvable and unsolvable problems and to play games that will help them develop coping strategies for "unsolvable" problems. The third block, consisting of the last two sessions of FCIP, encourages positive self-esteem and family appraisals as well as empathy for others. The children review their thoughts and feelings about the group and are asked to talk about some of the positive aspects of their families.

Program Evaluation   In the final sessions of FCIP, the children are evaluated to test their knowledge of the program material and how the program has affected their perceptions and feelings about interparental conflict. For example, the children are asked how they feel about conflicts between parents as well as how they might act when witnessing marital conflict. Parents and group leaders also complete pre- and posttest measures regarding the behaviors and coping mechanisms of the children. In general, the results indicate that children improve significantly on a number of variables after taking part in the sessions (e.g., verbal expressiveness, emotional reactivity, problem solving, efficacy) (Lindsay, 2002).

Critical Analysis of Treatment Characteristics FCIP has many positive aspects, including comprehensiveness and an ability to involve children in meaningful activities. Each session focuses on different topics (e.g., emotion, family security) and offers children a wide variety of ideas. Many methods have proven successful in keeping children interested—for example, Terry the Turtle. The content of the program focuses on the effects of conflict and gives children the opportunity to recognize that parental conflict is normal and that it is not their responsibility to solve their parents' problems. However, the topic of marital conflict is not introduced until the fourth session, half way into the program. This is unusual, because one of the main goals of this program is to help children cope more adaptively with marital conflict. Also, some of the language and activities used in the curriculum of this program may be too advanced for the children involved. Many of the children have trouble distinguishing between a "solvable" and an "unsolvable" problem, which leads to some setbacks for participating children (Lindsay, 2002).

Critical Analysis of Design Characteristics The authors of FCIP reported that the program was effective in educating children about marital conflict and in helping children cope better with conflict by improving problem-solving skills and emotional reactivity. However, some of the measures used to evaluate the program are unreliable. Reports from parents, leaders, and children sometimes differed from one another, indicating that better measures of adjustment must be used (Lindsay, 2002; Lindsay et al., 2001). Furthermore, program effectiveness must be interpreted with caution because there was no comparison group and no preprogram measure used to assess children's improvement over the course of the sessions. Further evaluations with reliable measures would prove beneficial in evaluating the overall effectiveness of FCIP.

Finally, despite the evidence that marital conflict can have negative effects on the entire family system, FCIP did not include any sessions for parents. This prevention program focused entirely on children and their coping skills. Nothing was included to help parents better deal with conflict or to teach parents about the effects that conflict may have on children.

MODEL PROGRAM TO PREVENT HARMFUL CONSEQUENCES OF INTERPARENTAL CONFLICT

The model program to prevent harmful consequences of interparental conflict in intact families should incorporate all of the positive aspects of the previously reviewed programs into one comprehensive and theory-driven project, while improving on the previous programs' limitations. The goal of the model program is to make parents and children aware of the effects of conflict and to provide them with information and techniques that will improve their conflict and coping skills. An outline of the model program is presented in Table 9.2. This program's essential features include components for both children and parents; the inclusion of communication training for couples; information on the effects of conflict on other aspects of the couple's relationship, including co-parenting; and training for children regarding coping styles and emotion regulation in the context of marital discord.

The content is presented in group format for both parents and children. The former introduces parents to the important theory and research findings regarding the effects of marital conflict on spousal and parent–child relationships. Parents are taught that marital conflict differs from couple to couple in its intensity, frequency, content, and resolution strategies. Parents also are trained to recognize constructive and destructive conflict behaviors used during conflict and are taught specific communication skills that promote constructive conflict tactics. In addition, parents learn that their destructive conflicts are detrimental to the behavioral, emotional, and cognitive development of their children. A portion of the program focuses on child-rearing and parenting practices. Couples learn that parenting is a marital issue that should be approached cooperatively, with parents working together as a team. Co-parenting, behavioral control, and emotional availability are addressed, with emphasis placed on maintaining a united front and fostering optimal child development.

The child component of the model program operates in conjunction with the parent component. It consists of various games that focus on helping children

Table 9.2. Components of a model program to prevent harmful consequences of interparental conflict

	Model program	
	Parent component	Child component
Targets	Married or cohabitating couples	Children of intact families
Content	Education regarding the effects of marital conflict on the family The importance of co-parenting The importance of strong emotional bonds Communication skills training	Recognizing and labeling emotions Problem-solving skills Emotion focused coping Enhanced self-perceptions
Outcomes	Improves: Conflict tactics Parenting practices Child adjustment Reduces: Destructive interparental conflict	Improves: Expression of feelings Emotional reactivity Problem-solving skills Reduces: Fear of conflict Involvement in conflict

learn about different emotional states and recognizing the emotions of others. Children learn that all people experience emotions of various kinds and intensities. This component also teaches children how to better cope with emotions, especially in relation to interparental conflict. They are taught that all parents experience conflict and handle these conflicts in different ways. Most important, children learn that interparental fights are not their fault and that they are not responsible for solving disagreements between their parents. They are continually instructed that no matter how severe an argument may be, their parents will continue to love them.

This model program builds and improves on the programs previously reviewed in this chapter. It combines the separate parent and child protocols into a single family-based project. The components are theory driven and serve to educate parents and children regarding the effects of conflict on family functioning and children's well-being. In addition to focusing on the negative impact of destructive conflict on the family, the program promotes healthy parent–child relations. The intriguing presentation methods for children and parents, including puppets and PowerPoint presentations, could be highly effective in educating families and improving communication skills.

❖

The Jackson Family

The Jacksons are a family that could benefit from participation in the model program. There are various issues within this family that lead to destructive and impaired communication between the parents, Jason and Beth, as well as between their child Steven and each of his parents. The disagreements between Beth and Jason about Jason's work hours and lack of free time are ongoing conflict topics. These disagreements are never resolved and are therefore continuously harmful to the functioning of the entire family system. Also, Steven is often a witness to his parents' arguments and becomes extremely distressed as a result. This distress may be contributing to his lack of positive social skills and academic success. The model program may open Jason and Beth's eyes to the importance of constructive and resolved conflict for the improvement of their relationship and for the sake of Steven. This program also may offer Steven optimal coping strategies for dealing with his parents' conflicts.

Beth and Jason are recruited to participate in the parent component of the model program while Steven participates in the child component. They are introduced to the effects their conflicts are having on their marriage and on their individual well-being. They learn the differences between constructive and destructive conflict and begin to recognize how their destructive communication styles may be causing ongoing and unresolved conflicts in their marriage. They are taught constructive communication skills and given opportunities to practice these skills. This helps Jason see that his work schedule is affecting Beth. The other sessions of the model program help Jason and Beth see the effects their conflicts are having on Steven. They now recognize the negative ways that Steven reacts to their fighting and are taught the importance of communication in regard to co-parenting so that their unity can help improve Steven's success in school and social settings. In addition, by continuing to improve their communication skills, Jason and Beth enhance the overall quality of their marital relationship.

An important benefit for Steven is that he comes to understand that his parents' fights are not his fault, even if they are about him. Although Jason and Beth may bicker about his grades, Steven is taught that it is not his job to intervene or attempt to fix his parents' arguments. Steven is now able to recognize the emotions that may arise during difficult situations and can generate solutions to his problems. This helps him identify the depressed feelings of his mother and see that he does not cause them. In addition, Steven can select adaptive responses to interparental conflict. The facilitators are continuously stressing to the children that their parents' arguments are grown-up problems, although there are other problems that the children can help to solve in their own lives. For Steven, this may include studying harder to improve his grades and seeking tutoring from a teacher or a peer.

The model program equips the Jackson family with new communication skills and coping strategies to help each person individually as well as the family overall. Working together, Jason and Beth are better able to parent Steven and discuss and resolve the issues in their marriage. The program helps Steven recognize that it is acceptable for him to be distressed when his parents have disagreements, but that they are not his fault and it is not his responsibility to solve them.

PROGRAMS TO PREVENT
THE NEGATIVE EFFECTS OF DIVORCE

Programs designed to diminish the risk associated with parental divorce should attempt to reduce levels of destructive interparental conflict, improve parenting practices, and build skills for coping with the stress of divorce. Unfortunately, few empirically validated programs address even one of these topics. Two exceptions stand out as exemplary programs for the prevention of the deleterious consequences of divorce on children: the NB program (Wolchik et al., 1993; Wolchik et al., 2000; see also Weiss & Wolchik, 1998) and the CODIP (Pedro-Carroll & Cowen, 1985; see also Pedro-Carroll, 1997).

The New Beginnings Program

The New Beginnings (NB) program targets parents with children between 9 and 12 years old who have experienced divorce within the past 2 years (Wolchik et al., 1993; Wolchik et al., 2000; see also Weiss & Wolchik, 1998). Training takes place during 11 weekly group sessions that are 1 hour and 45 minutes long and include brief lectures, discussions, demonstrations, practice, and homework assignments. In addition, 1-hour sessions after weeks 3 and 6 provide individual problem-solving instruction.

The primary goal of NB is to improve the quality of the custodial mother–child relationship. Specifically, the program seeks to increase maternal warmth, listening, and effective discipline. To achieve these goals, the program teaches three skills: Family Fun Time, One-on-One Time, and Catch 'em Being Good. During the first session, program leaders introduce Family Fun Time, an activity that mothers are asked to do every week. Children choose an activity the family can enjoy together. The purpose is to increase positive interaction between mothers and children and promote a sense of family cohesiveness. During the second session, program instructors introduce the concept of One-on-One Time, in which mothers schedule short periods of time to participate in an activity of their child's choice and offer undivided positive attention. Mothers also are taught to Catch 'em Being Good; that is, to identify when their children are well-behaved and reward them. Both of these activities are designed to increase the children's sense that they are loved and valued and to promote harmonious mother–child relations.

The next three sessions are devoted to listening skills. Good listening skills are presented as following a cycle of listening, thinking, and responding. Mothers are taught to listen to their children by paying attention to what they say, adopting a body language that signals they are interested, using open-ended questions, and asking children to elaborate. Mothers are taught to think about what their children say in order to assess the meaning of their communication and to determine whether they need them to elaborate. They are asked to paraphrase what their children say to ensure the accuracy of their perceptions and to generate solutions to problems when listening is not enough.

The program encourages child contact with the noncustodial father and addresses conflict between the parents. Session six is devoted to this goal. Mothers are provided with anger management training in which they are taught to effectively express and regulate their anger. They are taught about the importance of father involvement in children's lives and are encouraged to remove possible obstacles preventing their ex-husbands from maintaining contact with their children. The seventh session is designed to help mothers implement their listening skills with their child. The remaining sessions, devoted to disciplinary practices, address three skills: adopting clear and realistic expectations of children, monitoring children's misbehavior and its consequences, and increasing the consistency of discipline. During this part of the program, mothers are taught to identify problem behaviors and to develop, implement, and evaluate a plan for changing these behaviors.

Program Evaluation   Evaluations of NB include comparisons to individuals in a literature control group who have received no intervention after divorce. NB also has a low attrition or drop-out rate among participants in the program at posttest, 3 months after posttest, and 6 years after posttest. Results have indicated positive impacts on mother–child relationship quality, parental discipline, and children's mental health. These gains were greatest for families with the poorest initial functioning. At the 6-year follow-up (Wolchik et al., 2002), children whose mothers participated in NB had fewer symptoms of mental disorders, had less externalizing of problems, and used less alcohol and drugs than children in the control group.

Critical Analysis of Treatment Characteristics   NB is theory driven and based on a cognitive-behavioral framework and previous research indicating that poor parenting, parental maladjustment, and interparental conflict are important risk factors for children of divorce. In targeting multiple pathways that have been established between parental divorce and children's adjustment problems, including parenting, father involvement, and interparental conflict, NB is also comprehensive. Comprehensiveness is further increased by the multiple components within targeted domains, such as addressing parental warmth, communication, and discipline within the parenting domain. An additional strength is that the program uses varied teaching methods. Participants receive information and develop skills using lecture, discussion, demonstration, practice, and homework assignments. However, the portion targeting interparental conflict could be improved. Simply providing anger management techniques to one parent fails to address the complex nature of children's reactions to interparental conflict. It is important to distinguish between constructive and destructive conflict and to highlight how children's perceptions of conflict can lead to adjustment problems.

Critical Analysis of Procedural Characteristics   The attention paid to treatment fidelity and training staff sets NB apart from many prevention programs. The extensive efforts included 30 hours of training and weekly supervision of administrators. Data were collected to determine if fidelity was achieved; independent raters of videotaped sessions found that administrators were nearly perfect in their fidelity to the program. However, the program could have been more appropriately timed. Families were eligible if they had been granted a divorce as much as 2 years previous to participation. Children's adjustment problems may be even more effectively prevented if the program's initiation is closer to the family disruption.

Critical Analysis of Design Characteristics   A major advantage of NB is the high interpretive standards. The experimental group was compared with a literature control group that received books for parents and children about coping with divorce and syllabi to guide readings. NB included excellent outcome evaluation: Child adjustment was assessed both in the short term and the long term (6 years). The program also is internally valid in that the mechanisms through which program goals were to be achieved (improving parenting and reducing conflict) were evaluated.

Children of Divorce Intervention Program

The Children of Divorce Intervention Program (CODIP) began as a group program for fourth- through sixth-grade suburban children. Based on its success, it has since been adapted for use with fourth- through sixth-grade urban children (Pedro-Carroll, Alpert-Gillis, & Cowen, 1992), seventh- and eighth-grade children (Pedro-Carroll & Alpert-Gillis, 1997), second- and third-grade urban and suburban children (Alpert-Gillis, Pedro-Carroll, & Cowen, 1989; Sterling, 1986), and kindergarten and first-grade suburban children (Pedro-Carroll & Alpert-Gillis, 1997), with minor changes to reflect diverse cultural backgrounds as well as children's differing developmental needs. CODIP has five goals: 1) establish a supportive environment, 2) identify and express feelings, 3) foster understanding of divorce, 4) develop communication and problem-solving skills, and 5) promote self- and family-esteem. The programs vary in length, depending on the age group included. For example, CODIP for second- and third-grade urban school children includes 16 weekly 45-minute sessions, whereas the program for kindergarten and first-grade children consists of 12 weekly 45-minute sessions.

In the program developed for fourth- through sixth-grade suburban children, the first session focuses on achieving a supportive group environment. A name is selected for the group, confidentiality is explained, and some discussion about divorce-related feelings and coping strategies takes place. The second session helps children understand the changes that are taking place in their family, including custody arrangements and parental dating. The third session focuses on communication and coping strategies. The fourth, fifth, and sixth sessions teach social problem-solving skills using a six-step procedure for identifying problems, thinking of alternatives, considering consequences, choosing a solution, evaluating the solution, and implementing the solution. The seventh session is a review, and the eighth and ninth sessions focus on the causes and consequences of anger and ways of handling it. Session 10 promotes acceptance of diverse family structures. The goal of session 11 is to enhance children's self-esteem and explore the positive results of divorce. Session 12, the last session, considers termination issues such as feelings of loss and using alternative sources of support. Variations of CODIP developed for alternative populations have a similar format.

Program Evaluation　　Most evaluations of CODIP for the various age groups include comparisons to a wait-list control group and a nondivorced, intact family group. Studies report that children in the program for fourth and sixth graders are better able to express their feelings, communicate effectively, behave appropriately, and solve problems relative to control groups (Pedro-Carroll, 1997). Children in the experimental groups also experienced less anxiety. Teachers rated participants as more competent and less disruptive. The program designed for second- and third-grade urban children increased children's adjustment to divorce and decreased emotional and behavioral problems compared with the wait-list control group (Alpert-Gillis et al., 1989). The program adapted for kindergarten and first-grade children increased children's competencies and decreased their adjustment problems at posttest and at 2-year follow-up (Pedro-Carroll, Sutton, & Wyman, 1999).

Critical Analysis of Treatment Characteristics　　CODIP stands out in promoting positive relationships. The content of the program often focuses on developing relationships between the children as coping resources and on building a strong sense of self-esteem and family pride. Children are encouraged to talk to each other about their problems both during and outside of the program. CODIP employs varied teaching methods including instructional films, writing projects, role playing, participating on a "panel of experts," and modeling. CODIP also is a model program for ensuring sociocultural relevance. The designers have adapted the program to diverse populations. For example, the program for young urban children includes a greater focus on using extended family members as coping resources and a greater discussion of infrequent contact with non-custodial parents. However, CODIP does not address any of the mechanisms that research has identified as important reasons why children of divorce are at risk. Studies indicate that both parenting and interparental conflict are critical pathways through which divorce harms children. Although the evaluation of CODIP indicates its effectiveness, theoretically driven prevention programs for children of divorce must address these issues.

Critical Analysis of Procedural Characteristics   CODIP procedures ensure well-trained staff and treatment fidelity. First, the program is based on a detailed and structured protocol. Second, the administrators of the program include only professionals (psychologists, social workers, and nurses) or paraprofessionals (graduate students). Third, the creators provided 8 hours of training to the session leaders prior to the beginning of the program. Finally, the creators of the program met with the session leaders twice a month for the duration of the program. These training sessions and ongoing meetings provided background information about children of divorce, program goals, administration techniques, and review of past and upcoming sessions. One current weakness is a lack of attention to appropriate timing in sample recruitment. Participants include children whose parents divorced several years prior to enrollment in the program as well as children whose parents are currently in the process of divorcing.

Critical Analysis of Design Characteristics   The designers of CODIP have done an excellent job ensuring appropriate outcome evaluation and internal validation. Evaluations of CODIP typically include a large battery of assessments in child functioning and the targeted processes. However, there is a major weakness in the interpretive standards of CODIP: Evaluation typically does not include random assignment. Children of divorce self-select into the treatment or no-treatment control conditions. The result is sometimes significant group differences in outcome variables before treatment (Pedro-Carroll et al., 1999). Although program evaluations also included a nondivorced control group, there has been little discussion about differences between the treatment group and the nondivorced control group. Thus, CODIP is unique in being able to test whether children who have completed the program are functioning at the same levels as their counterparts in intact families, but researchers have yet to make full use of this advantage.

MODEL PROGRAM TO PREVENT HARMFUL CONSEQUENCES OF DIVORCE

The model program to prevent harmful consequences associated with divorce is designed to provide coping resources for children and to help parents protect their children. Thus, the model program includes a parent and child component. Both parents are eligible to participate in the program, but families in which only one parent wants to participate also are welcome. This type of flexibility in family recruitment recognizes the importance of mothers and fathers for successful child development while at the same time accommodating possible bitterness and acrimony between parents. An outline of the model program is presented in Table 9.3. Its main features include an inclusive program for parents and children, a

Table 9.3. Components of a model program to prevent harmful consequences of divorce

| | Model program | |
	Parent component	Child component
Targets	Families currently going through a divorce Mothers or fathers or both	Children currently going through a divorce
Content	Building supportive relationships Instruction on the possible effects of divorce and interparental conflict on children Coping skills and problem-solving training Instruction on the use of constructive conflict tactics Parent skills training	Building supportive relationships Improving understanding of divorce and interparental conflict Coping skills and problem-solving training Building self- and family-esteem Exploring divorce-related feelings
Outcomes	Improves: Understanding of children's perspectives Parenting skills Child adjustment Reduces: Destructive interparental conflict Parental stress and adjustment problems	Improves: Self- and family-esteem Coping skills Problem-solving skills Reduces: Stress Emotional problems Behavioral problems Social problems Academic problems

focus on problem solving and cooperative relationships among divorcing couples, education about the reasons why divorce occurs and coping techniques for dealing with it, and building supportive networks among participants.

The specific goals of the parent component include improving understanding of children's perspective on divorce, parental adjustment to the divorce, parenting skills, and interparental conflict strategies. These goals are met by fostering positive relationships between participants as a coping resource; for example, families share their own stories, thoughts, and concerns about their experiences. This teaching method serves the additional goal of ensuring sociocultural relevance by emphasizing the uniqueness of each family. Participants from diverse backgrounds are likely to have different stories, and allowing them to share these stories will help them feel integrated and respected. Leaders emphasize that parents must make choices about what is best for their family, noting that all families are different and choices may vary.

Group discussion is combined with presentations about the effects of divorce and opportunities for participants to practice skills. Early sessions provide information about why divorce might be harmful for children. These sessions help parents understand their children's perspectives on divorce, especially their mixed emotions and their "acting out." In addition, they provide the rationale for the remaining sessions in the program by encouraging parents to think about aspects of their family that are in particular need of change for the benefit of the children. Later sessions provide the skills parents need to make those changes.

The model program targets parental stress and adjustment to a new lifestyle. Program leaders talk and lead discussions about the wide range of possible problems that individuals experience during and following a divorce. They develop strategies for coping with stress and solving problems. Parents are trained in the differences between constructive and destructive conflict and learn techniques to better handle their conflicts with each other. Emphasis is placed on avoiding lengthy, acrimonious custody battles and on not using children to communicate or spy on each other. The program is also designed to provide skills on parenting children through a divorce. Program leaders explain the importance of sensitive, warm, and consistent parenting and have parents practice these skills. Assistance also is provided in making plans for the family regarding housing and court visits following the divorce. Descriptions of some options available for families of divorce are provided and lead into discussions with parents about how children often react to changing schools or moving to new homes.

The goals of the child component are to improve children's self- and family-esteem, coping skills, and problem-solving strategies. Just as in the parent component, children are given opportunities to tell their own stories. The goal is for children with painful backgrounds to feel comfortable disclosing and seeking support. Early sessions prevent children from feeling guilty about their parents' divorce and conflicts. Program leaders describe different reasons why adults have irreconcilable disagreements that lead to divorce and emphasize that children are not to blame. In addition, early sessions help children explore their feelings, including guilt, shame, sadness, and anger. Children learn to identify these emotions, understand that they are normal, and effectively cope with them. In later sessions, children prepare for their post divorce lives, including moving to a new home and school. These sessions focus on building coping and problem-solving skills. Children also are encouraged to consider how going through a divorce can make them stronger individuals.

❖

A Prevention Program for Keisha Smith

The Smith family has long suffered the effects of destructive, even violent, marital conflict. They chose to divorce in the hope that the fighting would stop. Keisha complains of being put in the middle of her parents' disagreements, and the discord eventually reaches an intensity great enough to prompt a restraining order against Keisha's father. Keisha is forced to change schools and move to a new home, and she misses having contact with her father. As a result, she is showing signs of academic and behavioral problems.

Keisha could benefit from a well-designed prevention program. The model program includes families like Keisha's in which children are particularly at risk, yet the participation of both parents is impossible. Keisha's mother, Debra, could benefit by gaining the skills necessary to deal with stress and create an environment that will best foster her child's development. From the very first session of the program, Debra forms supportive relationships with other families going through divorce. She is able to share her story with others who have a good understanding of her experiences. By listening to the stories of others, she sees that she is not alone in her struggles. Debra learns about how the divorce may be affecting Keisha. Because Debra has been so concerned with separating from Gary and trying to create a new life, she is not aware of her daughter's feelings and concerns. Debra comes to understand that Keisha's growing academic and behavior problems are likely the result of family circumstances. Instead of blaming and harshly punishing Keisha, Debra's new understanding fosters a feeling of empathy. Debra also learns that although recent events have brought several risks to Keisha's development, there are ways in which Debra can counteract them and protect her daughter.

As she moves through the program, Debra realizes that the first thing she can do to help her daughter is to help herself. She gets a chance to let off some steam during a session by expressing all of her fear, anger, frustration, disappointment, and hurt. She comes to understand that these are normal emotions, and she gains skills for coping with these emotions and for dealing with her stress. She is instructed on ways of handling conflict with her ex-husband and effectively parenting Keisha as well as on the importance of not putting Keisha in the middle of interparental disagreements. Because Gary has been violent in the past, Debra learns a lot about the cycle of violence and how to stop it. The model program helps her understand that Gary has an important role as Keisha's father, but unless he learns to interact with family members without becoming violent, he should have very limited contact with Debra and Keisha. Overall, the model program motivates Debra to change her family circumstances, enhances her sense of self-efficacy about making those changes, and ensures that she has the tools needed to make them.

For Keisha, the program provides resources for coping with the changes in her life and her feelings of anger and sadness. She has the chance to talk to peers who share her experiences and begins to understand that there are others who have the same problems. She learns that her parents' divorce is not her fault, and the wide range of feelings she is experiencing is normal. During discussions, Keisha realizes that divorce was the only option for her parents because of her father's violence. She suddenly sees Debra's decision to leave as courageous and difficult and understands that her mother did it to keep Keisha safe. As a result, instead of blaming Debra for disrupting her life, Keisha appreciates her and wants to support her.

Keisha and the other children learn about interparental conflict and the process of divorce. Keisha develops some problem-solving skills as the children present sample problems and then practice solving them together. The children talk about what they like about their families, and Keisha relates how proud she is that her mother was able to leave her abusive father. She points out that her father has decided to get treatment for his problem.

One of the most important benefits of the model program for both Debra and Keisha is their increased sense of confidence and pride in their ability to cope with the divorce. Debra has a greater understanding of what her daughter is experiencing and now possesses the skills she needs to help Keisha. Keisha has become proud of her family and herself. She obtains skills in problem solving that she puts to use in her own life and when helping others. Together, Debra and Keisha deal with Keisha's anger and resentment with hopes of improving her academic functioning and behavioral problems. Instead of seeing themselves as victims, they see themselves as resilient survivors.

FUTURE DIRECTIONS: IMPROVING PROGRAMS FOR PREVENTING THE EFFECTS OF CONFLICT

Comprehensive prevention programs that focus on advancing the knowledge of parents and children about the effects of conflict and divorce should be a priority for both researchers and clinicians because the effects of conflict are often detrimental for the well-being and long-range development of children. How a married couple reacts to each other during conflict has implications not only for their marriage, but also for the functioning of the entire family system. To avoid the effects of conflict on marital and parent–child relationships, it is necessary to develop theory-based programs that educate parents about destructive conflict and that enhance communication and effective co-parenting. A goal should be to teach each member of the family, particularly children, to cope better with the actions of others as well as to control their own actions. By helping parents and children recognize how they affect one another, programs can aim to improve relations in families that are still together as well as those that are now apart.

The model programs presented in this chapter focus on improving the over-all well-being of married couples and the family systems in which they exist. It is important to note that due to the wide range of possible participants, these programs could be implemented in areas of varying risk levels, socioeconomic status, and potential need. These programs could be adapted by churches of different denominations as well as by university and community-based organizations aimed at helping to improve family life and child development. People in need of prevention programs for conflict and divorce, or those simply interested in participating, could take part at no cost. Because many approaches can be used to train parents and children, different methodologies could be adapted to accommodate the locations, funding needs, and religious affiliations of the centers in which these programs are run. This high adaptability also helps to lower the costs of such programs, enabling more people to benefit. Programs designed to help families avoid the negative consequences of destructive conflict before they begin can serve as effective tools in teaching parents to argue constructively and children to cope constructively. If divorce does occur, then parents and children can learn to handle it in mature and beneficial ways for the family as a whole. Whether designed for intact or divorced families, these programs can aid both parents and children in recognizing how their behaviors affect others and how they can improve these behaviors in order to ensure a healthier development over time for both themselves and the members of their families.

REFERENCES

Alpert-Gillis, L.J., Pedro-Carroll, J.L., & Cowen, E.L. (1989). The children of divorce intervention program: Development, implementation, and evaluation of a program for young urban children. *Journal of Consulting and Clinical Psychology, 57,* 583–589.

Amato, P.R. (1993). Children's adjustment to divorce: Theories, hypotheses, and empirical support. *Journal of Divorce and Remarriage, 55,* 23–38.

Amato, P.R. (2000). The consequences of divorce for adults and children. *Journal of Marriage and Family, 62,* 1269–1287.

Bagarozzi, D.A., & Rauen, P. (1981). Premarital counseling: Appraisal and status. *The American Journal of Family Therapy, 9,* 13–30.

Baruch, D.W., & Wilcox, J.A. (1944). A study of sex differences in preschool children's adjustment coexistent with interparental tensions. *Journal of Genetic Psychology, 64,* 281–303.

Behrens, B., & Halford, W.K. (1994, August). *Advances in the prevention and treatment of marital distress.* Paper presented at the Helping Families Change Conference, University of Queensland, Brisbane, Australia.

Burnett, C.K. (1994). *Communication skills training for marriage: Modification and evaluation of the Prevention and Relationship Enhancement Program (PREP).* Unpublished doctoral dissertation, University of North Carolina, Chapel Hill.

Cherlin, A.J., Furstenberg, F.F., Chase-Lansdale, P.L., Kiernan, K.E., Robins, P.K., Morrison, D.R., et al. (1991). Longitudinal studies of effects of divorce on children in Great Britain and the United States. *Science, 252,* 1386–1389.

Cox, M. J., Paley, B., & Harter, K. (2001). Interparental conflict and parent–child relationships. In D. Frank and J.H. Grych (Eds.), *Interparental conflict and child development: Theory, research, and applications* (pp. 249–272). New York: Cambridge University Press.

Cummings, E.M. (1997). Marital conflict, abuse, and adversity in the family and child adjustment: A developmental psychopathology perspective. In D. Wolfe (Ed.), *Child abuse: New directions in prevention and treatment across the lifespan,* (pp. 3–26). Thousand Oaks, CA: Sage Publications.

Cummings, E.M. (1998). Stress and coping approaches and research: The impact of marital conflict on children. *Journal of Aggression, Maltreatment and Trauma, 2,* 31–50.

Cummings, E.M., Ballard, M., & El-Sheikh, M. (1991). Responses of children and adolescents to interadult anger as a function of gender, age, and mode of expression. *Merrill-Palmer Quarterly, 37,* 543–560.

Cummings, E.M., & Davies, P.T. (1994). *Children and marital conflict: The impact of family dispute and resolution.* New York: Guilford Press.

Cummings, E.M., Simpson, K.S., & Wilson, A. (1993). Children's responses to interadult anger as a function of information about resolution. *Developmental Psychology, 29,* 978–985.

Davies, P.T., & Cummings, E.M. (1994). Marital conflict and child adjustment: An emotional security hypothesis. *Psychological Bulletin, 116,* 387–411.

Erel, O., & Burman, B. (1995). Interrelatedness of marital relations and parent–child relations: A meta-analytic review. *Psychological Bulletin, 118,* 108–132.

Gassner, S., & Murray, E.J. (1969). Dominance and conflict in the interactions between parents of normal and neurotic children. *Journal of Abnormal Psychology, 74,* 33–41.

Goeke-Morey, M.C. (1999). *Children and marital conflict: Exploring the distinction between constructive and destructive marital conflict behaviors.* Unpublished doctoral dissertation, University of Notre Dame, South Bend, IN.

Goodman, M., Bonds, D., Sandler, I., & Braver, S. (2004). Parent psychoeducational programs and reducing the negative effects of interparental conflict following divorce. *Family Court Review, 42,* 263–279.

Gottman, J.M., Notarius, C.I., Gonso, J., & Markman, H.J. (1976). *A couple's guide to communication.* Champaign, IL: Research Press.

Grych, J.H., & Fincham, F.D. (1990). Marital conflict and children's adjustment: A cognitive–contextual framework. *Psychological Bulletin, 108,* 267–290.

Grych, J.H., & Fincham, F.D. (1993). Children's appraisals of marital conflict: Initial investigations of the cognitive–contextual framework. *Child Development, 64,* 215–230.

Hahlweg, K., Markman, H.J., Thurmaier, F., Engl, J., & Eckert, V. (1998). Prevention of marital distress: Results of a German prospective longitudinal study. *Journal of Family Psychology, 12*(4), 543–556.

Halford, W.K., Markman, H.J., Kline, G.H., Galena, H., & Stanley, S.M. (2003). Best practice in couple relationship education. *Journal of Marital and Family Therapy, 29,* 385–406.

Hans, J.D., & Fine, M.A. (2001). Children of divorce: Experiences of children whose parents attended a divorce education program. *Journal of Divorce and Remarriage, 36,* 1–26.

Hawley, D.R., & Olson, D.H. (1995). Enriching newlyweds: An evaluation of three enrichment programs. *The American Journal of Family Therapy, 23,* 129–147.

Heatherington, E.M., Cox, M., & Cox, R. (1982). Effects of divorce on parents and children. In M.E. Lamb (Ed.), *Nontraditional families: Parenting and child development* (pp. 233–285). Mahwah, NJ: Lawrence Erlbaum Associates.

Heavey, C.H., Larson, B.L., & Carpenter, K. (1997). *Primary prevention of marital distress during the transition to parenthood: A test of PREP.* Manuscript under editorial review.

Hubbard, R.M., & Adams, C.F. (1936). Factors affecting the success of child guidance clinic treatment. *American Journal of Orthopsychiatry, 6,* 81–102.

Jouriles, E.N., Bourg, W.J., & Farris, A.M. (1991). Marital adjustment and child conduct problems: A comparison of the correlation across subsamples. *Journal of Consulting and Clinical Psychology, 59,* 354–357.

Lindsay, L.L. (2002). The family conflict intervention program: A pilot of school-based groups for second- and third-grade children. (Doctoral dissertation, Rochester University, 2002). *Dissertation Abstracts International, 62*(12-B), 5969.

Lindsay, L.L., Pedro-Carroll, J.L., & Davies, P.T. (2001). *The family conflict intervention program: Curriculum for support groups with second and third grade children.* Unpublished doctoral dissertation, University of Rochester, New York.

Markman, H.J., & Floyd, F. (1980). Possibilities for the prevention of marital discord: A behavioral perspective. *American Journal of Family Therapy, 8,* 29–48.

Markman, H.J., Floyd, F.J., Stanley, S.M., & Storaasli, R.D. (1988). Prevention of marital distress: A longitudinal investigation. *Journal of Consulting and Clinical Psychology, 56,* 210–217.

Markman, H.J., & Hahlweg, K. (1993). The prediction and prevention of marital distress: An international perspective. *Clinical Psychology Review, 13,* 29–43.

Markman, H.J., Jamieson, K., & Floyd, F. (1983). The assessment and modification of premarital relationships: Preliminary findings on the etiology and prevention of marital and family distress. In J. Vincent (Ed.), *Advances in family interventions, assessment and theory* (Vol. 3, pp. 41–90). Greenwich, CT: JAI Press.

Markman, H.J., Renick, M.J., Floyd, F.J., Stanley, S.M., & Clements, M. (1993). Preventing marital distress through communication and conflict management training: A 4- and 5-year follow-up. *Journal of Consulting and Clinical Psychology, 61,* 70–77.

National Center for Health. (2002, January). *National vital statistics reports: Births, marriages, divorces, and deaths.* Retrieved October 29, 2004, from National Center for Health Statistics via NCHS: http://www.cdc.gov/nchs

Pedro-Carroll, J.L. (1997). The children of divorce intervention program: Fostering resilient outcomes for school-aged children. In G.W. Albee & T.P. Gullota (Eds.), *Primary prevention works* (pp. 213–238). Thousand Oaks, CA: Sage Publications.

Pedro-Carroll, J.L., & Alpert-Gillis, L.J. (1997). Preventive interventions for children of divorce: A developmental model for 5 and 6 year old children. *The Journal of Primary Prevention, 18,* 5–23.

Pedro-Carroll, J.L, Alpert-Gillis, L.J., & Cowen, E.L. (1992). An evaluation of the efficacy of a preventive intervention for 4th–6th grade urban children of divorce. *Journal of Primary Prevention, 13,* 115–130.

Pedro-Carroll, J.L., & Cowen, E.L. (1985). The children of divorce intervention program: An investigation of the efficacy of a school-based prevention program. *Journal of Consulting and Clinical Psychology, 53,* 603–611.

Pedro-Carroll, J.L., Sutton, S.E., & Wyman, P.A. (1999). A two-year follow-up evaluation of a preventive intervention for young children of divorce. *School Psychology Review, 28,* 467–476.

Porter, B., & O'Leary, K.D. (1980). Marital discord and childhood behavior problems. *Journal of Abnormal Child Psychology, 8,* 287–295.

Renick, M.J., Blumberg, S.J., & Markman, H.J. (1992). The prevention and relationship enhancement program (PREP): An empirically based preventive intervention program for couples. *Family Relations, 41,* 141–147.

Rutter, M. (1970). Psychological development: Predictions from infancy. *Journal of Child Psychology and Psychiatry and Applied Disciplines, 11,* 49–62.

Sayers, S.L., Kohn, C.S., & Heavey, C. (1998). Prevention of marital dysfunction: Behavioral approaches and beyond. *Clinical Psychology Review, 18,* 713–744.

Schilling, E.A., Baucom, D.H., Burnett, C.K., Allen, E.S., & Ragland, L. (2003). Altering the course of marriage: The effect of PREP communication skills acquisition on couples' risk of becoming maritally distressed. *Journal of Family Psychology, 17,* 41–53.

Simons, R.L., Beaman, J., Conger, R.D., & Chao, W. (1993). Stress, support, and antisocial behavior trait as determinants of emotional well-being and parenting practices among single mothers. *Journal of Marriage and the Family, 55,* 385–398.

Simons, R.L., Lin, K.H., Gordon, L.C., Conger, R.D., & Lorenz, F.O. (1999). Explaining the higher incidence of adjustment problems among children of divorce compared with those in two-parent families. *Journal of Marriage and the Family, 61,* 1020–1033.

Stanley, S.M., Markman, H.J., Prado, L.M., Olmos-Gallo, P.A., Tonelli, L., St. Peters, M., et al. (2001). Community-based premarital prevention: Clergy and lay leaders on the front lines. *Family Relations: Interdisciplinary Journal of Applied Family Studies, 50,* 67–76.

Stanley, S.M., Markman, H.J., St. Peters, M., & Leber, B.D. (1995). Strengthening marriages and preventing divorce: New directions in prevention research. *Family Relations, 44,* 392–401.

Stanley, S.M., & Trathen, D.W. (1994). Christian PREP: An empirically based model for marital and premarital intervention. *Journal of Psychology and Christianity, 13,* 158–165.

Sterling, S.E. (1986). *School-based intervention program for early latency-aged children of divorce.* Unpublished doctoral dissertation, University of Rochester, New York.

Towle, C. (1931). The evaluation and management of marital situation in foster homes. *American Journal of Orthopsychiatry, 1,* 271–283.

Van Widenfelt, B., Hosman, C., Schaap, C., & van der Staak, C. (1996). The prevention of relationship distress for couples at risk: A controlled evaluation with nine month and two-year follow-ups. *Family Relations, 45,* 156–165.

Wallace, R. (1935). A study of the relationship between emotional tone of the home and adjustment status in cases referred to a travel child guidance clinic. *Journal of Juvenile Research, 19,* 205–220.

Weiss, L., & Wolchik, S.A. (1998). New beginnings: An empirically-based intervention program for divorced mothers to help their children adjust to divorce. In J.M. Briesmeister & C.E. Schaefer (Eds.), *Handbook of parent training: Parents as co-therapists for children's behavior problems* (pp. 445–478). New York: John Wiley & Sons.

Wolchik, S.A., Sandler, I.N., Millsap, R.E., Plummer, B.A., Greene, S.M., Anderson, E.R., et al. (2002). Six-year follow-up of preventive interventions for children of divorce: A randomized controlled trial. *Journal of the American Medical Association, 288,* 1874–1881.

Wolchik, S.A, West, S.G., Sandler, I.N., Irwin, N., Tein, J.Y., Coatsworth, D., et al. (2000). An experimental evaluation of theory-based mother and mother-child programs for children of divorce. *Journal of Consulting and Clinical Psychology, 68,* 843–856.

Wolchik, S.A., West, S.G., Westover, S., & Sandler, I.N. (1993). The children of divorce parenting intervention: Outcome evaluation of an empirically based program. *American Journal of Community Psychology, 21,* 293–331.

10

WHERE DO WE GO FROM HERE?

A Synthesis of Science and Art

John G. Borkowski and Chelsea M. Weaver

The coverage of effective programs in eight important domains of infant, child, and adolescent development was built around the importance of 15 principles of effective prevention research. This chapter provides an overview of the critical analyses in the preceding chapters, identifying those principles that have occurred most frequently in the best of past prevention research and suggesting principles that should occur with greater frequency in order to make more rapid advances of the existing research literature. After reviewing the utilization of essential principles, we develop arguments as to why effect sizes have been modest, even in the more successful prevention programs. The argument focuses on two somewhat interrelated points: 1) genetic vulnerability and program effectiveness and 2) toxic social environments and the need for more broad-based integrated, prevention programs. The chapter concludes with considerations about difficulties encountered in blending science and art in field settings and focusing on the importance of individual strengths rather than deficits.

PRINCIPLES OF SUCCESSFUL PREVENTION PROGRAMS

The development of a list of essential principles rests heavily on the scholarship of Nation and colleagues (2003), who analyzed four major areas of prevention research in an attempt to determine the most frequently occurring principles of effective prevention programs: 1) substance abuse, 2) risky sexual behavior, 3) delinquency and violence, and 4) school failures. Across these four content areas, 35 well-designed studies were used for qualitative and quantitative analyses.

In the areas of substance abuse and risky sexual behaviors, the most important principles were the comprehensiveness of the intervention, varied methods of teaching, appropriate timing of the program with respect to the participant's age or stage of development, and the sociocultural appropriateness and sensitivity of the program's contents. In the area of delinquency and violence, building positive relationships between participants and staff and the administration of sufficient treatment dosage also were important. All of the previously mentioned principles appeared in successful programs designed to prevent school failures; moreover, having a well-trained staff proved to be an important characteristic.

The thorough analysis of Nation et al. (2003) helped to form the conceptual and empirical foundation for the 15 principles listed earlier in Table 1.1 and again in Table 10.1. The principles can be grouped into three overlapping categories: *treatment principles, procedural principles,* and *design and evaluation principles.* Treatment principles corresponds to the specific curriculum and associated components of an intervention, procedural principles refers to how that intervention is implemented in the field, and design and evaluation principles relates to an appropriate and convincing assessment of program effectiveness. Chapter 1 noted that if endorsed in practice, the use of these principles, in combination, should produce sizeable effects and clear interpretations about the causal factors that produce meaningful outcomes following an intervention. In general, the review of *best practices* in eight content areas supports this contention. Table 10.1 contains a summary of the frequency with which each of the 15 principles appeared in the domains analyzed in this book.

Three principles stood out in the analyses of the 27 exemplar prevention programs covered in the preceding chapters: well-trained staff, systematic evaluation of clearly defined outcomes, and clinically or socially significant findings, with each being included in 25 of the 27 programs. The integration of these three components has implications for the quality of programs experienced by program participants as well as for documenting program outcomes: High levels of staff training indicated that participants were taught the curricula from individuals who were well versed in each program's contents. Interestingly, treatment fidelity, or the staff's adherence to program content during its implementation, was adequately addressed by only 17 of the 27 programs. In other words, there seems to have been a disconnect between the training received by staff and the quality of programming they delivered to program participants. In some cases, it may be that well-designed training procedures took the place of measures of treatment fidelity, with an assumption that adherence to the intervention protocol would be followed. In

Table 10.1. Number of programs in eight domains that addressed each of 15 essential principles

	Prevention domain (number of programs evaluated)								
	Infant health (4)	Developmental delay (3)	Child maltreatment (3)	Youth violence (3)	Substance use (4)	Risky sexual behaviors (3)	Dating violence (3)	Marital conflict (4)	Total (27)
Treatment principles									
Theory driven	3	2	3	3	4	2	2	4	23
Comprehensive	1	3	3	3	2	3	1	2	18
Varied teaching methods	2	1	2	3	4	3	3	4	22
Positive relationships	1	1	3	3	3	3	2	4	20
Sociocultural relevance	3	1	2	2	4	1	2	2	17
Procedural principles									
Sufficient dosage	3	2	2	3	4	3	3	3	23
Appropriate timing	4	1	2	1	4	1	2	2	17
Well-trained staff	3	2	3	3	4	3	3	4	25
Programmed generalization	0	1	1	3	4	1	2	4	16
Treatment fidelity	0	2	2	2	3	1	3	4	17
Design and evaluation principles									
Interpretive standards	0	3	1	2	3	3	2	4	18
Outcome evaluation	4	3	2	3	4	3	3	3	25
Adequate effect size	0	3	0	1	3	3	3	4	17
Clinical or social significance	4	2	3	3	4	3	2	4	25
Internal validation	0	0	3	3	4	2	2	4	18

addition, the measurement of treatment fidelity is expensive and time consuming. Under ideal conditions, high standards of staff training would be accompanied by the direct assessments of strict adherence to clearly outlined treatment protocols.

In addition to highly trained staff, most programs included clearly stated goals about targeted outcomes and appropriate analytical techniques, often leading to socially important findings. The magnitude of treatment effects must be weighed in light of the social significance of each program's major findings. For example, a small to moderate effect size may translate into a dramatic improvement in the quality of life for a few individuals, increasing the safety of neighborhoods or saving millions of federal dollars devoted to prevention programming. Strong experimental designs allow for the identification of important preventive programs as well as increase the likelihood that relevant findings will eventually be disseminated to the scientific and public communities. For example, programs that systematically evaluate clearly defined, socially relevant goals and related behavioral and psychosocial processes hold the potential to advance developmental science as well as gain access to funding sources that can be used to disseminate information and replicate findings in other settings with diverse groups.

The essentials of effective prevention efforts that were least likely to be integrated into the exemplar programs were promotion of generalization of newly acquired skills, sociocultural relevance of treatment content, appropriate timing of intervention, treatment fidelity, and reasonable treatment effect sizes. Only 16 of the 27 evaluated programs included components such as booster sessions or opportunities to practice skills across multiple settings in order to facilitate the maintenance and generalization of the program. From an ecological systems perspective, this omission is critical because children, along with adults and peers in their lives, must be treated within naturalistic environments to elicit meaningful changes that will be sustained over time. Relatedly, programs must be relevant to the sociocultural contexts in which participants live, providing opportunities to work on personally significant and important goals as well as to build permanent, supportive social networks.

The most critical deficit, found in 11 of the 27 evaluated programs, is poor timing related to program implementation. This is troublesome because inherent in the term *prevention* is the explicit goal of forestalling the onset of a target behavior, or cluster of behaviors, before it occurs. Implementing a prevention program before the manifestation of destructive problem behaviors is imperative. Some of the evaluated prevention efforts were designed to be secondary or tertiary programs (e.g., the Multisystemic approach of Henggeler, Schoenwald, Pickrel, Brandino, & Hall, 1994). Nevertheless, many primary prevention programs simply begin too late to produce large-scale effects. For example, a program designed to prevent risky sexual behaviors, such as sexual initiation at a young age, must begin before participants become sexually active. Similarly, dating violence prevention programs must reach older children and adolescents before they become perpetrators or victims. Related to adequate timing, the least scientifically rigorous prevention programs were in the area of promoting infant health and development. None of the three well-designed programs in this domain incorporated supports for the generalization of skills to other settings, steps to ensure treatment fidelity, experimental designs with high interpretive standards, tests of internal validation, or findings with adequate effects sizes.

It is clear from the synthesis of the strengths and limitations among the exemplar prevention programs in eight socially relevant domains that there has been a good deal of sophisticated and meaningful scientific work, especially with individuals at risk for social, emotional, and behavioral maladjustment. Despite these efforts, however, there is a clear need for better planned, designed, and executed prevention programs. Specifically, prevention researchers, in collaboration with school and community advocates, must be cognizant of the 15 essentials of effective programming, especially in terms of timing, ecological and sociocultural relevance, and treatment fidelity.

"HIDDEN LIMITATIONS" TO TREATMENT EFFECTIVENESS

Even if prevention programs adhere to all of the 15 principles emphasized in this book, treatment effectiveness may, in some cases, remain modest. One potential explanation is related to individual differences in genetic and/or biological factors that can impose a *hidden ceiling* on an otherwise successful prevention program. This point is made clear in the research on gene environment interactions (Caspi et al., 2002; Jaffe et al., 2005). A second limitation is the presence of toxic environments that can mitigate the effects of strong programs.

Genetic Vulnerability and Prevention Effectiveness

Caspi and colleagues (2002) published a widely cited study in *Science* that has attracted widespread scientific and media attention. The data revealed the influence of a monoamine oxidase A (MAOA) polymorphism on adolescent/adult antisocial behavior following a history of childhood maltreatment. A birth cohort of 1,037 New Zealand children were assessed from ages 3 to 21, at 2-year intervals, using a range of self-report, parent-report, and teacher-report measures to index antisocial behavior as well as child maltreatment. The MAOA gene moderated the impact of maltreatment on antisocial behaviors, such that high levels of expression neutralized the effects of severe maltreatment, whereas low levels and severe maltreatment magnified the effects.

Jaffee et al. (2005) assessed whether the effects of maltreatment on the elevation on the antisocial behaviors associated with conduct problems was strongest among children who were at genetic risk, using data from a representative cohort of 1,116 5-year-old British twin pairs and their families. Children's conduct problems were based on parent and teacher interviews, and diagnostic categories were formed using DSM-IV criteria. Degree of physical maltreatment was measured via parental reports. Genetic risks for conduct problems were estimated as a function of co-twin's conduct disorder status and the pair's zygosity. The effects of maltreatment on conduct problems were strongest among those at highest genetic risk. More specifically, the experience of maltreatment was associated with an increase of 2% in the probability of conduct disorder diagnoses among children at low genetic risk but an increase of 24% among children at high genetic risk. An implication of the findings of Jaffee et al. is that the prediction and treatment of behavioral problems will attain greater accuracy if both environmental and genetic risks are taken into account. Jaffee and colleagues hypothesized that it is unlikely that genes account directly for antisocial or conduct problems. That is, some genotypes (e.g., MAOA) may increase children's sensitivity to environmental adversities, such as physical maltreatment (abuse or neglect), whereas others may promote resistance to childhood trauma. Genes most likely do not have their influence directly on antisocial behaviors but rather act to alter children's susceptibility or resistance to stressful environmental experiences.

If this perspective on the role of genes and harmful environments is correct, then the search for the specific genes related to complex behavioral problems, such as adolescent conduct disorders and socioemotional behavioral problems, may be advanced primarily by assessing the gene-environment interaction rather than assuming a direct gene disorder correspondence (Hamer, 2002). It is likely that several genes are involved in the development of conduct problems and will eventually be related to complex gene-environment interplay, suggesting that purely environmental theories of teenage conduct problems are incomplete as are deterministic genetic accounts. In short, the prediction of behavioral disorders and antisocial behaviors, and their prevention, will likely attain greater accuracy and effectiveness if both harmful environments and genetic risks are measured and their interplay and reciprocity analyzed for a range of potentially harmful socioemotional outcomes during late childhood and adolescence.

The recent findings on gene-environment interactions are relevant to a number of important issues related to prevention research. Why are some children resilient in the face of maltreatment, whereas others are highly susceptible? How can the effects of antisocial behaviors be minimized, even in individuals with heightened genetic risk? Do epigenetic forces influence the interplay between genetic risks and environmental experiences? Can phenotypic or behavioral markers of genetic vulnerabilities be identified early in life, thus setting the stage for modifying the type, depth, and duration of individualized interventions? These are but a few of the major questions that are on the brink of being answered through the creation of a developmental science that integrates the dynamic contributions from biological, behavioral, and preventive sciences.

Toxic Social Environments

Harris (2002) has emphasized repeatedly the importance of negative peer groups in counteracting the positive effects of parenting on adolescent development. Peer pressures and unsafe home, school, and neighborhood environments often undermine the impact of well-intentioned community or school-based prevention programs. In fact, the more successful programs reviewed in this book generally attempted to include both peers and parents in their intervention programs to mitigate the effects of toxic social environments. However, small steps in this direction may not be enough. Because at-risk populations are typically found in impoverished communities, they face multiple social problems—not only from family functioning and destructive peer groups, but also from larger-scale, community problems, such as the lack of adequate support networks or access to health care. Although community-based prevention programming is limited in the funding currently available, social agencies that provide such services are in place in many disadvantaged neighborhoods. The problem is often with accessibility and overly complicated referral and delivery processes.

Effective prevention programs should not only target individuals in multiple locations (e.g., family, school) but also should help establish and extend formal and informal social networks that will be maintained well after each program terminates. For example, program participants should be evaluated and referred to agencies and programs for which they demonstrate an individualized need. These referrals should take into account sociocultural factors, such as involvement in religious support programs or ethnic social clubs. A child from a single-parent home without an extended family network should be referred to a mentoring program, where a lasting relationship with a positive, influential adult can be established and maintained. According to Nation et al. (2003), supportive relationships are especially important in protecting against substance use as well as academic failures and school dropout. Moreover, parents and children should be referred to community mental health services, if needed, and then given viable treatment programs.

The evaluations of prevention programs contained in this book elucidate the fact that similar processes are involved in many different domains of problematic development. Children who are at risk for violence victimization also are vulnerable to using alcohol and engaging in risky sexual behaviors. In addition, the presence of problem behaviors among their families and peer networks is likely. Programs should make every attempt to diminish the potential negative effects from toxic social environments that many children who are at risk are confronted with, and expected to negotiate, on a daily basis. Children involved in prevention programs can hardly be expected to succeed when their family and community systems are not actively included in programming or when they are not being simultaneously treated for existing problems in the very areas that prevention programs are attempting to target.

Peer Influences

The influence of peers on the development of children's attitudes and behaviors is important, especially during adolescence. Among teenagers, the desire for independence and autonomy leads to an increased dependence on peers, as opposed to parents, for support, especially in stressful times even in the context of strong, positive family relationships (Allen & Land, 1999). There is much debate about the potential influence of parents versus peers. For example, Harris (1995, 1998) has asserted that parents have little to no long-term impact on their children's development, especially in the personality domain. Instead, she believes that peers have a stronger influence on adolescents, with group socialization theory explaining how this process operates. Harris (2002) has argued that children will use behaviors that were learned at home in a peer context only if they are useful in this realm. If they are not, these behaviors will be dropped, and new, and often harmful, behaviors will develop.

Dodge, Dishion, and Lansford (2006) argued that interventions with high-risk teens should carefully form the treatment conditions, ensuring that participants with varying levels of risky behaviors are included. Generally, youth with histories of bad behavior (e.g., delinquency or drug abuse) should not be placed in the same group, where they would associate only with deviant peers. Instead, children and adolescents at risk should be seen individually or in groups composed of a variety of teens, including some who show appropriate behaviors. In a sense, group composition is the 16th principle of effective intervention research: Do not place children or adolescents with major psychopathologies or addictions in the same condition (Dodge et al., 2006).

In contrast, research on parenting has documented the long-term effects that parents have on their children in multiple domains, such as cognitive functioning, academic achievement, and socioemotional adjustment (cf. Borkowski, Ramey, & Bristol-Power, 2002). Parents lay the foundation on which a child's framework for future relationships and social decision-making skills is built. It seems clear that both parents and peers are important sources of influence on academic, social, and emotional development and should both be the targets of well-integrated prevention programs. In addition, programs need to be embedded within the larger cultural context of school and community systems. Finally, by measuring multiple process variables (e.g., social competency, self-regulation), the effects of prevention programs can actually help to inform developmental science (Cicchetti & Hinshaw, 2002), shedding light on the differential contributions of family and peer networks on children's growth and adjustment.

Administering Prevention Programs Under Difficult Circumstances

A final difficulty encountered in program implementation is the complexity of real-life environments. Particularly demanding are the experiences of staff members implementing home-based interventions to children and families who are at risk for maladjustment. The challenge of delivering reliable programs to participants with diverse backgrounds requires service delivery personnel who are both flexible in the presentation of key information and cognizant of the circumstances of each family unit at the time of the visit. For example, a staff member (e.g., Family Coach) must determine when a mother is unable to understand and process the message and then be flexible enough to present the information in another way or at a different time. The staff must also adapt the presentation of the material to the learning style and attention span of the participant. Many families are in a state of crisis when the Family Coach arrives at the home to do a scripted intervention session. Crises may include the death of a family member, illness, evictions, and/or involvement of a child protective service agency. As a result, prevention personnel must have the latitude to adapt in-home sessions in such a way that the family's unfortunate circumstances are acknowledged and addressed before the program contents are presented.

Family conflicts represent another challenge for home-based staff and their delivery of a full, intact intervention module. In chaotic families, sessions sometimes must be postponed or rescheduled in search of a quieter time. Frequent conflict between family members can interrupt the delivery of the curriculum, and appointments may need to be rescheduled for a time when fewer people will be present. Rescheduling, however, is costly and extremely difficult to achieve in practice. The net result is that the full program may be compromised due to a chaotic home environment. From a scientific perspective, it is essential to document which components were and were not delivered as well as the reasons why the program was modified. Furthermore, these variables should be included in analyses as possible predictors, mediators, or moderators of program outcomes.

There are other reasons for needing to be flexible in program delivery, including mental health problems, lack of immediate financial resources, and issues that arise when mothers must juggle child care to accommodate their work or school schedules. If home-based staff are not flexible, then participants will be lost through attrition or take part in sessions only when they think they can meet the demands of the project as dictated by their schedules. Decisions regarding the delivery of treatment components must be relevant to each family's needs, should be made within the context of supervision, and always documented in the data base.

Being flexible in meeting scheduling needs, being stood up for home visits, and being in the midst of family crises and conflict all take their toll on the staff and may influence their performance, thereby compromising treatment fidelity as well as the program's impact on participants. It is clear that constant supervision of the staff is critical not only to maintain the integrity of the program's procedures, but also to provide a safe forum for unloading stress. Supervision must be readily available for the home-based prevention staff to talk about difficult cases, to offer guidance and support, and to promote staff adherence to the research protocol.

THE NEED FOR INTEGRATED, COMPREHENSIVE PROGRAMS

Effective prevention programs must be comprehensive in nature, meaning that they must employ varied teaching methods that aim to elicit changes on multiple levels (e.g., attitude change as well as behavioral change), in multiple domains (e.g., communication, problem solving), and in multiple settings (e.g., home, work, school). Nation and colleagues (2003) defined *comprehensive* as "providing an array of interventions to address the salient precursors or mediators of the target problem" (p. 451). This definition highlights the need for effective programming to identify the mechanisms that are involved in eliciting lasting change in specific domains. For example, prevention researchers must not conceptualize risk and resilience as static traits that children either do or do not possess, but instead as dynamic processes that change within and between individuals over time and across contexts (cf. Egeland, Carlson, & Sroufe, 1993). The identification of mechanisms that are involved in the manifestation of problem behaviors as well as those that serve to protect children in the face of varying levels of risk allow for the development and implementation of effective prevention programs. It is evident from the evaluation of exemplar prevention programs that the most effective are those that target skill building, such as social competency, and provide opportunities for participants to practice these skills in realistic and supportive environments. Not only can developmental theory serve as a foundation for informing prevention research, but well-designed, methodologically rigorous prevention trials also can advance developmental science by shedding light on the processes involved in the manifestation of specific pathologies and problem behaviors (Cicchetti & Hinshaw, 2002).

The evaluation of prevention programs must include not only an assessment of targeted outcomes but also theoretically related process-oriented variables such as problem solving, decision making, and communication skills. Equally important to *what* a program was able to change is *how* the program was able to elicit that change. If the mechanisms responsible for bringing about lasting, positive changes are identified, then more specific, focused, and cost-effective preventions can be developed. It is not feasible to incorporate every domain of a child's life into prevention programs. As a result, program developers must make theoretically grounded choices as to which subsystems of the child's ecological environment will be targeted and why. By espousing a process-oriented approach to prevention science, more precisely targeted, comprehensive, and theoretically driven programs, aimed at reducing risk and promoting resilience among children, their families, and their communities, will be developed and implemented on a widespread basis.

The Systems Perspective

Prevention programs must be ecologically valid, keeping in mind that each child is part of a larger familial, community, and cultural context. According to Bronfenbrenner (1977), the developing child's environment is characterized by nested subsystems, each of which influences change and growth over time. To promote lasting change among children and adolescents, multiple domains must be incorporated into prevention programs. From a general systems perspective (Sameroff, 1995), each social system is self-organizing and self-stabilizing, meaning that its components need equilibrium and integration to become established and maintained. Relationships among a system's components are thought to be transactional in nature. In other words, an individual is not only affected by his or her environment, but the environment is also affected by the individual. For example, a child may be exposed to severe marital conflict, which then leads to behavioral problems. In turn, aggressive behavior may elicit harsh, ineffective parenting strategies as well as cause further friction in the marital relationship. It is evident how these cyclical relationships may quickly lead to a pattern of negative functioning; however, transactions within the social system also can be capitalized on by facilitating patterns of positive, supportive interactions among peers, parents, and teachers as replacements for destructive patterns.

In the case of prevention programming, treating a child in only one context (e.g., school) will likely fail to reorganize a family system, thereby falling short in producing desired outcomes. Furthermore, without an assessment of the entire system's needs, whether it is a family or an entire community, prevention programs run the risk of lacking individual and sociocultural relevance, which most likely will result in a lack of participant motivation and program failure. By treating multiple family members as a unit and addressing demonstrated needs that are deemed important to the participants, the likelihood of positive change is enhanced. Even better, multicomponent, communitywide prevention efforts have the potential to create shifts in attitudes and behaviors on a much larger scale, influencing the attitudes and values of society as a whole (Wandersman & Florin, 2003).

Strength-Based Approaches to Prevention

An effective prevention program must not only be comprehensive and well integrated, but it also should be individually tailored to build on participants' existing unique strengths (Maton, Schellenbach, Leadbeater, & Solarz, 2004). Many prevention programs approach treatment from a deficit model, with an emphasis on identifying and ameliorating weaknesses. The major problem with this approach is its focus on limitations rather than strengths; a more subtle problem, however, is that of teaching novel skills that individuals may have difficulty mastering or that may have no personal or sociocultural relevance. Thus, the agenda of a prevention researcher may not be in line with what is meaningful to a specific participant or group of participants. According to Dunst, Trivette, and Mott (1994), all individuals and families have strengths that are unique to their cultural and ethnic backgrounds. Furthermore, the failure to display competence in a specific domain must be viewed as a failure of the social systems to provide opportunities for success. By building on existing strengths, prevention programs will become more focused on promoting resilience and optimal development, thereby empowering families, building self-esteem, strengthening motivation, and fostering independence and success (cf. Maton et al., 2004).

In addition to building on an individual's abilities rather than focusing on his or her deficits during the planning and implementation phases, prevention programs should also incorporate a strengths-based approach in outcome evaluations. The U.S. Department of Health and Human Services (2004) called for more qualitative, participatory methods of outcome analyses that focus on the measurement of positive capacities of both children and their families. Moreover, these assessments should involve not only the program staff and other essential members of the prevention team, but also the participants themselves. By espousing an active role for participants in the evaluation and future development of intervention programs, their opinions and experiences will be heard and valued, thereby leading to more positive relationships with the staff and producing more optimal, relevant outcomes. Comprehensive, well-integrated prevention programs that are developed, implemented, and evaluated using a strengths-based approach should lead to meaningful and lasting changes not only in targeted domains but also in the social, emotional, and academic well-being of children and adolescents.

REFERENCES

Allen, J.P., & Land, D. (1999). Attachment in adolescence. In P.R. Shaver & J. Cassidy (Eds.), *Handbook of attachment: Theory, research, and clinical applications* (pp. 319–335). New York: Guilford Press.

Borkowski, J.G., Ramey, S.L., & Bristol-Power, M. (Eds.). (2002). *Parenting and the child's world: Influences on academic, intellectual, and social-emotional adjustment.* Mahwah, NJ: Lawrence Erlbaum Associates.

Bronfenbrenner, U. (1977). Toward an experimental ecology of human development. *American Psychologist, 32,* 513–530.

Caspi, A., McClay, J., Moffitt, T., Mill, J., Martin, J., Craig, I. W., et al. (2002). Role of genotype in the cycle of violence in maltreated children. *Science, 297,* 851–854.

Cicchetti, D., & Hinshaw, S.P. (2002). Prevention and intervention science: Contributions to developmental theory. *Development and Psychopathology, 14,* 667–671.

Dodge, K.A., Dishion, T.J., & Lansford, J.E. (2006). Deviant peer influences in intervention and public policy for youth. *Social Policy Report* (Volume XX, No.1). Ann Arbor, MI: Society for Research in Child Development.

Dunst, C.J., Trivette, C.M., & Mott, D.W. (1994). Strengths-based family-centered intervention practices. In C.J. Dunst, C.M Trivette, & A.G. Deal (Eds.), *Supporting & strengthening families: Methods, strategies, and practices* (pp. 115–131). Cambridge, MA: Brookline Books.

Egeland, B.R., Carlson, E., & Sroufe, L.A. (1993). Resilience as process. *Development and Psychopathology, 5,* 517–528.

Hamer, D. (2002). Rethinking behavior genetics. *Science, 298,* 71–72.

Harris, J.R. (1995). Where is the child's environment? A group socialization theory of development. *Psychological Review, 102,* 458–489.

Harris, J.R. (1998). *The nurture assumption: Why children turn out the way they do.* New York: The Free Press.

Harris, J.R. (2000). Context-specific learning, personality, and birth order. *Current Directions in Psychological Science, 5,* 174–177.

Harris, J.R. (2002). Beyond the nurture assumption: Testing hypotheses about the child's environment. In J.G. Borkowski, S.L. Ramey, & M. Bristol-Power (Eds.), *Parenting and the child's world: Influences on academic, intellectual, and social-emotional adjustment* (pp. 3–20). Mahwah, NJ: Lawrence Erlbaum Associates.

Henggeler, S.W., Schoenwald, S.K., Pickrel, S.G., Brandino, S.J., & Hall, J.A. (1994). *Treatment manual for family preservation using multisystemic therapy.* Charleston: South Carolina Health and Human Services Finance Commission.

Jaffee, S.R., Caspi, A., Moffitt, T.E., Dodge, K.A., Rutter, M., Taylor, A., et al. (2005). Nature x nurture: Genetic vulnerabilities interact with physical maltreatment to promote conduct problems. *Development and Psychopathology, 17,* 67–84.

Maton, K.I., Schellenbach, C.J., Leadbeater, B.J., & Solarz, A.L. (Eds.). (2004). *Investing in children, youth, families, and communities: Strengths-based research and policy.* Washington, DC: American Psychological Association.

Nation, M., Crusto, C., Wandersman, A., Kumpfer, K., Seybolt, D., Morrissey-Kane, E., et al. (2003). What works in prevention: Principles of effective prevention programs. *American Psychologist, 58,* 449–456.

Sameroff, A. (1995). General systems theories and developmental psychopathology. In D. Cicchetti & D. Cohen (Eds.), *Developmental psychopathology: Theories and methods* (Vol. 1, pp. 659–695). New York: John Wiley & Sons.

U.S. Department of Health and Human Services. (2004, April). *Evaluating your prevention program.* Washington, DC: Author.

Wandersman, A., & Florin, P. (2003). Community interventions and effective prevention. *American Psychologist, 58,* 441–448.

Index

Page numbers followed by *t* indicate tables.